# Lipids, Malnutrition & the Developing Brain

*The Ciba Foundation for the promotion of international cooperation in medical and chemical research is a scientific and educational charity established by CIBA Limited – now CIBA-GEIGY Limited – of Basle. The Foundation operates independently in London under English trust law.*

*The Nestlé Foundation for the study of the problems of nutrition in the world is an independent foundation established by Nestlé Alimentana S.A. of Vevey.*

*Ciba Foundation Symposia are published in collaboration with Associated Scientific Publishers (Elsevier Scientific Publishing Company, Excerpta Medica, North-Holland Publishing Company) in Amsterdam.*

Associated Scientific Publishers, P.O. Box 3489, Amsterdam

# Lipids, Malnutrition & the Developing Brain

A Ciba Foundation Symposium
jointly with the Nestlé Foundation
in memory of Sir Norman Wright

1972

Elsevier · Excerpta Medica · North-Holland
Associated Scientific Publishers - Amsterdam - London - New York

ISBN Excerpta Medica 90 219 4003 5
ISBN American Elsevier 0-444-10372-4

Library of Congress Catalog Card Number 72-76 008

Published in 1972 by Associated Scientific Publishers, P.O. Box 3489, Amsterdam, and 52 Vanderbilt Avenue, New York, N. Y. 10017.
Suggested series entry for library catalogues: Ciba Foundation Symposia.

Printed in the Netherlands by Royal VanGorcum, Assen

# Contents

# Contributors

*Symposium on Lipids, Malnutrition and the Developing Brain, held jointly with the Nestlé Foundation at the Ciba Foundation, London, 19th-21st October 1971*


A. VON MURALT (*Chairman*) Nestlé Foundation, 4 Place de la Gare, PO Box 1051, 1001 Lausanne, Switzerland

H. AEBI Universität Bern Medizinisch-Chemisches Institut, Bühlstrasse 28, 3000 Bern, Switzerland

G. B. ANSELL Department of Pharmacology, The University of Birmingham Medical School, Birmingham B15 2TJ, England

NICOLE BAUMANN Laboratoire de Neurochimie, Clinique des Maladies du Système Nerveux, Hôpital de la Salpêtrière, Paris 13e, France

J. BERNSOHN Neuropsychiatric Research Laboratory, Veterans Administration Edward Hines, Jr., Hospital, Hines, Illinois 60141, USA

D. BOVET Laboratorio di Psicobiologia e Psicofarmacologia, Consiglio Nazionale delle Ricerche, Via Reno 1, 00198 Roma, Italy

D. CHAPMAN Department of Chemistry, The University, Sheffield S3 7HF, England

F. COBOS Harvard University School of Public Health, Bogota Project Office, Direccion de Nutricion, ICBF, Apartado Aereo 15609, Bogota, Colombia

M. A. CRAWFORD Nuffield Institute of Comparative Medicine, The Zoological Society, Regent's Park, London NW1 4RY, England

A. N. DAVISON Department of Biochemistry, Institute of Neurology, Queen Square, London WC1N 3BG, England

J. DOBBING Department of Child Health, University of Manchester, Clinical Sciences Building, York Place, Manchester 13 OJJ, England

N. HERSCHKOWITZ Department of Neurochemistry, Universitäts-Kinderklinik, Inselspital Bern, Freiburgstrasse 23, 3008 Bern, Switzerland

DOROTHY F. HOLLINGSWORTH The British Nutrition Foundation Limited, Alembic House, 93 Albert Embankment, London SE1 7TY, England

U. M. T. HOUTSMULLER Unilever Research, Olivier van Noortlaan 120, Vlaardingen/Duiven, The Netherlands

R. E. KLEIN Human Development Division, Instituto de Nutricion de Centro America y Panama, Carretera Roosevelt Zona 11, Guatemala

P. D. LEATHWOOD Biology Department, Nestlé Products Technical Assistance Co. Ltd., 1814 La Tour de Peilz, Switzerland

JUNE K. LLOYD Department of Child Health, University of London Institute of Child Health, 30 Guilford Street, London WC1N 1 EH, England

J. F. MEAD University of California, Los Angeles, Laboratory of Nuclear Medicine and Radiation Biology, 900 Veteran Avenue, Los Angeles, California 90024, USA

J. H. MENKES Division of Pediatric Neurology, University of California Center for the Health Sciences, Los Angeles, California, 90024, USA

R. PAOLETTI Institute of Pharmacology and Pharmacognosy, University of Milan, Via A Del Sarto 21, 20129 Milan, Italy

E. ROSSI Universitäts-Kinderklinik, Inselspital Bern, Freiburgstrasse 23, 3008 Bern, Switzerland

L. SVENNERHOLM Department of Neurochemistry, Psychiatric Research Centre, University of Göteborg Faculty of Medicine, Medicinaregatan 9, Göteborg SV, Sweden

M. J. WINICK Institute of Human Nutrition, Columbia University, 511 West 166th Street, New York, NY 10032, USA

F. G. YOUNG Department of Biochemistry, University of Cambridge, Tennis Court Road, Cambridge CB2 1QW, England

*Editors:* KATHERINE ELLIOTT and JULIE KNIGHT

# Nomenclature

In this volume the unsaturated fatty acids are designated by the carbon atom where the first double bond appears, counting from the methyl end of the molecule. For example:

| | | |
|---|---|---|
| *n*–9 series: | 18:1 (*n*–9) | oleic acid |
| | 20:3 (*n*–9) | eicosatrienoic acid |
| | 22:3 (*n*–9) | docosatrienoic acid |
| *n*–6 series: | 18:2 (*n*–6) | linoleic acid |
| | 20:4 (*n*–6) | eicosatetraenoic acid |
| | 22:4 (*n*–6) | docosatetraenoic acid |
| | 22:5 (*n*–6) | docosapentaenoic acid |
| *n*–3 series: | 18:3 (*n*–3) | linolenic acid |
| | 20:5 (*n*–3) | eicosapentaenoic acid |
| | 22:5 (*n*–3) | docosapentaenoic acid |
| | 22:6 (*n*–3) | docosahexaenoic acid |

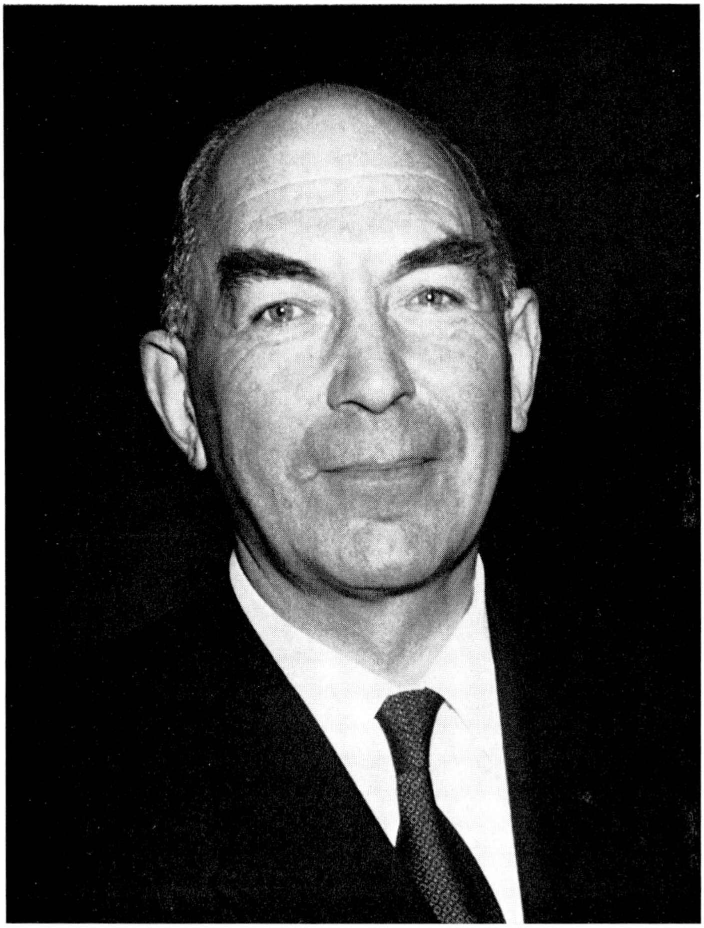

*Reproduced by permission of*
*Chemical Age*

SIR NORMAN WRIGHT, FRSE

*1900-1970*

Plans for this symposium had from the beginning the encouragement and interest of Sir Norman Wright, Deputy Director-General of the Food & Agriculture Organization of the United Nations from 1959 to 1963. With his help the idea for a joint meeting with the Nestlé Foundation (of whose Council he was a member) became reality. At his death in 1970, both Foundations grieved to lose a wise and valued friend. With sincere affection and respect we offer this book in honour and remembrance of Norman Wright, whose life was given to the struggle against malnutrition.

# The developing brain and the damage inflicted by malnutrition: an introduction

ALEXANDER VON MURALT

*Nestlé Foundation, Lausanne*

Wherever malnutrition prevails—and unfortunately this happens in vast areas of our world—the children are always most severely affected. Children are so dependent on the insight of their mothers, on the socio-economic background, and on the hygienic conditions of their small world, that they easily get caught by a vicious circle beginning with malnutrition and ignorance, leading up to a premature death. Malnutrition is the primary cause of the high rates of infant mortality in developing countries, even if the ultimate cause which the death certificate states may be something else, often an infectious disease like measles, which in malnourished children is apt to take a dangerous turn.

In recent years we have become more and more aware of the high vulnerability of infants, mainly for protein-calorie malnutrition. From animal experiments we have learned that growth is not only retarded by early malnutrition, but even stunted (see Widdowson and McCance 1960; Widdowson and Kennedy 1962; McCance and Widdowson 1962; Winick and Noble 1966, 1967; and also Miller 1969). What happens to the brain of a malnourished infant and what are the chances for the later intellectual development of a child who has been subjected to malnutrition at a critical period in his early life?

Our symposium deals with one aspect only, the lipids and the developing brain, but the problem has such an overwhelming importance for developing countries that it should be the *Leitmotiv* of the symposium!

## *Vulnerability*

Prolonged starvation of human adults, leading finally to death, had the following effects on the weight of the various organs: brain and heart lost only 3% of their bulk; the muscles, liver and spleen lost 31%, 54% and 67%, respectively. Wright (1945) concluded that 'the essential organs are thus spared as far as possible', or to put it in another way, that the tissues are sacrificed in inverse proportion to their importance. Is one entitled to conclude from these sad experiences of World War II that the brain of the adult is less vulnerable towards starvation than other organs? One can argue just as convincingly that special homeostatic mechanisms protect the brain during starvation, so-called 'brain sparing', just because it has a high vulnerability.

It appears that one must distinguish between intrinsic causes and extrinsic causes of vulnerability. Let me mention an example to explain this. Babies are vulnerable to water deprivation. Intrinsic cause: the immature kidney produces a hypotonic urine (in the adult it is hypertonic) and the baby loses comparatively more water. Extrinsic cause: the baby is unable to mobilize the fluid reserves in its tissue spaces in order to replace the loss of water because the homeostatic mechanisms of water balance have not yet been developed. This example may illustrate the two aspects of vulnerability.

## *Critical periods*

As long as organogenesis goes on, the developing organism is much more defenceless against harmful external factors, such as malnutrition, than when it has reached maturity. During the period where the brain grows faster than any other organ of the body—the period Dobbing (1968*a*, *b*) called 'the growth spurt'—brain vulnerability is critical. But the timing of critical periods varies from animal to animal, and since we have to rely on animal experimentation the extrapolation of such results to the human brain is loaded with uncertainty. As far as we can guess now, the critical period for human babies begins with the second half of foetal life and ends about 18 months after birth.

Research has to go a long way before we can connect biochemical or structural abnormalities, due to malnutrition, with any specific dysfunction of the brain. Apathy of the children is one of the most constant signs of protein-calorie malnutrition; the loss of curiosity and the lack of desire for exploration, a progressive withdrawal from the environment, are other symptoms of acute protein deficiency. How can they be connected with deficiencies in the assembly of molecules into relevant brain structures or with a failure of forces that stabilize molecular conformations in the brain? There is a very deep gap between our knowledge of biochemical and structural brain maturity and what we call the process of achieving mental maturity—in a way the same gap that exists between the perfection of a computer at delivery from the factory and its performance after having been programmed.

Considering this example it becomes clear that what we want to know is this: does damage, inflicted on the brain of an infant at a critical period, heal with time and nutritional rehabilitation, or does it leave persistent effects which produce below-age-norm scores in all fields of behaviour 6-10 years later? Cravioto (1970) summarizes the situation as follows: 'From all quoted studies we can conclude that the existence of an association between protein-calorie malnutrition in infancy and retardation in mental development has been established beyond reasonable doubt'. A similar statement was made by Monckeberg (1971): 'Various studies made on both man and animals confirm that there really exists a critical period during the first months of life, when the damage produced by malnutrition has more serious and permanent consequences, which persist even when environmental conditions improve later on'.

### *Socio-economic influence*

In animal experiments one can confirm the persistence of damage caused by early malnutrition after rehabilitation by chemical, structural and electrophysiological analyses over a lapse of time which is relatively short. Not so in human studies! There, the infants are exposed to poor housing, low levels of educational achievement, high infection rates and all sorts of taboos—nutritional and educational— during many years. The establishment of a truly causal relationship between malnutrition and deficient mental function is a very difficult task. Poor socio-economic conditions are almost always coupled with malnutrition, and both can have a significant deleterious effect on the growing child. This conjunction of factors makes it so difficult to determine the part which malnutrition may have played at the critical period—and yet, we should be able to overcome this ambiguity.

Two approaches seem to me of special interest: the study of siblings and the study of intersensory development.

*Siblings*. Cravioto and co-workers (1969) have carried out a study in a group of school-children who had suffered from severe protein-calorie malnutrition before their 30th month of life. The influence of the socio-economic factor was reduced by examining a group of siblings of similar age and identical sex. The children who had suffered from protein-calorie malnutrition in their early life scored consistently lower in all tests than their siblings who had no nutritional damage.

A similar study on siblings, but on a much larger scale, is now underway in Bogotà (Harvard—I.C.B.F.—Cornell Research Project). Dr Cobos is going to tell us about it in this symposium.

*Intersensory development.* Cravioto, together with Birch and collaborators (Cravioto, De Licardie and Birch 1966; Cravioto, Espinosa-Gaona and Birch 1967), studied the effect of early malnutrition on auditory-visual integration in school-age children of shorter stature, age by age. They showed poorer intersensory development than their taller equals in age. Such studies should be extended, especially with children who have been followed up from their critical period of early malnutrition until reaching school-age, in a vertical study. Intersensory disturbances are certainly more closely connected to internal factors due to malnutrition than to environmental influences.

*Separation of the influence of early malnutrition from environmental factors*

A clear experimental separation of the consequences of early nutritional damage of the brain from the disturbing socio-economic factors is of primary importance, because in the course of advising agencies or governments about the appropriate measures against mental retardation we must stand on solid ground with regard to its causes. Nutrient deficiencies during the critical period, together with low socio-economic factors, produce retardation of growth and of development of the intellect, and difficulties in learning and behaviour. This is not only true for infants who have passed through an attack of kwashiorkor or marasmus, but also for those who have suffered from moderate malnutrition, which is so abundant in developing countries. What we must know is whether malnutrition *per se* is sufficient to induce persistent effects on the functioning of the brain.

*Lipids and their functional role in the brain*

One of the events in the maturation of the brain that has evoked a considerable amount of attention is myelination. Our knowledge of the structure of the myelin sheath was gained by studies on peripheral nerve, based on the pioneering work of Schmitt, Bear and Clark (1935), Fernández-Morán (1952), Geren (1954) and Geren and Schmitt (1955). These and other studies provide the following picture. The myelin sheath is a highly ordered, concentric and spiral layered structure, surrounding the axon in the internode. The lipids form a bilayer with their axes in radial orientation, between two protein sheaths, which originate from an invagination of Schwann cell membranes, wrapped around the axon in many layers (up to 100 and more). The axon at the centre is surrounded by its own axonal membrane, which at the node, where the myelin sheath is interrupted, is excitable. In the brain, myelin deposition is more complicated and the glial cells (oligodendroglia) produce the myelin 'coating'.

The electrophysiologist considers myelin as an insulating material of high importance, ensuring the correct functioning of the complicated electrical network of nerve cells, axons and dendrites, and he is rather surprised to hear that a deficiency in essential fatty acids has consequences not only for the myelin composition, but also for the functioning of the brain! Between nerve cells and glial cells there is a 'symbiotic contact', much more intimate and functionally important than the contact of our insulator and a conducting element.

## *The excitable membrane*

This membrane creates the nervous impulse and is thus the basic element of the activity of the peripheral and central nervous system. The excitable membrane is the carrier of information.

Our conceptions of the structure of membranes have recently changed quite a lot and the Danielli-Davson (1935) and Robertson (1962) model is in conflict with recent new findings. No evidence could be found for the presence of proteins in β-conformation, as postulated by the model. On the contrary, in erythrocyte membranes half of the proteins are in α-helical conformation, the rest are coiled (see Zahler 1969). In most membranes studied, hydrophobic bonds could be demonstrated between lipids and proteins (see Chapman 1968; Chapman and Kamat 1968; Wallach and Gordon 1968; Zahler 1969; Zahler and Weibel 1970). It seems evident that the loosely bound lipids (cholesterol and portions of the phosphatides) are held within the membrane by hydrophobic bonds with the helical proteins. Lecithin and sphingomyelin are probably more tightly fixed by polar interaction with protein. How is this high degree of organization of the lipids achieved? There is a strong mutual interaction between the lipids and the protein backbone of the membrane. The assumption that the great variety of lipids of a given membrane are selected and incorporated by the membrane proteins seems plausible.

Changes of the membrane potential in squid and *Maia* axons produce rapid, reversible changes of the birefringence of the radially oriented lipoproteins of the membrane (see Cohen, Keynes and Hille 1968, 1971). In the olfactory nerve of the pike this optical change is very marked, due to the large proportion of radially oriented lipoproteins in this nerve (see von Muralt 1972).

*Conclusions*

Recalling the *Leitmotiv* of our symposium, the problem of intellectual development of a child who has been subjected to malnutrition at a critical period in early life, it is obvious that protein deficiency and deficiency of essential fatty acids can have persistent effects on the biochemical maturity of the brain. Since proteins act as the backbone of lipid incorporation in the brain and are probably responsible for the highly complicated lipid substructure, a protein deficit should have a longer-lasting deleterious effect on the brain than a transient deficit in essential fatty acids. It is hoped that the contributions to this symposium will shed new light on this fascinating subject.

## References

CHAPMAN, D. (1968). In *Membrane Models and the Formation of Biological Membranes*, pp. 6-18, ed. L.Bolis and B. A. Pethica. North-Holland, Amsterdam
CHAPMAN, D. and KAMAT, V. B. (1968) In *Regulatory Functions of Biological Membranes*, p. 99, ed. J. Järnefelt. Elsevier, Amsterdam
COHEN, L. B., KEYNES, R. D. and HILLE, B. (1968) *Nature (Lond.)* **218**, 438-441
COHEN, L. B., KEYNES, R. D. and HILLE, B. (1971) *J. Physiol. (Lond.)* **211**, 495-515
CRAVIOTO, J. (1970) In *Malnutrition is a Problem of Ecology*, ed. P. György and O. L. Kline Bibl. *Nutritio et Dieta*, no 14, pp. 7-22. Karger, Basel
CRAVIOTO, J., DE LICARDIE, E. R. and BIRCH, H. G. (1966) *Pediatrics* **38**.2, 319-333
CRAVIOTO, J., ESPINOSA-GAONA, C. and BIRCH, H. G. (1967) *J. Spec. Educ.* **2**. 1, 75-82
CRAVIOTO, J., PIÑERO, C., ARROYO, M. and ALCALDE, E. (1969) In *Nutrition in Preschool and School Age* (Swedish Nutr. Fdn. Symp. VII) pp. 85-98, ed. G. Blix. Almqvist & Wiksell, Uppsala
DANIELLI, J. F. and DAVSON, H. (1935) *J. Cell Comp. Physiol.* **5**, 495-508
DOBBING, J. (1968*a*) In *Malnutrition, Learning and Behavior*, p. 181, ed. N. S. Scrimshaw and J. E. Gordon. M.I.T. Press, Cambridge, Mass.
DOBBING, J. (1968*b*) In *Applied Neurochemistry*, pp. 287-316, ed. A. N. Davison and J. Dobbing. Blackwell, Oxford
DOBBING, J. (1970) *New Sci.* **46**, 636-637
FERNÁNDEZ-MORÁN, H. (1952) *Exp. Cell Res.* **3**, 282-359
GEREN, B. B. (1954) *Exp. Cell Res.* **7**, 558-562
GEREN, B. B. and SCHMITT, F. O. (1955) In *Proceedings of the 8th Congress of Cell Biology, Leiden*. Interscience, New York
MCCANCE, R. A. and WIDDOWSON, E. M. (1962) *Proc. R. Soc. B* **156**, 326-337
MILLER, S. (1969) In *Mammalian Protein Metabolism*, vol. 3, pp. 183-233, ed. H. N. Munro. Academic Press, New York and London
MONCKEBERG, B. F. (1971) *FAO/WHO/UNICEF Protein Advisory Group Bulletin* **11**, 9-17
MURALT, A. VON (1972) *Pflügers Arch. Gesamte Physiol.* in press
ROBERTSON, J. B. (1962) *Res. Publ. Assoc. Res. Nerv. Ment. Dis.* **40**, 94-158
SCHMITT, F. O., BEAR, R. S. and CLARK, G. L. (1935) *Radiology* **25**, 131-151
WALLACH, D. F. H. and GORDON, A. S. (1968) In *Regulatory Functions of Biological Membranes*, p. 87, ed. J. Järnefelt. Elsevier, Amsterdam
WIDDOWSON, E. M. and MCCANCE, R. A. (1960) *Proc. R. Soc. B* **152**, 188-206

WIDDOWSON, E. M. and KENNEDY, G. C. (1962) *Proc. R. Soc. B* **156**, 96-108
WINICK, M. and NOBLE, A. (1966) *J. Nutr.* **89**, 300-306
WINICK, M. and NOBLE, A. (1967) *J. Nutr.* **91**, 179-182
WRIGHT, S. (1945) *Applied Physiology*, p. 808. Oxford University Press, London
ZAHLER, P. (1969) *Experientia* **25**, 449-456
ZAHLER, P. and WEIBEL, E. (1970) *Biochim. Biophys. Acta* **219**, 320-338

# Vulnerable periods of brain development

JOHN DOBBING

*Department of Child Health, University of Manchester*

The manner in which the brain develops during the earlier stages of organogenesis and subsequently grows towards the mature state has always attracted much interest from neurobiologists. In recent years there has been increasing concern to investigate the possibility that there may be certain periods of brain development during which comparatively mild interference with growth may produce irreversible alterations in its final form, and whether these may be of consequence to higher mental function. In spite of the increasing attention which these ideas are attracting, the field remains extremely nebulous, a situation partly due to the technical difficulties of its proper investigation, but more particularly to our negligible knowledge of the physical basis of such important and less tangible brain functions. The existence and significance of 'critical' or 'vulnerable' periods is central to the discussion and forms the subject of the present paper.

## CRITICAL OR VULNERABLE PERIODS

The idea of critical periods of brain development probably took root from two hitherto separated disciplines. The developmental behaviourists have described 'imprinting' phenomena in newly hatched birds and possibly analogous periods of 'socialization' in the postnatal development of mammals (Scott 1967; Fox and Stelzner 1966), while neurobiologists, more interested in the less behavioural aspects of brain development, have described a 'critical' period (Flexner 1955), when a large number of physical events are alleged to happen suddenly and in a meaningfully related way.

The critical period concerned with imprinting is more helpfully and more usually described as a 'sensitive' period, implying that developing behaviour is more *susceptible* at this particular stage to certain lasting modifications of future performance, and the behavioural literature is full of similar, if less dramatic, examples of such periods of susceptibility in all species including man.

By contrast the 'critical' period of physical brain development (Flexner 1955) is much more diffusely described and may be thought to stand up less well to detailed scrutiny. Furthermore it did not (at least originally) imply sensitivity, but merely a collection of sudden, dramatic and simultaneous events. In retrospect it may now only appear to have been the first awareness of the phenomenon of the brain 'growth spurt' to be described later, and much of the suddenness may be an artefact due to the use of animals having short lifespans with a very compressed growth programme.

Certainly at this distance of time the original accounts now read rather incoherently as a catalogue of processes examined in only one small area of cerebral cortex in the period from 41 to 45 days of gestation in the guinea-pig, corresponding to the 10th day or so of postnatal life in the rat. There seems to be little similarity in the direction being taken by these processes. Some of them are coming to an end at this time (e.g. the maturation of neuronal nuclear volume); some are in full spate (the growth of dendritic processes and the arrival of Nissl substance); some are beginning their upward journey towards adult levels (the activity of certain enzymes); some are beginning to fall from their elevated immature levels (the chloride space); and some are only detectable for the first time (cortical electrical activity). The latter presumably depends on the sensitivity of the electronic apparatus of detection.

In fact, as we know from much less sophisticated investigations, this 'critical' period from 41 to 45 gestational days is merely the earlier part of the brain growth spurt which is at its height in this species from 45 to 50 days. If earlier workers had looked at other parts of the brain for other processes at other times, they would have detected equally dramatic phases of glial cell division occurring at about 55 days and of myelination just before term (66th day of gestational period) (Dobbing and Sands 1970*a*).

From the point of view of neurobiology having an application to human populations, the older concept of critical periods has little relevance. It is more profitable to investigate the *sensitivity* or *vulnerability* of developmental phases to interference, and especially to look for long-term evidence of such susceptibility in the shape of detectable distortions of structure and function in the adult brain. The best-known examples of such vulnerable periods are in the field of teratology, where there are a number of examples of very precise moments of susceptibility during that period of organogenesis when the organ is acquiring its shape. Non-specific insults at this time may result in very gross disturbances of shape and form, which by their nature are irreversible. In humans such disastrous events are probably confined to the first trimester of gestation and it must be conceded that their detailed aetiology is often at best only suspected. In experimental animals viral disease, drugs, nutritional (vitamin) imbalance, X-irradiation and even mild pyrexia of short duration will produce deformities in the central nervous system, dependent on the precise timing of the insult in relation to embryological events.

Very little is known of any possibility of vulnerability during the second human trimester, although this is the period during which there seems to be a distinct phase of neuroblast proliferation, and adult numbers of neurons are virtually achieved by the time it is over (Dobbing and Sands 1970*b*). Perhaps within limits the number of neurons is functionally less important than their later dendritic development and the establishment of synaptic interconnections which are probably laid down during the third trimester and later. Perhaps the physiological circumstances of the second trimester render it less subject to foetal deprivation. Alternatively, it may even be that our academic ignorance of second trimester neuropathology is associated causally with our total ignorance of the nature and pathogenesis of vast numbers of cases of so-called unclassified mental retardation, whose brains the traditional neuropathologist finds such unrewarding objects of study.

The neuropathology of the third trimester of human gestation has until recently been mainly a matter of focal lesions, or patterns of focal lesions, inflicted by the circumstances of abnormal birth such as hypoxia, hypoglycaemia, or kernicterus. The consequences of these common lesions are just as lasting as the deformities of teratology, but their primary aetiology lies outside the nervous system and we need not postulate any particularly vulnerable period of brain development to account for them. Indeed, the brain is a great deal more susceptible to many of these insults in adult life than in the perinatal period.

## THE BRAIN GROWTH SPURT

More recently the brain growth spurt has been identified as a period of vulnerability. This is the transient period during which increase in brain weight and a number of other important developmental processes proceeds at very high velocity. The nature of the vulnerability is different from that already described at other periods. There are no true deformities, nor is there any focal tissue destruction. However it seems that it is only necessary to retard growth during the period of the brain growth spurt for there to be irrecoverable distortions of pattern as well as quantitative deficits which are detectable in the adult brain. In the human this growth spurt period appears to correspond to the last trimester of gestation and the first 18 months or so of postnatal life.

These ideas arose from testing the hypothesis that the vulnerability of the developing brain (in the present sense) may be related to its rate of growth. Thus the period of slow growth *preceding* the growth spurt should be as relatively invulnerable as is the mature brain when the growth period is over. In very general terms this proposition, even though it takes far too simple a view of the growth of such a complex organ, can indeed be shown to be true. When one considers the heterogeneity of brain structure compared with most other parenchymatous tissues, as well as the complicated temporal sequence and spatial distribution of most of its developmental processes, it is surprising how well such a hypothesis can be tested using such crude indices as estimates of cell number, degree of myelination and fresh weight of large complex regions.

Fortunately the general pattern of events in brain development seems to be similar from one mammalian species to another, so that the hypothesis can be tested experimentally in animals, provided the species differences in the timing of birth are taken into account (Fig. 1). Unlike the respiratory and cardiovascular systems, normal birth is of no significance to brain development, and it matters little that the growth spurt is foetal in guinea-pigs, perinatal in pigs,

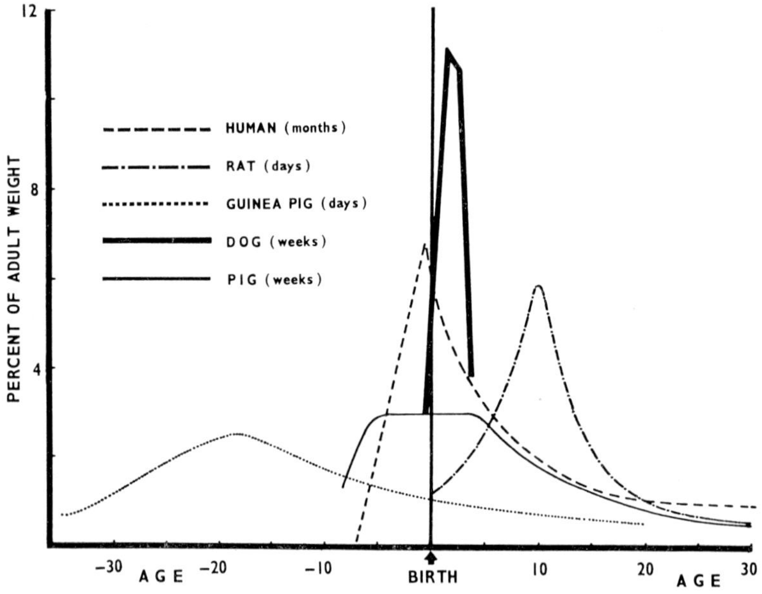


FIG. 1. Rate curves of brain growth in relation to birth in different species. Values are calculated at different time intervals for each species.

predominantly postnatal in humans and entirely so in rats (Davison and Dobbing 1968). It is only necessary to abandon such expressions as 'foetal brain' or 'neonatal brain', unless the species be specified and the brain growth characteristics of that species known.

The major brain growth spurt may be said to begin in all species at about the time the adult number of neurons is virtually achieved: by the end of the second human trimester or at birth in the rat. There is some neurogenesis later than this time, especially amongst microneurons in the cerebellum.

Among the major identifiable processes during the brain growth spurt period are the following:

(1) Very considerable *glial* cell multiplication. This in terms of numbers is much greater than the pre-growth spurt multiplication of *neurons* (Dobbing and Sands 1970*b*, 1972*a*) and it is therefore quite wrong to regard the end of cell multiplication in, for example, the rat as occurring at birth, as is often stated (Davison and Dobbing 1968).

(2) Myelination (Dobbing and Sands 1972*a*).

(3) The development of several enzyme systems (Adlard and Dobbing 1971*a*, *b*, 1972).

(4) Changes in brain carbohydrate metabolism (Gaitonde and Richter 1966).

(5) Development of certain reflex patterns (Smart and Dobbing 1971*a*, *b*).

(6) Changes in water and cation content (de Souza and Dobbing 1971).

## EVIDENCE FOR SELECTIVE VULNERABILITY OF THE BRAIN GROWTH SPURT PERIOD

This has accumulated from a number of different experimental designs, mostly exploiting the postnatal timing of the growth spurt in rats during their suckling period.

In the first and most widely used design, growth is retarded by increasing the size of the suckling litter, so that rats are weaned at about half the normal weight. They are then given food *ad libitum* until maturity and the mature brains of permanently stunted animals are examined (Fig. 2). These are compared with brains of animals well fed until weaning and undernourished later, or with those of severely undernourished adult rats. Deficits and distortions are confined to those animals underfed in the suckling period. It is noteworthy that growth retardation confined to the bodily growth spurt (which occurs later than that of the brain) does *not* induce permanent stunting of either whole body or brain (Dobbing 1968; Dobbing and Sands 1972*a*).

A second experimental design which may be more satisfactory, especially from the behaviourist's point of view, involves underfeeding the mother during

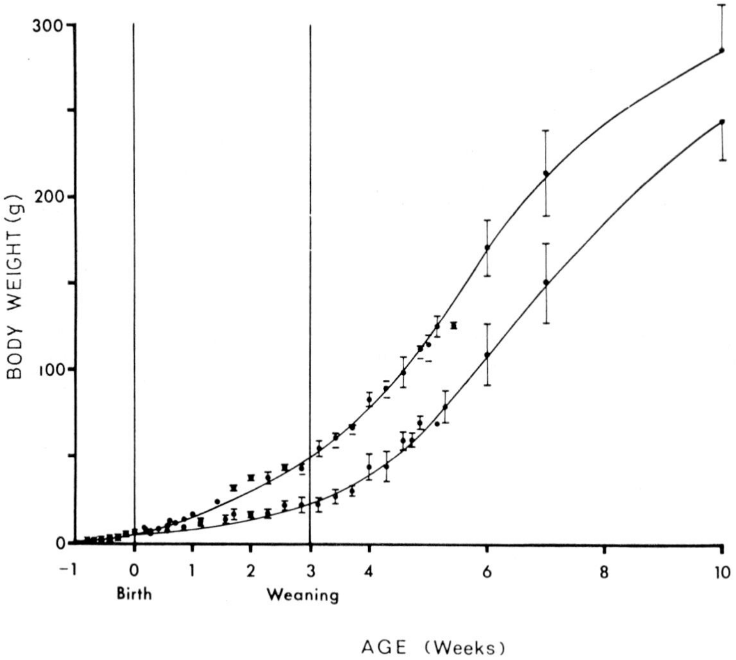


FIG. 2. Body weights of rats reared in two sizes of litter until weaning and fed *ad libitum* thereafter (Dobbing and Sands 1972*a*). Upper curve, small litters.

the pregnancy. Stunted offspring as well as normal control newborns are then cross-fostered at birth to well-fed and undernourished lactating females, *the litter size being standardized.* Thus there are four groups according to whether the gestational period or the suckling period or both or neither was nutritionally restricted. Any of these groups can be weaned to a restricted or an adequate diet, and in this way all combinations and permutations of growth restriction can be imposed in the pre-growth spurt, growth spurt or post-growth spurt periods. Figs. 3*a* and *b* show the bodily growth curves when this is done and emphasize the dominating influence of growth during the brain growth spurt on ultimate attainment.

In experiments at present in progress an attempt is being made to imitate the case of the human baby of low birth weight for its gestational age, known to clinicians as 'small-for-dates'. On the assumption that a 5-day-old rat is at a comparable stage of brain development to the human full-term newborn, animals from underfed mothers are left with their mothers until 5 days after birth and then cross-fostered in the same manner as in the previous design.

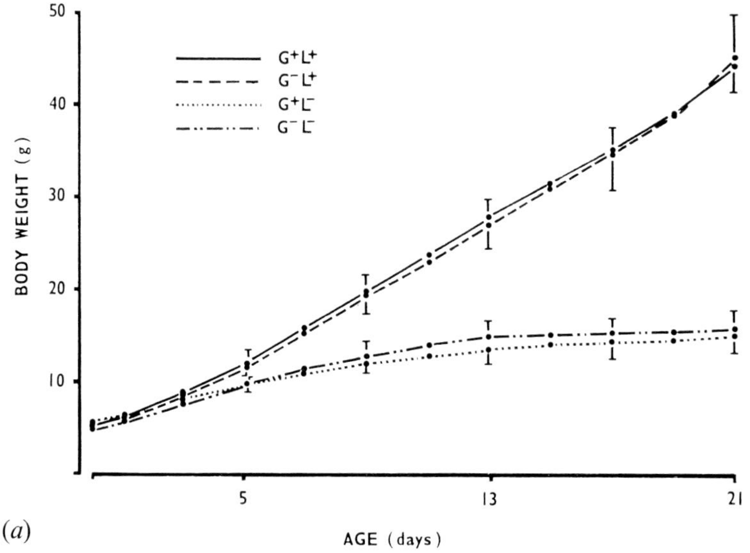


(*a*)

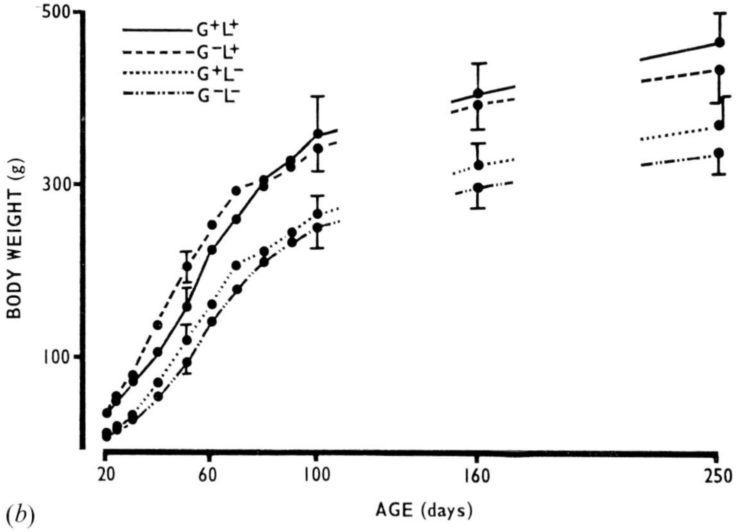


(*b*)

FIG. 3 (*a*) and (*b*). Body weights of rats (*a*) before and (*b*) after 21 days of age reared in standardized litter sizes from mothers underfed during gestation (G-) and/or lactation (L-) and cross-fostered at birth. Diet was *ad libitum* from 21 days onwards. The birth weight was significantly less in progeny from underfed mothers (Smart and Dobbing 1971*b*).

Preliminary results again show (Figs. 4*a* and *b*) the dominance of the brain growth spurt period in deciding the final outcome.

The results of all these experimental manipulations have led to the general conclusion that permanent, irrecoverable distortions and deficits can be prod-

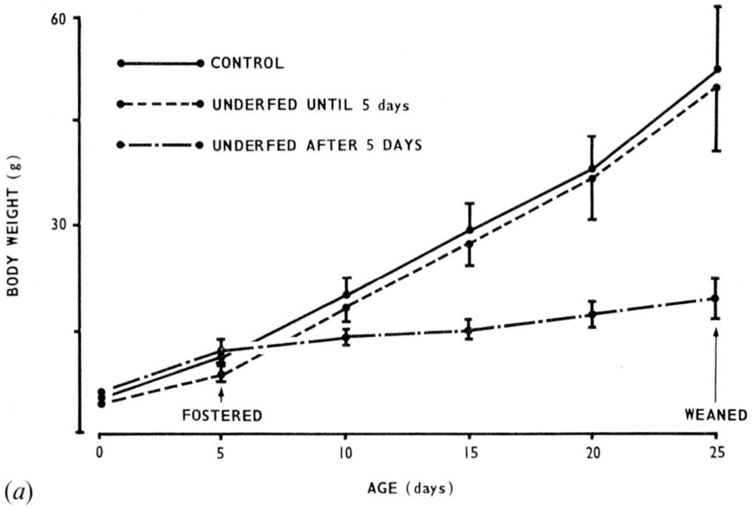


(*a*)

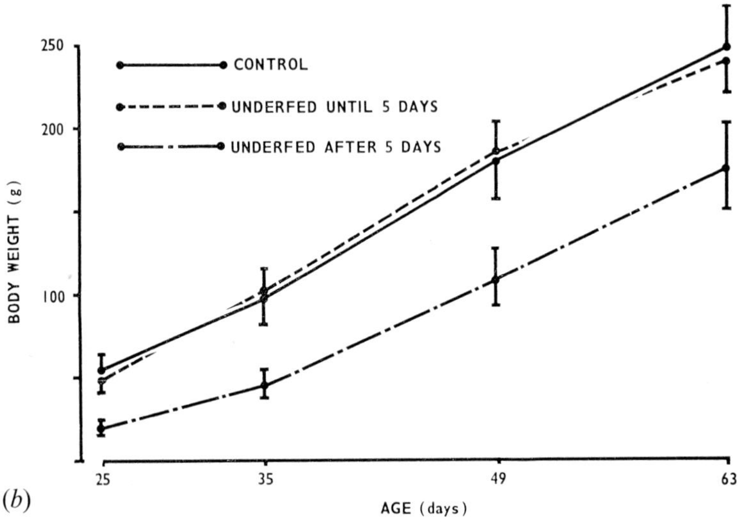


(*b*)

FIG. 4 (*a*) and (*b*). Body weights of rats (*a*) before and (*b*) after 25 days of age reared as in Fig. 3 except that cross-fostering and standardization of litter size occurred at 5 days after birth, to provide a model for human 'small-for-dates' babies (B. P. F. Adlard and J. L. Smart, in preparation).

uced in the brain, provided growth restriction has been imposed during the brain growth spurt, but not otherwise. In this sense, therefore, a vulnerable period has been demonstrated.

## EFFECTS OF RESTRICTIONS DURING THE BRAIN GROWTH SPURT

These effects have been described in detail elsewhere and will only be summarized here.

(1) There is a true, ultimate microcephaly. The adult brain is ultimately not only small for the age, but inappropriately small for the body weight (Dobbing and Sands 1972*a*). This is in spite of the high brain weight:body weight ratio during the growing period, sometimes ambiguously known as 'brain sparing'.

(2) The reduction in brain size is not uniform. For example, the cerebellum is much more reduced than other parts (Dobbing 1970*a*).

(3) Not only is there a permanent reduction of the total cell number of whole brain, but this too occurs selectively in certain areas and among certain cell types (Dobbing, Hopewell and Lynch 1971).

(4) The amount of brain cholesterol is reduced more than would be predicted from the reduced brain size (Dobbing and Sands 1972a), and specifically myelin lipids appear to be selected for reduction (Dobbing 1968).

(5) Brain enzyme patterns are distorted (Adlard and Dobbing 1971*a*, *c*, 1972; Adlard, Dobbing and Smart 1970).

(6) Reflex ontogeny and some aspects of late behaviour (Smart 1971; Smart and Dobbing 1971*a*, *b*, *c*) are altered.

## CHRONOLOGICAL DETERMINATION OF BRAIN GROWTH

It has recently been shown that the timing of several of the major components of the brain growth spurt is determined by chronological rather than by developmental age. Vulnerability of the growth programme may thus reside in a failure, in growth-retarded animals, to accomplish proper growth at the fixed chronological age which is their only opportunity.

The demonstration of this concept involved the construction of reliable velocity curves for brain growth in control and growth-retarded animals. These cannot be convincingly drawn without very detailed primary data from very large numbers of animals reared under standard conditions and sampled at very frequent intervals. Smooth, 'best fit' lines are drawn using a computer curve-fitting procedure in order to eliminate personal bias, and velocity curves are then calculated. Velocity curves for brain growth, cell multiplication, and cholesterol accumulation in rats reared in abnormally large litters all show the same phenomenon (Dobbing and Sands 1972a). The *timing* of the peak velocity is not altered by the growth retardation, only its *extent*; and since there is no facility for 'catch-up' on restoration to an *ad libitum* diet at weaning, an ultimate deficit results. Fig. 5 shows this finding for whole brain DNA content.

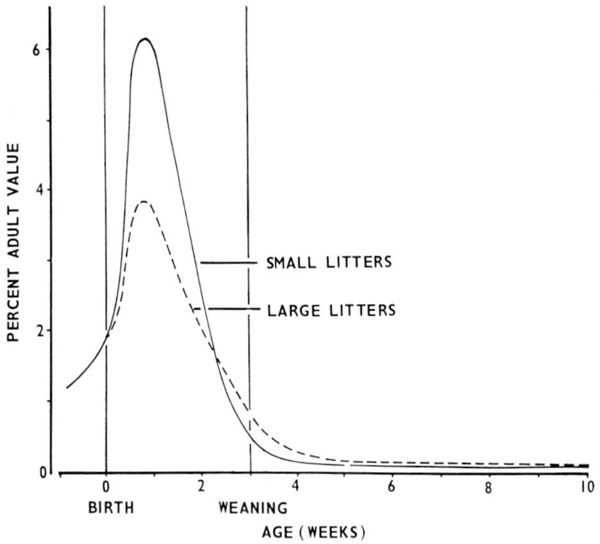


FIG. 5. Velocity curves of the increment in DNA in the brains of rats reared as shown in Fig. 2. Growth retardation has not delayed the timing of the peak velocity (Dobbing and Sands 1972*a*).

## THE HUMAN BRAIN GROWTH SPURT

Any attempt to transfer these ideas to man of course involves some important assumptions which may be unjustified. However, it is possible that this demonstration that rats have a once-only opportunity to grow their brains properly during the brain growth spurt may also apply to man. If so, the timing of the vulnerable period will have to be defined in humans, and this has been attempted (Dobbing 1970*b*; Dobbing and Sands 1972*b*). The human brain grows much more slowly than that of the small laboratory animals. The human growth spurt appears to extend throughout the last trimester of pregnancy and well into the 2nd year of postnatal life, and by analogy similar harm would be expected in the brains of humans growth-retarded during this time.

CONCLUSIONS AND SUMMARY

There is no question but that the transient period of brain growth, known as the brain growth spurt, is more vulnerable to growth restriction than the periods both before and afterwards. Vulnerability in this sense means that quite mild restriction leads in experimental animals to permanent, irrecoverable reduction in the trajectory of bodily growth and to easily detectable distortions and deficits in the adult brain. This vulnerable period is quite separate from the earlier better-known teratological period during which minor insults may result in gross and lasting deformity. Neither is there any detectable focal destruction or lesion. In the present case the 'damage' consists of permanent but non-uniform reduction in the extent of brain growth. There is accumulating evidence that it has functional importance. An important feature of this type of vulnerability is that it is highly dependent on the timing of the insult, although not as finely so as the earlier teratology. The question remains open whether these effects on the physical brain are analogous to similar sensitivities of developing behaviour.

ACKNOWLEDGEMENTS

I wish to acknowledge a grant from the Medical Research Council, with additional help from the National Fund for Research into Crippling Diseases, and the Spastics Society. I especially thank my colleagues Dr B.P.F. Adlard, Miss J. Sands, Dr J. L. Smart and Dr S. W. de Souza for their continuing help with this work.

# References

ADLARD, B. P. F. and DOBBING, J. (1971*a*) *Brain Res.* **28**, 97-107
ADLARD, B. P. F. and DOBBING, J. (1971*b*) *J. Neurochem.* **18**, 1299-1303
ADLARD, B. P. F. and DOBBING, J. (1971*c*) *Brain Res.* **30**, 198-199
ADLARD, B. P. F. and DOBBING, J. (1972) *Pediatr. Res.* in press
ADLARD, B. P. F., DOBBING, J. and SMART, J. L. (1970) *Biochem. J.* **119**, 46P
DAVISON, A. N. and DOBBING, J. (1968) In *Applied Neurochemistry*, pp. 253-286, ed. A. N. Davison and J. Dobbing. Blackwell, Oxford

DOBBING, J. (1968) In *Applied Neurochemistry*, pp. 287-316, ed. A. N. Davison and J. Dobbing. Blackwell, Oxford
DOBBING, J. (1970*a*) In *Developmental Neurobiology*, pp. 241-261, ed. W. A. Himwich. Thomas, Springfield, Ill.
DOBBING, J. (1970*b*) *Am. J. Dis. Child.* **120**, 411-415
DOBBING, J., HOPEWELL, J. W. and LYNCH, A. (1971) *Exp Neurol.* **32**, 439-447
DOBBING, J. and SANDS, J. (1970*a*) *Brain Res.* **17**, 115-123
DOBBING, J. and SANDS, J. (1970*b*) *Nature (Lond.)* **226**, 639-640
DOBBING, J. and SANDS, J. (1972*a*) *Biol. Neonat.* in press
DOBBING, J. and SANDS, J. (1972*b*) *in preparation*
FLEXNER, L. B. (1955) In *Biochemistry of the Developing Nervous System*, pp. 281-294, ed. H. Waelsch. Academic Press, New York
FOX, M. W. and STELZNER, D. (1966) *Anim. Behav.* **14**, 273-281
GAITONDE, M. K. and RICHTER, D. (1966) *J. Neurochem.* **13**, 1309-1318
SCOTT, J. P. (1967) *Ann. Rev. Psychol.* **18**, 1-40
SMART, J. L. (1971) *Psychiatr. Neurol. Neurochir.* **74**, 443-452
SMART, J. L. and DOBBING, J. (1971*a*) *Brain Res.* **28**, 85-95
SMART, J. L. and DOBBING, J. (1971*b*) *Brain Res.* **33**, 303-314
SMART, J. L. and DOBBING, J. (1971*c*) *Dev. Psychobiol.* in press
SOUZA, S. W. DE and DOBBING, J. (1971) *Exp. Neurol.* **32**, 431-438

# Discussion

*Herschkowitz:* Dr Dobbing, you do not include neuronal proliferation in the critical or vulnerable period. This statement is presumably based on the knowledge that early severe malnutrition during the period of neuronal multiplication does not affect the final number of neurons?

*Dobbing:* I am quite agnostic about this. The phase of neuronal multiplication certainly antedates, or is at the very beginning of, what we call the brain 'growth spurt'. The difficulty is how to investigate whether there is an ultimate deficit in neurons. Estimating the amount of DNA is useless, because there are seven or eight times as many glial cells as neurons, and a 20% or even 50% deficit of neurons wouldn't show up in the total. We know that after malnutrition there is a deficit in those comparatively few neurons which divide postnatally in the rat, in the cerebellum and perhaps even in the cortex. I wouldn't say that we don't include neuronal proliferation in the vulnerable period; we don't know whether to include it or not. Nothing short of a thoroughly detailed neuronal count will tell us.

*Winick:* You referred to the distortions of pattern which result from retardation of growth during the brain growth spurt. The data suggest that the distortion, or selective reduction, in certain brain areas is not really dependent on the area or even on the cell type, but rather on the rate at which the cells are dividing. If this is so, what is happening is that a quantitative difference is being converted into a qualitative difference, as a result of the fact that cells are dividing at different times in different areas. This seems to be a fundamental process in all cells, not only brain cells, and the question is whether the growth-retarding stimulus, in this case a nutritional stimulus, is interfering with DNA synthesis, so that it retards cell division only when DNA is being synthesized, and since DNA is synthesized at different times in different areas, the differential effects are produced. If so, a fundamental question to be investigated concerns the mechanisms by which these stimuli interfere with DNA synthesis. Would you agree with that?

*Dobbing:* It's perfectly true that cell multiplication alone could cause the distortions, because cell multiplication occurs in different regions at different times, and in a well-ordered sequence. So if the hypothesis has anything to it, it will be a question of relating the timing of cell multiplication in one particular area, and the ultimate deficit, to the timing of the growth restriction. This could also lead to a study of what controls DNA synthesis or cell division. I would extend your point even further and say that if other processes such as myelination are vulnerable (which we know not to occur throughout the whole system as crystallization does in a solution, but stepwise, tract by tract, and in another well-ordered sequence), one might expect that if one had the analytical techniques one could impose deficits in different areas according to the timing of that process. One could go even further and suppose that if the growth of dendritic branches and the establishment of connections also has a regional time sequence of this kind, that too would have consequences in the adult brain, related to the timing of the growth retardation.

What puzzles me is why the *rate* of growth is what makes the brain vulnerable, and why there appear to be no permanent consequences of growth retardation during *bodily* growth. Of course the body as weighed is the sum of a large number of different tissues, but it must have very large tissue masses conforming in pattern to general bodily growth. If you retard *them* there is a complete catch-up later. If you retard at the brain growth spurt, not only does the brain fail to catch up, but the body doesn't either.

*von Muralt:* Rats reared in large litters attained smaller body size than those reared in reduced litters. Is it possible that this is an adaptation to the low calorie supply? In keeping the body size small, the calorie requirement is in balance with the supply. The counter-argument to this view is the observation that the deficit in weight persists even if these rats subsequently are fed adequately. It is known, however, in physiological experiments that once such an adaptation has taken place there is a tendency to maintain it.

*Dobbing:* If a human being is growth-retarded in these early years of the brain growth spurt, the evidence suggests that the consequent stunting is permanent over the human lifespan. It has even been demonstrated recently that in such a comparatively mild growth retardation as occurs in the last trimester of some pregnancies and results in babies who are rather small for their gestational age, detectable differences in head circumference are found 5 or 6 years later, compared with both the normal baby and the prematurely born baby, provided that the premature baby has grown well after birth (Davies and Davis 1970). The suggestion that all nutritional growth retardation is an adaptation to the food shortage in order to reduce metabolic rate is interesting, but of course the surface area to mass ratio is increased in the small animal, and the relative loss of heat would therefore be greater.

*Winick:* B. Chow (unpublished observations 1967) and others have data which indicate that permanent metabolic changes are induced by malnutrition during the gestational and lactational period in rats. These changes consist of an abnormal handling of nitrogen, so that these animals actually eat *more* for the rest of their lives, no matter how they are fed thereafter, and excrete more nitrogen, so that this also persists. One could look at this as an adaptation to a previous environment which persists, or as a metabolic abnormality which has been induced. I don't know how to look at it, but these data support the kinds of ideas Professor von Muralt is suggesting.

*von Muralt:* Dr Dobbing, how do you explain the fact that, in Japan, the population began to increase in size beginning with government measures improving the nutritional value of rice?

*Dobbing:* There is good evidence that the Japanese birth weight has increased in the last 20 years (Gruenwald *et al.* 1967). This is very easy to show in Japan where records are meticulously kept. It is a reasonable assumption that during the last 20 years general socio-economic conditions, including nutrition, have so far improved as to give rise to a better rate of foetal as well as adult growth, and having given rise to that increased foetal growth in what I think is the vulnerable period, as a consequence, adult growth attainment is the better for it.

What is interesting to me is that the vulnerable period for bodily growth appears to be when the *brain* is growing fast. This suggests that the brain has some controlling influence over somatic growth. Against that, if you decapitate a foetal rabbit *in utero*, somatic growth of the foetus proceeds normally until birth, and it is indeed born alive until it discovers that it lacks a central nervous system to operate a postnatal existence. However, that might be too early, according to our hypothesis, since the brain growth spurt in the rabbit is probably postnatal, like the rat. At present we are decapitating foetal guinea-pigs, whose brain growth spurt is in the foetal period, to see if this affects somatic growth.

*Rossi:* Children with kwashiorkor have normal or high concentrations of growth hormone and insulin in the blood, according to Godard and Zahud (1971). Are you sure that it is only a question of nutrition? Secular acceleration is not only due to improvement of nutrition. In Sardinia, people growing up in the last 30 years have increased in height from 162 cm to 165 cm with the same type of food. Other factors must be involved.

*Dobbing:* Nutrition is one of many factors that can retard growth. Infectious disease interacts with this effect on growth, as it probably does on mental development. Thus, if there are better hospitals in Sardinia and a better public health service, this itself would lead to better growth achievement.

*Paoletti:* Has growth hormone been measured in the pituitary and in plasma of animals fed on a calorie-deficient diet? Professor Rossi's comment recalls a recent investigation by Dr James Iacono, a nutritionist working for the U.S. Department of Agriculture (personal communication). Being of Sicilian origin, he is very interested in the rate of growth of Sicilians during the first and second generations in the United States. The first generation and especially the second is several centimetres taller than the parents of the same genetic background. He feels that the diet is important because the population of Sicily eats a great deal of 'longlasting' carbohydrates, mainly pasta (spaghetti). These are slowly absorbed. This means that for many hours in the day there is a high concentration of glucose in plasma, which is enough to reduce the output of growth hormone. As soon as they change to a more caloric diet, especially a diet rich in proteins and low in carbohydrates, or containing different kinds of carbohydrates, the output of growth hormone may be more prolonged during the 24 hours. Dr Iacono has data that demonstrate this.

*Mead:* The opposite experiment to the Japanese and Sicilian experiments has actually been done. Greenland was colonized by people from Iceland who were subsequently cut off because of the lack of wood and the inability to build boats. They began to suffer from malnutrition. Apparently the last boat that visited Greenland in the 16th century found a race of dwarfs (Hermann 1954). This is the opposite experiment, and I don't know how reliable the information is, but perhaps something can be gleaned from that!

*Winick:* Growth hormone does not seem to be necessary during foetal or neonatal life for either normal growth or normal cell division. There is a strain of mice which are born without the anterior pituitary (Snell-Smith) and which have no growth hormone at all. For the first 10 days of life they grow normally and have a normal number of cells in all organs. Then the growth rate suddenly falls and cell number no longer increases, which suggests that growth hormone becomes necessary for normal rates of cell growth at 10 days of life (Winick 1968). In man, growth hormone becomes necessary at around 6 months of age.

We have studied some of the mechanisms involved in cell division in the rat, for example, the activity of the enzyme DNA polymerase, which may be involved in DNA synthesis (Brasel, Ehrenkranz and Winick 1970). In the normal rat in most organs the activity of this enzyme very nicely mirrors the rate of DNA synthesis, but in the hypophysectomized rat the activity of this enzyme drops immediately to almost undetectable levels. If we then inject this rat with growth hormone the activity of the enzyme increases and 48-72 hours later cells start to divide. We are now investigating what happens when we give growth hormone to the hypophysectomized rat when it has been kept as a dwarfed animal throughout life and has passed the time when somatic cells ordinarily stop dividing; can enzyme activity be turned on again? In other words, is the effect of hypophysectomy an example of what Dr Dobbing described, of reducing the rate of DNA synthesis but not changing the time at which such synthesis stops, or does this in a sense maintain the animal as a baby rat and could DNA synthesis be resumed at any time after administering growth hormone?

*Dobbing:* One certain way of obtaining adult rats with stunted brains but normal body weight is to X-irradiate the whole head with about 600 R in the first few days of life (Dobbing *et al.* 1970). This presumably reaches the pituitary and thyroid and profoundly affects brain development, which is very sensitive, particularly the cerebellum. If the pituitary or the thyroid or both were also radiosensitive at this time, it would suggest that neither is very important for subsequent development of the body.

*Cobos:* The frequency with which delayed physical growth is associated with malnutrition, as reported in the literature, suggests that perhaps other, non-nutritional factors may also result in deterioration of physical growth. A number of reports (Elmer 1960; Patton and Gardner 1963; Blodgett 1963; Feigenbaum, Fishhoff and Weiss 1967; Powell *et al.* 1967) have suggested that the 'failure to thrive syndrome', a condition in which the availability of food is not decreased, presents a clinical picture very similar to the one typical of malnutrition.

Furthermore, Rosenzweig (1969) has shown that lack of handling in the developing rat will result in alterations of the central nervous system similar to those described as a result of early malnutrition (Winick and Noble 1966). This suggests that perhaps the anthropometric changes observed in rats reared in litters with different numbers of littermates also have some relationship to the different amounts of maternal care that must occur under such conditions.

*Dobbing:* Yes. Miss Widdowson studied two orphanages in postwar Germany in which quite independently of the nutrition, the emotional climate was shown to affect the rate of growth. This was a very nicely controlled experiment which simply happened (Widdowson 1951).

*Cobos:* Spitz (1965) reported similar findings in studies of deprivation of children in Mexico. These children died not really from lack of food but from lack of maternal care. The clinical picture is very similar to the one observed in cases in which the infants died of malnutrition. Clearly, the 'emotional' factors should be kept in mind.

*Menkes:* But such emotionally deprived children have a lowered growth hormone secretion. Children with psychosocial dwarfism tend to have impaired growth hormone release before recovery (Powell *et al.* 1967). This is associated with a subnormal plasma cortisol response to hypoglycaemia. In infants with the maternal deprivation syndrome, serum growth hormone tends to be elevated, however (Krieger and Mellinger 1971).

*Cobos:* It is unfortunate that observations and studies such as those of Spitz could not include measurements of growth hormone. However, it should be remembered that demonstration of abnormally low growth hormone levels is extremely difficult, particularly in malnourished children.

*Winick:* There is some disagreement here. Certainly children with kwashiorkor who are malnourished and don't grow do *not* have low levels of growth hormone; if anything they have higher levels, as Professor Rossi said. The controversy is in marasmus, but I do not think that either group investigating this would ascribe the failure to grow to a growth hormone deficiency.

To return to the problem of environmental deprivation, Levitsky and Barnes (1969) have studied the interaction of environmental stimulation and malnutrition in animals, and the effects on the developing brain both chemically and developmentally. They find a synergistic effect: both malnutrition and environmental deprivation reduce the rate of cell division, affect RNA metabolism and elevate certain enzymes such as acetylcholinesterase in the long-term, and these two factors operate synergistically. Frankova (1970) has shown that the under-nourished rat and the so-called over-nourished rat (the litter of 18 and the litter of 3) both show decreased exploratory behaviour and other abnormalities which are similar. They both develop differently from rats reared in litters of 10 or 12. So there is a complicated interaction of environment and nutrition and it is becoming as difficult to isolate this in animals as it is in man.

*Young:* Nearly 40 years ago Philip Smith found that hypophysectomized baby rats grow to around 80–90 g in the absence of the pituitary gland. He also observed that the skull failed to keep pace in its growth with the brain and that considerable pressure on the brain developed.

*Dobbing:* The plasma level of growth hormone may not be the only factor; what about the sensitivity of the target tissues to the hormone? If we could get enough human growth hormone to administer, it would be interesting to see what response there was.

*Winick:* Monckeberg and co-workers (1963) studied this in Chile. They injected human growth hormone into malnourished children and found some improvement in growth. That doesn't answer the fundamental question, however, because it doesn't say that the administered growth hormone is reversing the mechanism by which malnutrition caused the growth abnormality. In fact the evidence suggests that another mechanism is being stimulated and is giving a little more growth.

*Young:* When one speaks of growth in animals or in humans under the influence of administered growth hormone one must be careful about the criteria of growth, because there are disproportionate influences on different organs. In growth-hormone-treated rats the growth of skeletal muscles, the lengthening of the long bones and the increase in body weight may not go hand in hand. Normal growth cannot be inferred from a body weight increase.

*Bovet:* Psychological factors such as appetite may be important in influencing what people will eat, and should be remembered when changes in body size in populations are discussed, such as the Sicilians already mentioned.

*Crawford:* C. H. Waddington showed that in fruit flies reared at high temperature, morphological changes occur, and subsequent generations show the same morphological changes although they are bred at the lower temperature. Have you looked at your underprivileged rats reared in large litters to see whether changes are continuing to be transmitted in the second generation?

*Dobbing:* We haven't done this. The only relevant experiments that I know are those of Cowley and Griesel (1963), who looked at the behaviour of second and third generation progeny of malnourished rats. In spite of there being no undernutrition in the succeeding generations, it was claimed that there were traces of behavioural changes in the third generation, following grandmaternal undernutrition. This interested us very much until we learned from our behavioural colleagues that the phenomenon of grandmaternal effects in developmental behaviour is not a new one and doesn't imply the physical handing down of impaired physical growth of the brain or any other part of the body; behavioural effects can be handed on from mother to progeny. Whether one can select small rats by going on rearing them small, in large litters, is not really known. My guess is that for a few generations you might, but that like the Japanese and Sicilians they would gradually revert to normal size with successive generations on the rehabilitation regime.

*von Muralt:* We are using the concept of 'adaptation' in two different senses: one has to distinguish between 'genetic adaptation', induced by mutation and selection, and the adaptations a physiologist observes as a reaction of the body to a change in environment.

*Crawford:* If the blood supply to the foetus is restricted a small foetus is produced, and so if you have a smaller animal, it's likely that it will again produce a smaller foetus.

*Dobbing:* There is some tendency of a smaller animal to go on producing a smaller foetus, from experiments with horses and ponies (see McCance 1962).

*Aebi:* Your experiments remind me in a way of earlier studies by McKay (1947). He investigated the effect of restricted food intake on growth rate and lifespan of rats and observed that the lifespan can be significantly increased by slowing growth. What are the average lifespans of rats from large and small litters?

*Dobbing:* Remarkably few people have studied this. Widdowson and Kennedy (1962) have summarized the position, and I think their feeling is that the rats which grew fastest, in the smaller litters, suffer ultimately from less respiratory pathology and may have a longer life. That may be quite different from allowing an adult rat to eat *ad libitum*, which results in a decreased lifespan and a greater incidence of cardiovascular and respiratory pathology. A very important question therefore arises: what is optimum growth in a child? Could it be suggested that the optimum growth rate in children, as it appears to be in rats, is the maximum rate of growth in terms of lean body-mass? Is this the optimum growth rate from the point of view of longevity or pathology?

*Mead:* Did you make any behavioural studies in the adult rats that had been reared in the large and small litters?

*Dobbing:* Many behavioural studies have been done on previously undernourished rats, but those made on the progeny of the large and small litters are open to the grave objection that behavioural development may have been affected by modifying the litter size. In the design where the litter size is standardized at birth, this objection is to some extent met.

When it comes to higher mental function, we're in trouble. There *are* differences in 'higher mental function' between previously underfed and normal animals, but these are differences which I am unable to see as 'deficits' or as anything else but differences. There are distinct differences, however, in tests which *appear* to be tests for fine motor coordination, and we think these may be related to the small ultimate cerebellar growth. In one such test a rat is made to walk around the rim of a large beaker. A normal rat can do it, whereas a rat previously mildly growth-retarded stumbles. But this isn't higher mental function. The whole subject of the behavioural testing of rats to my mind is hopelessly *sub-judice* at present, in spite of the fact that differences can quite certainly be shown.

*Ansell:* When you divide the rats into small or large litters, are there any alterations in the environment other than the availability of and access to food?

Were there any differences, for example, in the degree of illumination or in the size of cage?

*Dobbing:* The physical environment of the animal house is very carefully regulated. Temperature, humidity, ventilation and lighting are kept as uniform as possible. The behavioural environment is, as you suggest, considerably different. There are a limited number of feeding stations, for example; the larger family has to feed in relays. The others meanwhile go to sleep or find something else to do. The maternal attention which is given other than feeding and which is very considerable, particularly in the first few days with regard to bladder function, must be very different in the large and small litters. This design is a bad one if you are interested in investigating behaviour; it happens to be very convenient for 'physiologically' altering the physical growth of the brain.

*Leathwood:* Biochemical studies on the effects of deprivation during vulnerable periods of brain development in the rat have demonstrated clear and long-lasting deficits. In contrast, behavioural studies on early malnutrition and subsequent 'learning ability' have produced inconsistent results and have often shown little or no effect. Would Dr Dobbing care to comment further on the problems of behavioural testing and why the behavioural results are so confusing?

*Dobbing:* From my colleague Dr Smart (1971) I gather that there have been 12 or 15 studies on the adult behaviour of animals reared in this sort of way; in about eight or nine studies no changes were found; of the remainder, about half showed changes in one direction ('better' performance in tests) and the other half, changes in the 'opposite' direction. Smart has produced behavioural differences in rats, but the ease with which they can be produced depends on the sensitivity of the test regime or on the extent to which you push the animals. If you push them very hard, you bring to light differences on the edges of their performance that aren't apparent by simply observing them. The whole question of how you interpret this is very confused, to my mind.

## References

BLODGETT, F. M. (1963) In *Modern Perspectives in Child Development*, ed. A. J. Solnit and S. A. Provence. International Universities Press, New York

BRASEL, J. A., EHRENKRANZ, R. A. and WINICK, M. (1970) *Dev. Biol.* **23**, 424-432

COWLEY, J. J. and GRIESEL, R. D. (1963) *J. Genet. Psychol.* **103**, 233

DAVIES, P. A. and DAVIS, J. P. (1970) *Lancet* **2**, 1216

DOBBING, J., HOPEWELL, J. W., LYNCH, A. and SANDS, J. (1970) *Exp. Neurol.* **28**, 442-449

ELMER, E. (1960) *Pediatrics* **25**, 717

FEIGENBAUM, D., FISHHOFF, J. and WEISS, H. (1967) American Orthopsychiatric Association Conference, Washington, D.C. March 1967

FRANKOVA, S. (1970) *Nutr. Metab.* **12**, 228-239

GODARD, C. and ZAHUD, G. R. (1971) *Helv. Paed. Acta* **26**, 266-275

GRUENWALD, P., FUNAKAWA, H., MITANI, S., NISHIMURA, T. and TAKEUCHI, S. (1967) *Lancet* **1**, 1026-1029

HERMANN, P. (1954) *Conquest by Man.* Harper, New York

KRIEGER, I. and MELLINGER, R. C. (1971) *J. Pediatr.* **79**, 216

LEVITSKY, D. and BARNES, R. H. (1969) *Fed. Proc. Fed. Am. Soc. Exp. Biol.* **28**, 555

MCCANCE, R. A. (1962) *Lancet* **2**, 621-626

MCKAY, C. M. (1947) *Am. J. Public Health* **37**, 521

MONCKEBERG, F., DONOSO, G., OXMAN, S., PAK, N. and MENEGHELLO, J. (1963) *Pediatrics* **31**, 58-64

PATTON, R. G. and GARDNER, L. I. (1963) *Growth Failure in Maternal Deprivation.* Thomas, Springfield, Ill.

POWELL, G. F., BRASEL, J. A., RAITI, S. and BLIZZARD, R. M. (1967) *New Engl. J. Med.* **276**, 1279

ROSENZWEIG, M. R. (1969) In *Symposium on the Biopsychology of Development.* The American Museum of Natural History, New York

SMART, J. L. (1971) *Psychiat. Neurol. Neurochir.* **74**, 443-452

SPITZ, R. A. (1965) *The First Year of Life.* International Universities Press, New York

WIDDOWSON, E. M. (1951) *Lancet* **1**, 1316

WIDDOWSON, E. M. and KENNEDY, G. C. (1962) *Proc. R. Soc. B* **156**, 96-108

WINICK, M. (1968) *J. Nutr.* **94**, 121-124

WINICK, M. and NOBLE, A. S. (1966) *Am. J. Nutr.* **89**, 300

# The role of fatty acids in myelin and other important brain structures

D. CHAPMAN

*Department of Chemistry, Sheffield University*

At this conference we are concerned to examine the role of lipids in the developing brain. We are also interested in whether malnutrition during the critical stage of brain growth can cause irrevocable changes or defects in brain organization and if so, what is the molecular basis of these changes. It seems to me that before we ask questions about the role of lipids in the developing brain we need first to discuss the role of lipids, including the fatty acids, in the 'normal' fully developed brain. The following initial questions can therefore be posed:

(*a*) Where are lipids situated in the brain?

(*b*) Which lipid classes and which fatty acids occur in these regions?

(*c*) What are the possible roles of these different lipid classes and also of the different fatty acids in the structure and function of the 'normal' brain?

(*d*) How could the brain structure and function be modified by alterations in lipid class or fatty acid composition?

If we can answer these initial questions satisfactorily, even in the broadest terms, we may be able to proceed to the next stage and consider the consequences of molecular abnormalities arising from nutritional factors. We need to remember that concentrating on one component such as the lipids, despite their considerable diversification, in a structure as complicated as the brain may be somewhat myopic, as far as the conclusions are concerned, since balancing factors using protein may operate to provide a slightly different but functioning structure.

## LIPIDS AND FATTY ACIDS PRESENT IN THE BRAIN

The brain structure on gross anatomical inspection is seen to consist of grey and white regions. The differentiation between the grey and white matter is not

TABLE 1

Lipid composition of myelin from the central nervous system and peripheral nervous system of different species. Values expressed as µmoles of lipid per µmole of cholesterol unless otherwise stated (From Dickerson 1968, by permission of the publisher)

| | Central nervous system | | | | | | | | Peripheral nervous system | |
|---|---|---|---|---|---|---|---|---|---|---|
| | *Man* | *Ox* | *Rat* | *Rabbit* | *Guinea-pig* | *Pigeon* | *Dogfish* | *Frog* | *Rat* | *Guinea-pig* |
| Protein (mg/100 mg dry wt. myelin) | 47.3 | 29.5 | 36 | 38 | — | 47.4 | 56 | 39 | — | — |
| Cholesterol (µmoles/mg lipid) | 0.700 | 0.622 | 0.670 | 0.665 | 0.640 | 0.758 | 0.558 | 0.660 | — | — |
| Cerebroside | 0.354 | 0.454 | 0.331 | 0.315 | 0.50 | 0.388 | 0.214 | 0.203 | 0.4 | 1.8 † |
| Sulphatide | 0.073 | — | 0.066 | 0.075 | | 0.059 | 0.131 | — | | |
| Total phospholipid P | 0.82 | 0.93 | 0.94 | 0.96 | 0.97 | 0.640 | 1.35 | 1.16 | 1.21 | 1.56 |
| Phosphatidylinositol | 0.013 | 0.029 | 0.042 | 0.024 | 0.028 | 0.016 | 0.034 | 0.026 | 0.23 | 0.53* |
| Serine phospholipid | 0.154 | 0.174 | 0.146 | 0.146 | 0.123 | 0.069 | 1.13 | 0.088 | | |
| Cardiolipin, phosphatidic acid | 0.004 | — | 0.025 | 0.074 | 0.019 | 0.057 | 0.088 | 0.021 | — | — |
| Sphingomyelin | 0.160 | 0.143 | 0.080 | 0.159 | 0.12 | 0.051 | 0.199 | 0.107 | 0.24 | — |
| Lecithin | 0.172 | 0.180 | 0.246 | 0.178 | 0.25 | 0.164 | 0.334 | 0.454 | 0.29 | 0.33 |
| Ethanolamine phospholipid | 0.425 | 0.330 | 0.421 | 0.346 | — | 0.288 | 0.600 | 0.462 | 0.45 | 0.7 |
| Total plasmalogen | 0.252 | 0.274 | 0.462 | 0.326 | 0.247 | 0.323 | 0.686 | — | — | — |

* Value includes sphingomyelin.
† Authors say that this value was confirmed by 5 determinations on 3 preparations.

completely clear but is mainly related to the presence of nerve cells and unmyelinated fibres in grey matter and the presence of mainly myelinated fibres in white matter. Lipids occur in *both* grey and white matter and occur as integral parts of membrane structures of mitochondria, nerve ending particles, nuclei, synaptic vesicles and particularly myelin. Approximately half of the lipid of the adult nervous system is present in the myelin membranes.

Analysis of these various membranes reveals that a variety of lipid classes make up their structure. If, for example, we look at an analysis of myelin membranes of several vertebrate species, shown in Table 1, we see a fairly consistent pattern, with a molar ratio of about 2:2:1 for cholesterol:total

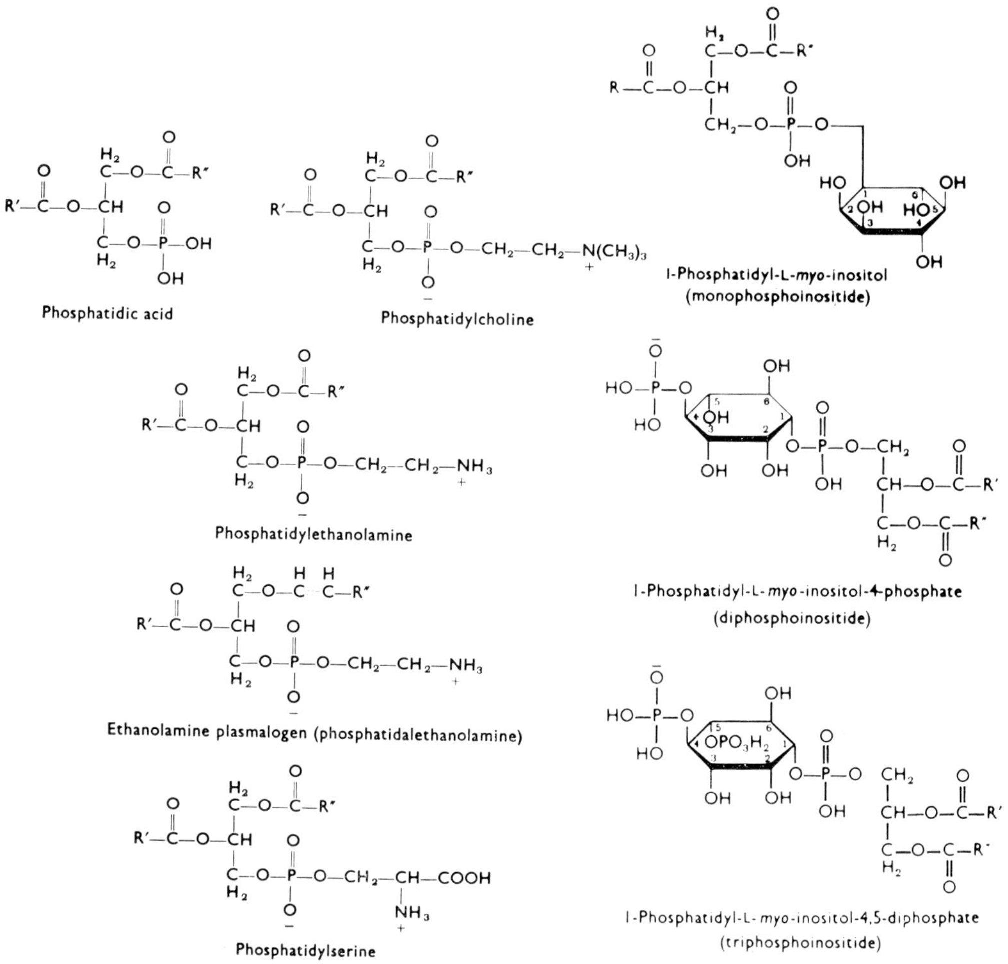


FIG. 1. The phospholipids.

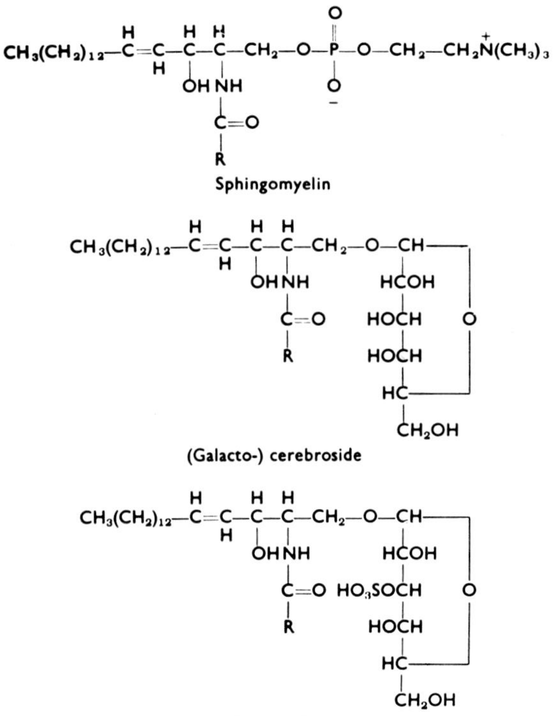


FIG. 2. The sphingolipids.

phospholipid:total galactolipids. The ratio of cholesterol to protein appears to be somewhat species-dependent (Dickerson 1968).

The individual lipids present include various sphingolipids and phospholipids, such as cerebroside, sphingomyelin, lecithin (phosphatidylcholines), phosphatidylethanolamines, plasmalogen and phosphatidylserines. The structures of these different lipid classes are shown in Figs. 1 and 2. Associated with each of these lipid classes in the membrane is a distribution of fatty acids. The structures of commonly occurring fatty acids appear in Fig. 3.

The cerebrosides and sulphate esters (Fig. 2) appear to be typical constituents of myelin, whilst gangliosides (Fig. 4) are primarily located in neurons, plasma membranes and synaptic membranes (see Table 2). Small quantities of gangliosides are reported to occur in myelin but the reported values vary considerably.

An interesting comparison of the lipid composition of myelin and grey matter from four humans at various ages has been made by O'Brien (1965). This shows that myelin contains higher proportions of cholesterol, cerebroside,

FATTY ACIDS

| **Common name** | **Systematic name** | *Formula* |
|---|---|---|
| | | Saturated |
| **Palmitic** | *n*-Hexadecanoic | $CH_3(CH_2)_{14}COOH$ |
| **Stearic** | *n*-Octadecanoic | $CH_3(CH_2)_{16}COOH$ |
| **Lignoceric** | *n*-Tetracosanoic | $CH_3(CH_2)_{22}COOH$ |
| **Cerotic** | *n*-Hexacosanoic | $CH_3(CH_2)_{24}COOH$ |
| | | Unsaturated |
| Oleic | 9-Octadecenoic | $CH_3(CH_2)_7CH{=}CH(CH_2)_7COOH$ |
| Linoleic | 9,12-Octadecadienoic | $CH_3(CH_2)_4CH{=}CHCH_2CH{=}CH(CH_2)_7COOH$ |
| Linolenic | 9,12,15-Octadeca-trienoic | $CH_3CH_2CH{=}CHCH_2CH{=}CHCH_2CH{=}CH(CH_2)_7COOH$ |
| Arachidonic | 5,8,11,14-Eicosa-tetraenoic | $CH_3(CH_2)_4(CH{=}CHCH_2)_4(CH_2)_2COOH$ |
| Nervonic | *cis*-15-Tetracosenoic | $CH_3(CH_2)_7CH{=}CH(CH_2)_{13}COOH$ |
| | | Hydroxy-acids |
| Cerebronic | 2-Hydroxytetra-cosanoic | $CH_3(CH_2)_{21}CHOH\ COOH$ |
| Hydroxy-nervonic | 2-Hydroxy-9-tetra-cosenoic | $CH_3(CH_2)_7CH{=}CH(CH_2)_{12}CHOH\ COOH$ |

STEROLS

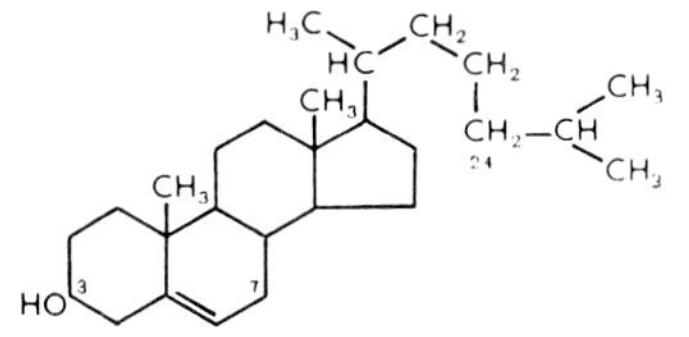


Cholesterol

*Desmosterol* has a double bond in the $C^{24}$ position.
*Esters* are formed by reaction of OH in position 3 with a fatty acid.

FIG. 3. Unconjugated lipids.

plasmalogens, and cerebroside sulphate than grey matter. The proportions of sphingomyelin and of phosphatidylserine are about the same in myelin and grey matter. Myelin contains lower proportions of ceramide, phosphatidylethanolamines and lecithins.

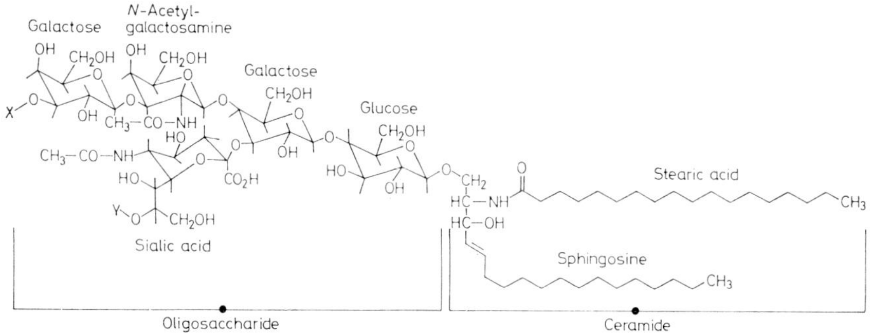


FIG. 4. The structure of a ganglioside.

TABLE 2

Lipid composition of synaptosomes and synaptic vesicles of guinea-pig brain
Values are μmoles constituent per 100 mg non-diffusible solids except for phospholipid fractions which are expressed as a percentage of the total lipid P
(From Dickerson 1968, by permission of the publisher)

| | *Synaptosomes* | *External* synaptosome membranes* | *Synaptic vesicles* |
|---|---|---|---|
| Cholesterol | 20.4 | — | — |
| Cerebroside + sulphatide | 0.66 | — | — |
| Ganglioside as *N*-acetyl neuraminic acid | 1.33 | — | — |
| Total lipid P | 47.5 | — | — |
| Phosphatidylcholine | 39.3 | 24 | 41.3 |
| Phosphatidylethanolamine | 17.6 | 10 | 14.8 |
| Phosphatidylserine | 12.9 | 3 | 11.3 |
| Phosphatidylinositol | 4.0 | 1 | 5.0 |
| Ethanolamine plasmalogen | 16.0 | 20 | 15.2 |
| Sphingomyelin | 5.3 | 6 | 11.2 |

* Values quoted by V. P. Whittaker (1966) from a personal communication from A. Sheltawy.

TABLE 3

Composition of mitochondria (From Dickerson 1968, by permission of the publisher)

| | *Rat* | *Guinea-pig* |
|---|---|---|
| Total protein (mg/g wet) | 10.22 | |
| | 13.4 | |
| Cholesterol | 25.3 [1] | |
| Cerebroside | 0.14 [1] | |
| Total phospholipid | 74.2 [1] | |
| Phosphatidylinositol | 3.7 [1] | 5.5 [2] |
| Phosphatidylserine | 4.7 [1] | 5.9 [2] |
| Cardiolipin | 5.8 [1] | |
| Sphingomyelin | 1.4 [1] | 3.7 [2] |
| Lecithin | 28.3 [1] | 40 [2] |
| Ethanolamine phospholipid | 30.3 [1] | 23.3 [2] |
| Acetylcholine (bound) | 0.025 [4] | |
| γ-Aminobutyric acid | 0.037 [3] | |
| Glutamic acid | 0.093 [3] | |
| Acetylcholinesterase | 2.1 [5] | |
| Succinic dehydrogenase | 27.5 [5] | |

[1] Moles per 100 moles lipid.
[2] % total lipid P.
[3] μmoles/mg protein.
[4] nmoles/mg protein.
[5] Units/mg protein.

TABLE 4

Lipid composition of microsomes from various species
Values expressed as μmoles lipid per μmole of cholesterol
(From Dickerson 1968, by permission of the publisher)

| | *Man* | *Rat* | *Rabbit* | *Pigeon* | *Dogfish* | *Frog* |
|---|---|---|---|---|---|---|
| Cholesterol (μmoles/mg lipid) | 0.590 | 0.562 | 0.700 | 0.645 | 0.980 | 0.830 |
| Cerebroside | 0.171 | 0.137 | 0.160 | 0.180 | 0.017 | trace |
| Sulphatide | 0.031 | 0.017 | 0.012 | — | — | — |
| Total phospholipid P | 1.40 | 1.37 | 1.18 | 1.20 | 0.71 | 0.85 |
| Phosphatidylinositol | 0.101 | 0.044 | 0.229 | — | 0.059 | 0.075 |
| Serine phospholipid | 0.179 | 0.146 | | 0.238 | 0.094 | 0.094 |
| Cardiolipin, phosphatidic acid | 0.032 | 0.044 | 0.075 | — | 0.014 | 0.049 |
| Sphingomyelin | 0.198 | 0.100 | 0.154 | 0.118 | 0.087 | 0.094 |
| Lecithin | 0.608 | 0.472 | 0.328 | 0.439 | 0.286 | 0.338 |
| Ethanolamine phospholipid | 0.284 | 0.458 | 0.390 | 0.434 | 0.161 | 0.270 |
| Total plasmalogen | 0.222 | 0.192 | 0.230 | — | 0.077 | — |

The fatty acid compositions also differ. Grey matter phospholipids contain very high proportions of highly unsaturated fatty acids, while myelin contains much less of these acids. As well as this, myelin contains ten times more very long-chain fatty acids (19 to 26 carbon atoms) than grey matter. Whereas in myelin, only one in every 17 fatty acids is polyunsaturated, in grey matter one in five is unsaturated. In myelin, one in five fatty acids has a chain longer than 18 carbon atoms; for grey matter the value is only one in 100.

The lipid composition of mitochondria is shown in Table 3 and of microsomes in Table 4. These distributions of the various classes of lipids can be contrasted with that in myelin.

## THE ROLE OF LIPIDS AND FATTY ACIDS IN MEMBRANE STRUCTURE

When we come to consider the role of lipids in the brain membranes, it is necessary to say that considerable work is in progress to try to deduce the detailed role of the different lipid classes and their associated fatty acids in cell membranes in general.

The overall structure of cell membranes themselves has long been debated but the application of new physical techniques is beginning to clarify the situation. Recent evidence has tended to strengthen the belief that a lipid bilayer is an important component of many cell membranes (Wilkins, Blaurock and Engelman 1971), although the position of the protein remains uncertain. In myelin it seems certain that a bilayer structure (see p. 44) is the dominant organizational feature of the membrane (Caspar and Kirschner 1971).

*Lipid–water systems*

Before we consider the details of membrane structure, let us first summarize what we now know of the physicochemical properties of the various lipid classes, the effect on these properties of variation in fatty acid content, and the effects of other components such as cholesterol. This will show us the possible ways in which the components can interact to form the functioning membrane structure.

The lipids composing cell membranes all have the property of possessing both a hydrophobic and a hydrophilic group within the molecule. They therefore orientate themselves in water so that the polar group is in the water and the hydrophobic group is away from the water. As we can see from Fig. 1, the polar groups of the different classes may have a nett neutral charge, as in lecithins, or a nett negative charge, for example phosphatidylserines, at pH 7.5. The phosphoinositides can have varying degrees of negative charge corresponding to structures containing one, two or three phosphate groups.

We are still uncertain of the precise reasons for the existence of the different lipid polar groups within a membrane system. It may be that these different polar groups are important for different types of interaction with protein or various types of ion binding; for example, the phosphoinositides have been implicated in the flux of cations in nervous tissue, but we are still uncertain about this.

The effects of variation in fatty acids can be illustrated by recent physical studies on phospholipids. Similar effects are also found with the sphingolipids.

When a pure phospholipid such as dimyristoyl phosphatidylethanolamine, which contains two saturated acyl moieties, is heated from room temperature to the final melting point, it first reaches a transition point at which a marked endothermic change occurs (Chapman 1968). At this temperature (sometimes more than 200°C below the final melting point), the aliphatic chains 'melt' and exhibit a very high degree of molecular motion. Above the endothermic transition temperature a given phospholipid is in a highly mobile condition with its aliphatic chains flexing and twisting (with greater motion at the methyl end of the lipid chain than in regions nearer to the polar group).

When water is added to the system, the marked endothermic transition temperature for a given phospholipid falls and reaches a limiting value. Quite high temperatures are still required to counteract the dispersion forces between the chains and to cause the chains to 'melt'. The limiting transition temperatures of individual phospholipids parallel the melting point behaviour of their constituent fatty acids and are lower with increasing unsaturation. At the temperatures common in biological systems, the phospholipids which contain highly unsaturated chains *are in a highly mobile and fluid condition.* The transition temperature for dipalmitoyl lecithin is 42°C, whereas stearoyl oleoyl lecithin has a transition temperature of 3°C.

When a phospholipid in water is raised in temperature above its transition temperature, what are termed myelin figures form spontaneously. These myelin figures contain concentric arrangements of bilayers of lipid separated by layers of water. Thus above the transition temperature a lecithin is arranged in a bilayer system with mobile fluid chains.

It is important to note that the polar group of a lipid affects the transition temperature of that lipid, so that the transition temperature of one lipid class can differ by many degrees from that of another even when they both *contain the same fatty acids.* Furthermore, ions interacting with the polar group can also influence the transition temperature of the lipid (J. Urbina and D. Chapman, unpublished observations 1971).

This endothermic transition is an important property of lipid–water systems. It is illustrated in the phase diagram of Fig. 5 for dipalmitoyl lecithin–water

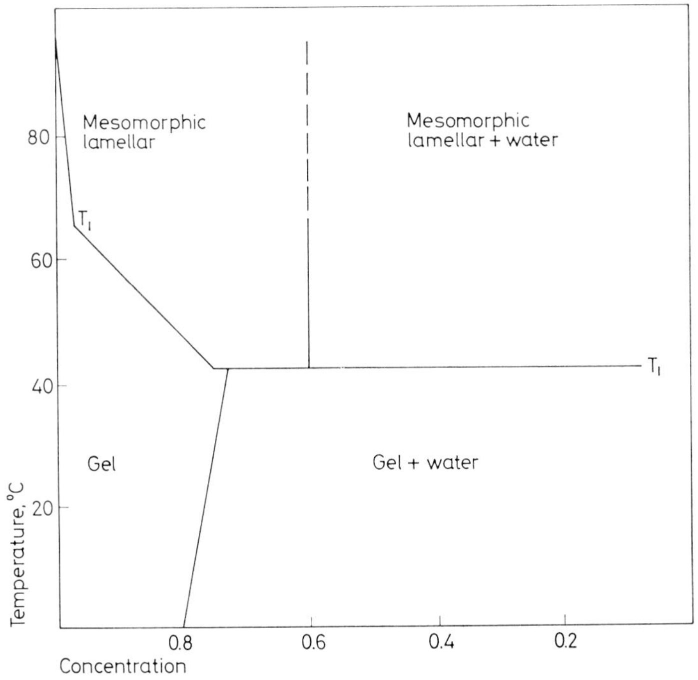


FIG. 5. Phase diagram of the 1,2-dipalmitoyl-L-phosphatidylcholine–water system. Concentration is in g of lipid per g of lipid/water mixture. (After Chapman, Williams and Ladbrooke 1967.)

(Chapman, Williams and Ladbrooke 1967). Below the transition temperature the lipid chains are packed in a crystalline manner and the lipid is in a gel condition. Above the transition temperature the lipid chains are in a fluid condition and the lipid is in a liquid crystalline condition. Endothermic transitions similar to these have even been observed with some membrane systems.

*Bound water.* Some added water in phospholipid appears to be *bound* to the lipid; dipalmitoyl lecithin binds about 20% water. This water does not freeze at 0°C, and calorimetric studies made with lipid–water mixtures have shown that only after more than 20% water has been added can one observe an ice melting peak at 0°C.

*Monolayers.* At room temperature, the saturated phospholipids form monolayers which are more condensed than those of unsaturated phospholipids containing *cis* double bonds; that is, the saturated phospholipids occupy a smaller area at low surface pressures than the corresponding unsaturated compounds. The monolayer behaviour of the phospholipids reflects their transition temperatures. Thus, at room temperature, a phospholipid which has a high transition temperature, such as distearoyl lecithin, forms a condensed film; a phospholipid having a lower transition temperature, such as stearoyl-oleoyl lecithin, exhibits an expanded film, or greater area per molecule.

*Phase polymorphism.* Phospholipids in the presence of water can also form different liquid crystalline phases. In some cases, as the concentration of water varies, transitions from lamellar to hexagonal phases occur. These transitions have been fully discussed by Luzzati and Husson (1962).

*Bilayers.* Recently there has been great interest in the formation of phospholipid bilayer systems. The transition temperatures of phospholipids are also relevant to the production of model bilayers. When a suitable phospholipid is heated above its transition temperature, satisfactory bilayers can be made. The same is true with sphingomyelins and cerebrosides; for example, ox-brain cerebroside has a transition temperature beginning about 50-55°C which is completed at about 65°C and bilayers are only formed at high temperatures (Clowes, Cherry and Chapman 1971). When cerebroside and lecithin are mixed together, which reduces the transition temperature of the cerebroside, bilayers can be formed at room temperature.

*Phospholipid–cholesterol interactions*

We have seen that cholesterol occurs in myelin and to a lesser extent in other cell membranes. The interaction between lipid and cholesterol may therefore be an important one.

For almost fifty years it has been known that cholesterol, when mixed with certain phospholipids in monomolecular films on water, reduces the area occupied by the fatty acids. This has received a great deal of attention and discussion. It has been suggested that this condensation effect is related to the presence of a *cis* double bond in the 9:10 position of the fatty acid of the phospholipid molecule. It was also thought that short-chain saturated phospholipids which give expanded monolayers do not interact with cholesterol.

However, studies in our laboratory show that an interaction between cholesterol and phospholipids occurs even when the double bond is not in the 9:10 position, provided the monomolecular film of the phospholipid is expanded. Thus, phospholipids containing chains with a double bond in the 6:7 position, or the 10:11 position, also show a condensation effect. Monolayers of the saturated phospholipids are usually condensed in type and so there is no further condensing effect in the presence of cholesterol. However, a condensing effect is found with saturated phospholipids if they are heated above room temperature (Chapman *et al.* 1969). Thus, the presence of a kink in the molecule due to a *cis* double bond at the 9:10 position is *not* a necessary condition for condensation. This condensation effect can be explained in terms of the inhibition of movement of the fatty acid chains by the adjacent bulky cholesterol molecule. This has been shown by nuclear magnetic resonance and electron spin resonance spectroscopy.

Cholesterol has an important effect on the lipid endothermic transition temperature. This has been shown in recent calorimetric studies. In Fig. 6 are shown the calorimetric curves between 7 and 87 °C for a series of dipalmitoyl lecithin–cholesterol mixtures (Ladbrooke, Williams and Chapman 1968), each containing 50 % by weight of water and varying ratios of lecithin to cholesterol. As the concentration of cholesterol increases, the main endothermic transition at first remains sharp, and a small peak at 35 °C disappears. Higher concentrations of cholesterol cause a profound change in which the main transition becomes broad and decreases in area. When the concentration reaches 50 mole % of cholesterol, no endothermic peak is observable. The same is also found with the sphingolipids.

In summary, we can say that various experimental techniques including nuclear magnetic resonance spectroscopy (Chapman and Penkett 1966) and electron spin resonance spectroscopy (Hubbell and McConnell 1969) have

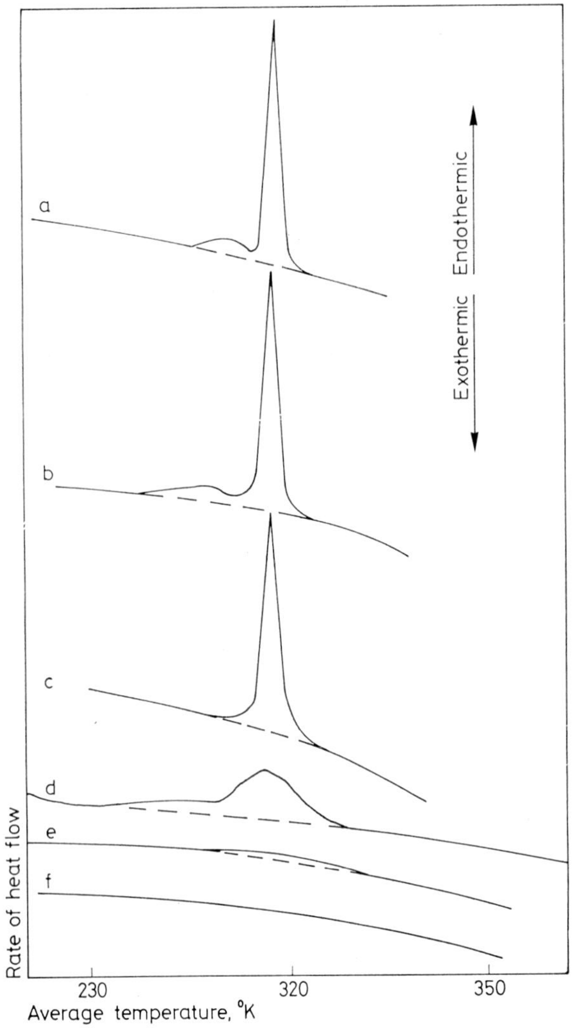


FIG. 6. Differential scanning calorimetry curves of dispersions in water (50% by weight) of 1,2-dipalmitoyl-L-phosphatidylcholine–cholesterol mixtures containing (*a*) 0.0 mole %, (*b*) 5.0 mole %, (*c*) 12.5 mole %, (*d*) 20.0 mole %, (*e*) 32.0 mole % and (*f*) 50.0 mole % cholesterol. (From Ladbrooke, Williams and Chapman 1968.)

shown that when cholesterol is added to a phospholipid (and also sphingolipids) in its liquid crystalline condition, some inhibition of chain motion can take place, *dependent* upon the *degree* of *unsaturation of the lipid.* The inhibition of chain motion is greatest at the end of the chain nearest the polar group.

However, when cholesterol is introduced into a phospholipid which at that temperature would normally be in its gel condition, the cholesterol prevents the lipid chains from crystallizing. In addition to this, cholesterol will also prevent the lateral movements of the lipid chains, and thereby prevent information transfer along the membrane by this mechanism.

### *Permeability studies in model systems*

Permeability properties are affected by the degree of unsaturation of the fatty acids present in the lipids. Finkelstein and Cass (1968) report that an increase in permeability to water is observed in model membrane systems with more unsaturated lipids.

It has also been shown with liposome systems (de Gier, Mandersloot and van Deenen 1968) that there is a pronounced increase in the rate of penetration of glycerol with an increase in unsaturation of the lipid. This has also been shown with glycol and erythritol (de Gier *et al.* 1971). The liposomes containing saturated lipids exhibit abnormal temperature effects, but this effect is removed by the presence of cholesterol.

It is concluded that these alcohols cross the lipid barrier as single, fully dehydrated molecules, and the activation energies are consistent with this concept.

Experiments with liposome systems containing lecithins from rats deficient in essential fatty acids and from normal rats (Chen, Lund and Richardson 1971) show that glucose permeability is *less* with the lecithin from the essential fatty acid-deficient rats. The passive diffusion rate of glucose is 50% of that of lecithin from normal rats. This is clearly related to the greater degree of unsaturation of the fatty acids in the lecithin from the control rats.

With this background of information on lipid-water and lipid-cholesterol-water systems, let us turn to the membranes themselves.

## MEMBRANE STRUCTURE

The study of membrane structures is now very active, and a variety of techniques is being used. The myelin membrane has received particular attention.

The molecular order in the nerve myelin sheath was characterized by Schmitt, Bear and Palmer (1941) from the results of their X-ray diffraction and optical studies. With the development of electron microscope techniques, Geren (1954) demonstrated that the periodic lamellar structure of the myelin sheath is formed from a spirally wrapped cell membrane. Analyses of X-ray patterns of myelin have been based on diffraction data to about 30 Å (3 nm) spacing. Recently the electron-density profiles of three types of myelin membrane have been made by comparing intensity measurements on their diffraction patterns with 10 Å (1 nm) spacing. These studies have been made with rabbit and frog sciatic nerves and rabbit optic nerve (Caspar and Kirschner 1971).

The conclusion from the many techniques applied to myelin is that the myelin membrane is essentially a bilayer of lipid, although there may be a small amount of protein extending across it, and the structure is arranged so that a pair of membranes lie with their cytoplasmic surfaces opposed.

Electron density does not carry a chemical label and so identification of features in the electron-density profile with a particular arrangement of the molecules in the myelin membrane is made on other arguments.

A schematic illustration of the structure of the myelin membrane based upon diffraction data out to 10 Å spacing is shown in Fig. 7 (Caspar and Kirschner 1971). Particular features of the *interpretation* of the data are that protein and water are distributed in the spaces between the membrane bilayers but the concentration of protein may be higher near the lipid surface. The cholesterol and polar lipid are present in equimolar ratio in the external side of the bilayer. It is suggested that there is about half as much cholesterol in the inner side of the hydrocarbon region (see Fig. 7). The asymmetrical distribution of cholesterol by Caspar and Kirschner is presumed to result from specific interactions with protein; however, the protein does not seem to modify significantly the local packing arrangement of the lipid. It is suggested from the electron-density profile that the methyl ends of the lipid chain are more disordered than the part of the chain near to the polar group, as observed in model lipid-cholesterol systems using nuclear magnetic resonance and electron spin resonance spectroscopy.

The hydrocarbon thickness of the myelin membranes is estimated at 38 Å (3.8 nm) for rabbit myelin and 35 Å (3.5 nm) for frog myelin.

Myelin membranes have also been studied with calorimetric techniques (Ladbrooke *et al.* 1968). We have seen that cholesterol removes the endothermic transition observed with lipids in model lipid–cholesterol systems at molar-molar ratios. Since myelin membranes contain considerable quantities of cholesterol, it is interesting to study myelin isolated from white matter of ox brain in a similar manner. The results of such experiments show that:

(*a*) With wet myelin, thermal transitions are not detectable. In this case the cholesterol and other lipids appear to be organized in a single phase. The

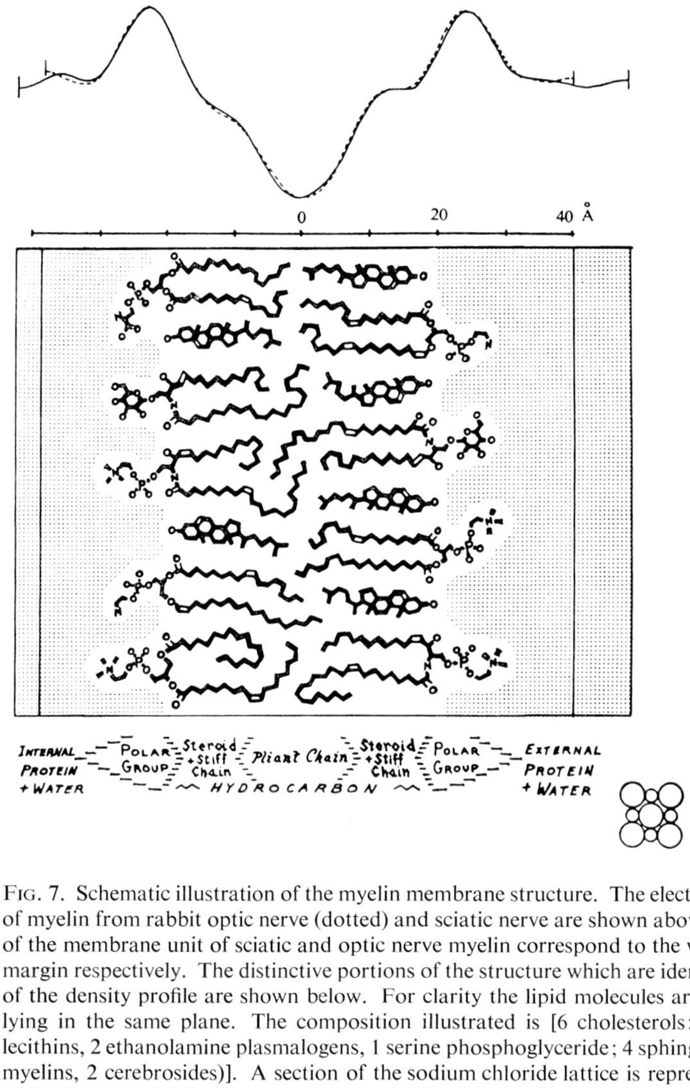


FIG. 7. Schematic illustration of the myelin membrane structure. The electron-density profiles of myelin from rabbit optic nerve (dotted) and sciatic nerve are shown above. The boundaries of the membrane unit of sciatic and optic nerve myelin correspond to the wider and narrower margin respectively. The distinctive portions of the structure which are identified with features of the density profile are shown below. For clarity the lipid molecules are represented as all lying in the same plane. The composition illustrated is [6 cholesterols: 5 glycerolipids (2 lecithins, 2 ethanolamine plasmalogens, 1 serine phosphoglyceride; 4 sphingolipids (2 sphingomyelins, 2 cerebrosides)]. A section of the sodium chloride lattice is represented at the same scale (bottom right). (From Caspar and Kirschner 1971 by permission of the Editor of *Nature*.)

organization of cholesterol in the membrane appears to prevent the lipids from crystallizing.

(*b*) To maintain the organization of the lipid in myelin a critical amount of water appears to be required. This water is unfreezable at 0 °C and may correspond to 'bound' water.

(c) When myelin membranes are dried, the cholesterol and other lipid crystallizes and precipitates. Endothermic transitions associated with cholesterol and other lipids can then be observed.
(*d*) The total lipid extract in water does not show a detectable endothermic transition but the cholesterol-free lipid does. In the absence of cholesterol, part of the myelin lipid is crystalline at body temperature.

## THE ROLE OF THE FATTY ACIDS

The composition of myelin shows that the phospholipids contain predominantly 18:0 and 18:1 fatty acids and the sphingolipids contain predominantly 24:0 and 24:1 fatty acids, both unsubstituted and in the hydroxy fatty acid form.

Let us consider the consequences of this composition in conjunction with the structure determined by X-rays and the physicochemical properties of the lipid–water systems already described. The situation is clearly complicated by the number of components present, and therefore the deductions are the more speculative.

Recent experiments using the bilayer system (Clowes, Cherry and Chapman 1971) show that in mixtures of lecithins and cerebrosides containing similar fatty acids an increased electrical resistance and breakdown voltage and a decrease in a.c. capacitance occur, compared to a lecithin control. Calorimetric studies show that the transition temperature of the cerebroside lipid moves from about 55 °C steadily downwards as the proportion of lecithin to cerebroside increases.

Thus we can infer that a lecithin-sphingolipid membrane would be more compact and electrically more stable with a greater width than a lecithin membrane alone. The effect of cholesterol on a lecithin membrane containing 18:0 and 18:1 fatty acids is to inhibit some of the molecular motion of the lipid chains and form a more compact structure. The diffusion of water through the membrane will be less and the permeability to other molecules, for example polyhydric alcohols, will also be affected.

Now the effect of cholesterol on the sphingolipids is to remove the gel phase, to produce a situation somewhat similar to that obtained with the lecithin-cholesterol system. It may be that some interdigitated cholesterol-sphingolipid is formed (Vandenheuvel 1963), but the chains are more mobile than they would be in the gel condition.

Thus we produce a fairly compact membrane structure having electrical insulation properties and good mechanical stability. There are a number of 'physical' consequences of this system. The phospholipids, for example the lecithins, because of their low transition temperatures could readily leave the membrane structure and form a separate bilayer, and could perhaps exchange with other membranes. The exchange of lipid molecules from one liposome system to another when they are in a liquid crystalline arrangement has been demonstrated by H. Träuble (personal communication). On the other hand, the cerebroside needs cholesterol or lecithin to disperse readily as a bilayer in water, so as to be able to leave the membrane.

This may be the reason for the low rate of turnover of these lipids in the myelin membrane. Thus cholesterol, cerebrosides, sphingomyelin and phosphatidylethanolamine are only slowly metabolized in brain, whereas lecithin turns over more rapidly. If the fatty acid in the cerebroside is for some reason reduced in chain length the transition temperature will then fall; this would enable the cerebroside to more readily leave the membrane structure. Other factors may also be important, such as ease of enzyme accessibility.

A case of disorder in myelin formation in metachromatic leucodystrophy, where such cerebrosides of reduced chain length occur as a result of failure to elongate the fatty acids beyond 18 carbon atoms, has been pointed out by O'Brien (1965). Other deficiencies of sphingolipids containing long-chain fatty acids have been observed, including multiple sclerosis (Gerstl *et al.* 1963), globoid cell leucodystrophy and infantile Gaucher's disease (Svennerholm 1963). The physical considerations that I have described may be relevant to these disease situations.

## OTHER BRAIN MEMBRANES

The remaining membranes of the brain have not yet received as much attention as myelin, as far as structure is concerned. The lipid classes are known (see Tables 2-4).

The separation of three homogeneous membrane fractions from brain has been described by Whittaker (1966). These are (*a*) myelin, (*b*) external neuronal membranes from the terminal region of the axon, and (*c*) synaptic vesicles. The detached nerve endings (synaptosomes) were resolved into external membranes, synaptic vesicles, intraterminal mitochondria and intraterminal soluble cytoplasm.

The external synaptosome membranes have a fairly high content of cholesterol (the molar ratio of cholesterol to phospholipid is 0.72:1), while the cerebroside content is very low. Synaptic vesicles contain considerably less cholesterol than the external membranes but have a similar phospholipid content. Mitochondria are characterized by a a very low content of cholesterol and negligible cerebrosides. Most of their lipid is phospholipid and includes about 11% cardiolipin. (This is a characteristic constituent of mitochondria from other tissues.)

The external synaptosome membrane is further characterized by its relatively large amount of ganglioside. Synaptic vesicles, myelin fragments and mitochondria all have a low ganglioside content. Recent studies in our laboratory (Clowes, Cherry and Chapman 1972) show that the addition of gangliosides to lecithin bilayers causes the electrical resistance of the membrane to fall by one to two orders of magnitude. There is, however, no change in breakdown voltage and no marked change in the a.c. capacitance, compared to a lecithin control. The presence of complicated sugar groupings in gangliosides and other lipid systems may be important in cell recognition.

Electron microscope studies of the isolated external membranes, synaptic vesicles and mitochondrial membranes show the usual 50-60 Å (5-6 nm) triple-layered unit membrane with permanganate fixation. Whittaker (1966) suggests that the synaptic vesicles may have a hydrophilic space in the centre of the bilayer.

Cotman and co-workers (1969) have analysed the fatty acid content of synaptic plasma membranes isolated from rat brain. These membranes consist primarily of synaptosomes. These authors observe that a distinguishable feature of the synaptic plasma membrane is the high proportion of long-chain fatty acids with a high degree of unsaturation. Thus the 22:6 acyl chains account for approximately 32% of the total fatty acids in phosphatidylethanolamine and phosphatidylserine + phosphatidylinositol. These membranes contain much fewer 18:1 chains in these particular phospholipids than in the whole brain. Some 60% of the fatty acids of phosphatidylethanolamine in the synaptic plasma membrane consist of 20:4 and 22:4–22:6 chains, whereas erythrocyte membranes have less than 44% of these acids in the phosphatidylethanolamine fraction. Kishimoto and co-workers (1969) report the presence of high quantities of 20:4, 22:4 and 22:6 fatty acids in phosphatidylethanolamine and phosphatidylserine lipids of synaptic vesicles (54%).

## CONCLUSIONS AND SUMMARY

Lipids are clearly a major component of brain structure and are associated with the brain membranes. Different lipid classes are present and the particular classes present vary from one type of membrane to the other; for example, cerebrosides are typical constituents of myelin whereas gangliosides are typical of synaptosome membranes. The fatty acids associated with the different lipid classes also vary from one membrane system to another. Thus myelin contains more saturated and longer chains than occur in the grey matter membranes.

Physical studies of lipid–water systems with and without cholesterol provide information about hydrocarbon chain fluidity and permeability properties. With this information it is possible to speculate about the role of the lipid classes and the effects of fatty acid variation. We can say that the myelin membrane is compact, will have good electrical insulation properties and that permeability to water and organic molecules will be extremely limited.

Those membranes of the brain which contain highly unsaturated lipids will exhibit greater ease of permeability to water and organic molecules than the membranes containing the more saturated lipids. Motion of the protein molecules within the membrane that are concerned with its electrical excitability may also take place more rapidly. When cholesterol is absent from a membrane we can expect greater possibilities for cooperative changes being transmitted as well as easier movement of lipid molecules along the length of the membrane.

The consequence of altering the distribution of fatty acids in some brain membranes, perhaps as a result of disease or undernutrition, can be broadly predicted from the physical data, provided that compensating factors involving other lipids and protein do not intervene. Compensatory effects are, however, known to occur in the membrane composition of some cell systems, such that the overall fluidity of the membrane remains the same.

Effects of the essential fatty acids are difficult to predict, as these molecules as well as having a structural role in membranes are concerned with the formation of prostaglandins. Another source of important effects connected with membranes and brain structure relates to differences, perhaps associated with disease or undernutrition, in the complicated sugar groupings of the sugar lipids. The sugar groups may be important for cell recognition purposes in general and in particular in interneuronal recognition in the brain.

ACKNOWLEDGEMENT

The Science Research Council is thanked for financial support.

# References

Caspar, D. L. D. and Kirschner, D. A. (1971) *Nature New Biol.* **231**, 46-52

Chapman, D. (1968) In *Biological Membranes*, pp. 125-199, ed. D. Chapman. Academic Press, London

Chapman, D., Owen, N. F., Phillips, M. C. and Walker, D. A. (1969) *Biochim. Biophys. Acta* **183**, 458-465

CHAPMAN, D. and PENKETT, S. A. (1966) *Nature (Lond.)* **211**, 1304-1305
CHAPMAN, D., WILLIAMS, R. M. and LADBROOKE, B. D. (1967) *Chem. Phys. Lipids*, **1**, 445-475
CHEN, L. F., LUND, D. B. and RICHARDSON, T. (1971) *Biochim. Biophys. Acta* **225**, 108
CLOWES, A. W., CHERRY, R. J. and CHAPMAN, D. (1971) *Biochim. Biophys. Acta* **249**, 301-317
CLOWES, A. W., CHERRY, R. J. and CHAPMAN, D. (1972) *J. Mol. Biol.* in press
COTMAN, C., BLANK, M. L., MOEHL, A. and SNYDER, F. (1969) *Biochemistry* **8**, 4606
DICKERSON, J. W. T. (1968) In *Applied Neurochemistry*, pp. 48-115, ed. A. N. Davison and J. Dobbing. Blackwell, Oxford
FINKELSTEIN, A. and CASS, A. (1968) *J. Gen. Physiol.* **52**, 1455
GEREN, B. B. (1954) *Exp. Cell Res.* **7**, 558-562
GERSTL, B., TAVASTSJERNA, M. G., HAYMAN, R. B., SMITH, J. K. and ENG, L. F. (1963) *J. Neurochem.* **10**, 889-902
DE GIER, J., MANDERSLOOT, J. G. and VAN DEENEN, L. L. M. (1968) *Biochim. Biophys. Acta* **150**, 666
DE GIER, J., MANDERSLOOT, J. G., HUPKES, J. V., MCELHANEY, R. N. and VAN BECK, W. P. (1971) *Biochim. Biophys. Acta* **233**, 610
HUBBELL, W. L. and MCCONNELL, H. M. (1969) *Proc. Natl. Acad. Sci. U.S.A.* **64**, 20-27
KISHIMOTO, Y., AGRANOFF, B. W., RADIN, N. S. and BURTON, R. M. (1969) *J. Neurochem.* **16**, 397
LADBROOKE, B. D., JENKINSON, T. J., KAMAT, V. B. and CHAPMAN, D. (1968) *Biochim. Biophys. Acta* **164**, 101-109
LADBROOKE, B. D., WILLIAMS, R. M. and CHAPMAN, D. (1968) *Biochim. Biophys. Acta* **150**, 333-340
LUZZATI, V. and HUSSON, F. (1962) *J. Cell Biol.* **12**, 207-219
O'BRIEN, J. S. (1965) *Science* **147**, 1099-1107
SCHMITT, F. O., BEAR, R. S. and PALMER, K. J. (1941) *J. Cell. Comp. Physiol.* **18**, 31-42
SVENNERHOLM, L. (1963) In *Brain Lipids and Lipoproteins and their Leucodystrophies*, pp. 104-119, ed. J. Folch-Pi and H. Bauer. Elsevier, Amsterdam
VANDENHEUVEL, F. A. (1963) *J. Am. Oil Chem. Soc.* **40**, 455-472
WHITTAKER, V. P. (1966) *Ann. N.Y. Acad. Sci.* **137**, 982
WILKINS, M. H. F., BLAUROCK, A. E. and ENGELMAN, D. M. (1971) *Nature New Biol.* **230**, 72-76

# Discussion

*Mead:* Professor Chapman has discussed the interesting question of why lipids have certain spatial configurations and how these affect the properties of membranes. We recently asked Dr D. R. Howton of our laboratory to consider the shape of a sphingolipid (e.g. a cerebroside) at a water–oil interface. We often tend to simplify the lipid structures in membranes by drawing the fatty acid chains (or one fatty acid chain and the hydrocarbon portion of sphingosine) as parallel lines. Conformational analysis of sphingolipids suggests that with all but one (the amide NH moiety) of the four (or five, in the case of α-hydroxy fatty acyl sphingolipids) highly polar groups of the molecule in contact with or immersed in the aqueous phase, the two lengthy hydrocarbon moieties are directed into the oil phase and *widely splayed* (rather than in close lateral register). Since membranous structures (such as myelin and the erythrocyte membrane) containing large amounts of sphingolipids are also usually rich in cholesterol, it seems conceivable that the two tend to be associated by hydrogen bonding between the sterol hydroxy group and the inward-oriented amide nitrogen of the lipid, the sterol thus serving to fill the 'void' between the splayed hydrocarbon moieties and making the assemblage much more compact (in close analogy with the surface-area conservation exhibited by mixed monomolecular films of lecithins and cholesterol, for example).

*Chapman:* The surface properties of sphingomyelin at the air–water interface have been studied and compared with dipalmitoyl lecithin (Shah and Schulman 1967). This shows that they both have approximately the same limiting area (42-44 $Å^2$ per molecule). Therefore in this case the two chains are not widely splayed out.

We know that cholesterol interacts with lecithins; for example, it inhibits some molecular motion of the lipid chains with an unsaturated lipid. In a liposome system at a molar-molar ratio, cholesterol with a saturated lipid such as dipalmitoyl lecithin prevents the lipid chains from crystallizing or packing together (Chapman 1968). Recent studies in our laboratory show a similar behaviour with beef-brain sphingomyelin and cerebrosides (E. Oldfield and D. Chapman, unpublished studies).

When we consider the possibility of hydrogen bonding between the hydroxy group of the sterol and the amide nitrogen of the sphingomyelin or with the phosphate group of lecithin, the following observations can be made:

(*a*) Hydrogen bonding between group A and group B in general is usually much weaker in the presence of water than in its absence. This is because of the competitive hydrogen bonding situations which arise between the water molecules and group A and group B;

(*b*) A recent nuclear magnetic resonance spectroscopic study of lecithin–cholesterol has been interpreted as indicating a hydrogen bond between the cholesterol hydroxy and lecithin phosphate groups (Darke *et al.* 1971);

(*c*) We have shown (E. Oldfield and D. Chapman, unpublished studies) in 220 MHz spectra of sphingomyelin–cholesterol mixtures that there is some slight restriction of motion of the $N(CH)_3$ group.

*Bernsohn*: Is the theme of your paper that one could modify membrane structure *ad infinitum*, for instance by substituting more unsaturated fatty acids for cholesterol, or *vice versa*, and yet retain essentially the same rotational properties of the myelin membrane and the same liquid-crystalline state of the membrane? This would imply that there isn't just one membrane of fixed composition but an infinite number of membranes, depending on the ratio of the components, which could carry on normal membrane functions.

*Chapman:* I don't envisage that one can replace cholesterol in a membrane by substituting unsaturated lipids and thereby fulfil all the functions that cholesterol normally carries out. However, it seems to me that some physico-chemical properties of a membrane can be mimicked by a variety of changes of lipid composition. Thus we can obtain a similar membrane fluidity by a cell using either unsaturated lipids or methyl branched lipids. There are also cases such as yeast cells (Myer and Block 1963) where, when the cell is grown under conditions which do not encourage the formation of double bonds (anaerobic conditions), a membrane is formed from short-chain and long-chain saturated fatty acids, producing thereby the same fluidity and chain-packing as is normally obtained in aerobic growth when the phospholipids contain long-chain unsaturated and long-chain saturated fatty acids.

We have taken a lecithin bilayer in the form of a model membrane system and added cerebroside (Clowes, Cherry and Chapman 1971). This increased the electrical resistance of the membrane system. Calorimetric studies showed that the transition temperature of the cerebroside is lowered by the presence of the lecithin. In a sense the unsaturated lecithin affects the transition of the cerebroside, so that you may to some extent have the same kind of fluidity produced as if cerebroside plus cholesterol were present. As a general point, perhaps I should say that we all tend to think that membranes are homogeneous, as far as lipid is concerned, but this may not be the case. It may be that one region is fluid and another region less fluid. We have found this recently with the *Acholeplasma laidlawii* system (Oldfield, Chapman and Derbyshire 1972)

*Bernsohn:* I was suggesting the possibility of a membrane having an infinite variety of composition, depending on the ratio of cholesterol to unsaturates, and of cerebroside to unsaturates, and at the same time retaining its normal physiological functions. This could have implications for nutrition.

*Chapman:* I think that for certain functions it may be possible to balance one component with another but one can envisage an out-of-balance situation in some cases. Let's take myelin as an example. We have this very complex structure with cholesterol fluidizing the cerebroside chains and inhibiting the motion of the unsaturated fatty acids. Supposing we now put highly unsaturated fatty acids into the lipids, *keeping everything else* the same, then I think that the membrane would become more permeable, more leaky to water and more easily diffused by organic molecules.

*Houtsmuller:* The work of van Deenen's group is interesting here, because they showed that in the erythrocyte small changes in cholesterol content alter the permeability of the erythrocyte membrane considerably, whereas if only the fatty acid composition of the red cells is altered, as in essential fatty acid deficiency, the permeability is not or only slightly affected (Bruckdorfer *et al.* 1969).

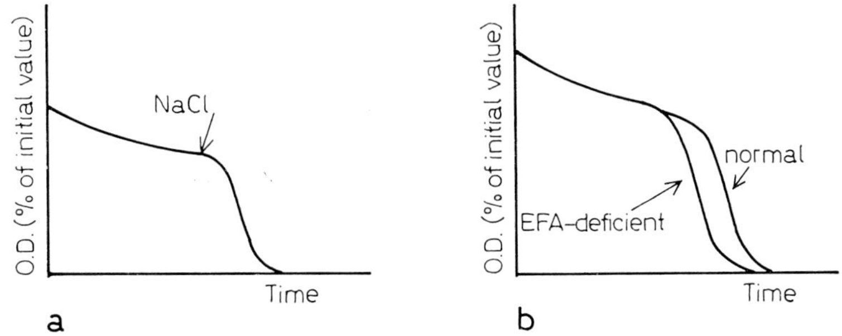


FIG. 1 (Houtsmuller). Red cell swelling and haemolysis in thiourea.

In our laboratory we have studied haemolysis in 0.3 osmolar thiourea. When the change in optical density—the parameter for the haemolytic process—is plotted against time, it becomes apparent that the process is biphasic (Fig. 1*a*). If sodium chloride is added (to a final concentration of 0.3 osmolar) at the moment indicated, the process can be stopped. It can subsequently be demonstrated, by centrifugation and measurement of haemoglobin in the supernatant, that no haemolysis occurred during this part of the process and therefore the change in optical density is entirely due to swelling. This swelling is related to the permeability of the red cell membrane for thiourea. The second, steeper, part of the curve represents the actual haemolytic process. Comparison of erythrocytes from rats deficient in essential fatty acids and normal rats (Fig. 1*b*) reveals that the swelling of both types of red cells is identical, which means that the permeability of the membranes is the same. The difference in the steeper part of the curves indicates that the relative volume increase is less for the EFA-deficient erythrocytes than for the normal ones, which could mean that the membranes are more fragile.

Therefore the permeability of membranes containing both cholesterol and phospholipids seems to be controlled primarily by cholesterol and the effect on permeability of unsaturation of the individual fatty acids is of minor importance. Van Deenen also showed that the whole lipid from the erythrocytes of the deficient rats had the same surface properties as the normal cells.

*Chapman:* Cholesterol does control the permeability of lipid systems, but permeability is also affected by the degree of unsaturation of the fatty acid. This has been shown with natural membranes and also in model experiments. In van Deenen's laboratory they have also been trying to correlate the permeability to glycerol and other polyhydric alcohols in liposome systems with the permeability of erythrocyte membranes (de Gier, Mandersloot and van Deenen 1968; McElhaney, de Gier and van Deenen 1970). In the model experiments they put liposomes of differing degrees of unsaturation into isotonic glycerol and measure the swelling rate; this is related to the way in which the glycerol can get through the lipid barrier. With an unsaturated lipid, glycerol passes through the system fairly readily, but when cholesterol is added it reduces the permeability of the liposome to glycerol, so cholesterol definitely affects the liposome permeability. With a saturated lipid the liposome has to be raised above its transition temperature before glycerol can penetrate the lipid bilayer. With unsaturated lipids with increasing unsaturation, glycerol molecules diffuse more easily through the bilayer; the lipid is then above its transition temperature. So in the absence of cholesterol, as the fatty acids in the membrane become more unsaturated, the permeability increases. In a very recent paper liposomes were made from lecithin taken from rats which were deficient in essential fatty acids (Chen, Lund and Richardson 1971) and the permeability for molecules like glycerol was compared with that of lecithins from normal rats. The permeability is greater for lecithin from normal rats than from the deficient rats.

*Menkes:* What is the effect of ions on the physical properties of lipid layers?

*Chapman:* If we take a simple lipid–water system, such as dipalmitoyl lecithin, and interact it with certain ions, say uranyl ions, which are known to have an electrostatic interaction with phosphate groups, the transition temperature increases by about 6-8°C. This idea of the ion affecting the transition temperature is also borne out by comparing the effects of sodium laurate and potassium laurate. The transition temperatures of sodium and potassium laurate may differ by some 20 to 30°C. We can envisage a lipid in the membrane having a certain fluidity and when an ion comes up and interacts with a polar group of the lipid, the 'local' fluidity may change quite dramatically. Regions of fluid and less fluid lipids could provide some memory process.

*Baumann:* What effect does the binding of calcium have on the physical properties of fatty acids in membranes?

*Chapman:* Calcium often raises the transition temperature of phospholipids, for example phosphatidylserine, and indeed can cause precipitation from water. Reorganization of a lipid in a membrane could certainly occur as a consequence of interaction with calcium.

*Baumann:* Is there specific binding of calcium to certain lipids?

*Chapman:* Yes. Calcium will interact with lipids such as phosphatidylserine, and with the phosphatidylinositols. I think that at low concentrations of calcium there is no interaction with the phosphatidylcholine. (There have been some monolayer studies where it has been suggested that calcium can interact more with saturated than unsaturated lecithins: see Shah and Schulman 1965.) The phosphoinositides can have one, two or three charges and can also interact with calcium ions.

*Ansell:* I believe that the total choline lipid content in a cell membrane is relatively constant and is sometimes made up of an excess of phosphatidylcholine and sometimes by an excess of sphingomyelin. Would you like to speculate that this might be relevant to the presence or absence of cholesterol in the membrane?

*Chapman:* My own speculation on this is that the phosphatidylcholine and the sphingomyelin lipids act as a bridge between lipoprotein regions where electrostatic interaction is occurring. If we have phosphatidylserine interacting electrostatically with protein in the membrane at a particular point, there may be hydrophobic interaction occurring in the surrounding regions as well. My feeling is that the sphingomyelin and phosphatidylcholine lipids, because of their internal charge neutralization, probably don't interact with ions to the same extent as does phosphatidylserine, and it may be that these choline lipids can interchange with each other. With regard to the absence or presence of cholesterol, it is interesting to note that cholesterol is usually present in membranes containing fairly saturated lipids rather than in, say, mitochondrial membranes, which usually contain highly unsaturated fatty acids.

*Crawford:* Sphingomyelin and the white matter in the brain carry with it a relatively small proportion of protein in relation to the lipid. Within the phospholids themselves, there is a considerable range of different electrical properties, as you have pointed out. There are quaternary amines, primary amines and amphoteric components, but generally speaking, in model systems we are working with fairly homogeneous lipid mixtures. Can you comment on the interaction that might occur with regard to liquid-crystalline properties if one mixed phospholipids of different polarity, for example, the quaternary amine and an amphoteric phospholipid? What effects are observed on the transition temperature?

*Chapman:* If you take, say, phosphatidylethanolamine and phosphatidylcholine of the same chain length and mix them, the different transition temperatures of each of the lipids can move, depending upon the ratio of one lipid to the other. Thus if you have one component with a high transition temperature and one with a low transition, say ox-brain cerebrosides and egg lecithin, the transition temperature of the cerebroside moves to lower temperatures.

*Crawford:* Is there any evidence of an electrical interaction between different phospholipid groups, perhaps analogous to protein binding? One always assumes from the Davson–Danielli picture of the membrane that there is a large amount of protein, but in myelin there is much more lipid than protein.

*Chapman:* I believe that many membrane structures will turn out to be ones in

which
and tl
so on
memt
betwe
becau
needs
impoı
put g
is low
lipid (
*Ber*
myeli
protei
*Ch*
magn
grour
wrapı
obser
of the
*Pa*
*Ch*
Just l
tion f
know
impo
perha
*Pa*
dehyc
myeli
Howe
and n

## Refe

BRUCK
*Bi*
CHAPN
Ne
CHEN,

# Types of fatty acids in brain lipids, their derivation and function

J. F. MEAD and G. A. DHOPESHWARKAR

*Laboratory of Nuclear Medicine and Radiation Biology, University of California, Los Angeles and Department of Biological Chemistry, UCLA School of Medicine, Los Angeles*

The derivation of the fatty acids of the brain lipids and their subsequent metabolism have been investigated by a number of scientists in several different laboratories. However, the results have often been confusing and at times contradictory. It has been difficult to determine, for example, if or how the fatty acids penetrate the blood–brain barrier and in what form. After their incorporation into lipids, moreover, good evidence has been found supporting both a rapid turnover and great stability (Davison and Dobbing 1959; Davison *et al.* 1959; Ansell and Spanner 1968; Smith 1968; Smith and Eng 1965).

Once the fatty acids have been incorporated into the brain lipids, it has been shown that they undergo many of the usual reactions such as chain shortening and elongation, desaturation and hydroxylation, but the nature of the enzymes effecting these changes and their location (in which types of cells and subcellular structures) is by no means clear.

In our laboratory a start has been made to find answers to all these questions, although it cannot yet be said with confidence that any of the problems are solved.

Although there are undoubtedly several sources of carbon for the synthesis of the brain fatty acids, we chose, for several reasons, to use carboxy-labelled acetate. The major reason was that it permitted us to predict the type of labelling that would be expected if carboxy-labelled long-chain fatty acids were degraded to acetate, which could then be used for fatty acid synthesis. The results obtained in rats (Dhopeshwarkar, Maier and Mead 1969) are shown in Fig. 1. It can be seen that acetate incorporation decreases precipitously from 9 to 30 days and then levels off at a low activity throughout adulthood, apparently in inverse relationship to the brain lipid content of the rats. Even in the adult, however, entry of acetate into the brain lipids is rapid. Experiments in which adult rats are decapitated 15 seconds after intracarotid injection of carboxy-

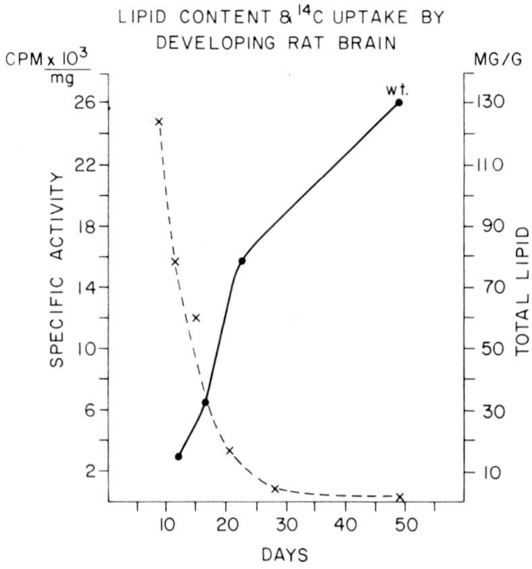


FIG. 1. Effect of age on total lipid content and uptake of [1-$^{14}$C]acetate into lipids of the rat brain. •——•, total lipid content; x-----x, specific activity. Each point represents the mean value for three rats each given 58 μCi of [1-$^{14}$C]acetate intraperitoneally and killed after 8 hours.

labelled acetate show incorporation into all the brain lipids, even those typical of myelin. Decarboxylation of the fatty acids revealed that at 15 seconds the distribution of $^{14}$C in the palmitate was close to the theoretical for total synthesis while that in stearate and other longer-chain acids indicated elongation (Dhopeshwarkar, Subramanian and Mead 1971*a*). Thus, both types of reaction occur readily in the adult brain. A similar distribution of activity was found 24 hours after injection (Table 1), indicating some stability of the synthesized fatty acids. The location of the fatty acids in the various lipids is also of interest. In Table 2, it can be seen that at 15 seconds, the highest activity is in serine phosphoglycerides (SPG) followed by cerebroside, whereas at 24 hours, choline phosphoglycerides (CPG) are most active. Ansell and Spanner (1962) failed to notice any appreciable amount of radioactivity going from [3-$^{14}$C]serine into ethanolamine phosphoglycerides (EPG) or CPG and concluded that decarboxylation of SPG to EPG is not a major pathway in the brain. Abdel-Latif and Abood (1966), however, did find that brain mitochondria are capable of decarboxylating SPG *in vitro*. *In vivo* experiments generally show uptake of the base only in the corresponding phospholipid (Ansell and Spanner 1968), indicating a minor role for the decarboxylation and methylation reactions in the brain.

Although the brain is obviously capable of supplying a good part of its fatty acid complement by synthetic processes, it could be surmised, from several

TABLE 1

Distribution of radioactivity (percentage relative carboxyl activity) in brain fatty acids 24 hours after administration of labelled fatty acids

| *Fatty acid administered* | *Fatty acid isolated from brain total lipids of rats 24 h after administration* | | | | | | |
|---|---|---|---|---|---|---|---|
| | *Palmitic acid* | *Oleic acid* | *Eicosaenoic acid* | *Linoleic acid* | *Linolenic acid* | *Arachidonic acid* | *Docosahexaenoic acid* |
| [1-$^{14}$C)acetate | 14.1 | 23.6 | 38.6 | — | — | 83.3 | 81.9 |
| [1-$^{14}$C]palmitic acid | 85.1 | 21.6* | — | — | — | — | — |
| [1-$^{14}$C]oleic acid | 74.5 | 58.1 | 10.1 | — | — | — | — |
| [1-$^{14}$C]linoleic acid | 19.6 | 48.3 | — | 88.0 | — | 3.5 | 72.4 |
| [1-$^{14}$C]linolenic acid | 13.8 | 32.9 | 94.3 | — | 92.4 | 81.7 | 12.4 |

* These values are for stearic acid instead of oleic acid.

TABLE 2

Incorporation of carboxy-labelled fatty acids into various polar lipids of the rat brain

| *Fatty acid administered* | *Specific activity c.p.m./mg* | | | | |
|---|---|---|---|---|---|
| | *Choline phosphoglycerides* | *Ethanolamine phosphoglycerides* | *Serine phosphoglycerides* | *Sphingomyelin* | *Cerebroside* |
| [1-$^{14}$C]acetate* | 86 | 45 | 239 | 59 | 138 |
| ]1-$^{14}$C]acetate† | 130 | 75 | 46 | 30 | 51 |
| [1-$^{14}$C]palmitic acid† | 304 | 116 | 83 | 14 | 22 |
| [1-$^{14}$C]oleic acid† | 266 | 156 | 71 | 42 | 67 |
| [1-$^{14}$C]linoleic acid† | 179 | 79 | 79 | 38 | 71 |
| [1-$^{14}$C]linolenic acid† | 101 | 84 | 76 | 23 | 100 |

* Incorporation after 15 seconds.
† Incorporation after 24 hours.

dietary studies involving essential fatty acids, that it is also capable of utilizing at least certain dietary lipids (Mohrhauer and Holman 1963). To those intrigued by the concept of the blood–brain barrier, however, this idea was not easy to accept. In order to settle this problem and also in an attempt to explain the mysterious dominance of *n*-3 (or linolenic family) fatty acids in brain as opposed to other tissues (Miyamoto, Stephanides and Bernsohn 1967), we embarked on a study of the passage of fatty acids of various sorts from blood to brain. These studies have involved both injection and feeding of the fatty acids and have been made at time intervals from 15 seconds to 24 hours. In each case, carboxy-labelled fatty acids have been used and the relative activities in the carboxyl and chain (relative carboxyl activity, RCA) have been compared with similar data from the experiments with acetate so that some idea could be gained of the proportion of fatty acids transported directly into the brain as opposed to those formed by degradation and resynthesis (Dhopeshwarkar, Subramanian and Mead 1971*b*). In some cases, results were compared with those from liver of the same animals; in others, the liver was functionally removed during the experiment (Dhopeshwarkar *et al.* 1972). A summary of the findings of these experiments is presented in Tables 1 and 3. In Table 3, it can be seen that at 24 hours after administration, the highest incorporation of the radioactivity of the administered acid is from linoleic acid, followed by linolenic acid*. This does not mean that the $^{14}C$ detected is still in the administered acids. As will be discussed below, these acids are rapidly transformed into their longer-chain more highly unsaturated derivatives. It is also interesting that the long-chain fatty acids appear to penetrate the brain even more efficiently than does acetate, possibly due to their lipid solubility (Davson 1967). In experiments in which the liver is functionally removed or the fatty acid given by direct intracarotid injection, it has also been shown that the fatty acid appears to be transported as the free fatty acid. There is no need to invoke transformation into complex lipids for passage into the brain.

In Table 1, the percentage RCA of the brain fatty acids after administration can be compared with that resulting from administration of acetate. There can be no doubt that the administered fatty acids were transported directly into the brain and were incorporated into the brain lipids without degradation to acetate and resynthesis.

In Table 2 is compared the incorporation of the administered fatty acid into the major polar lipids of the brain. Aside from the 15-second incorporation of acetate predominantly into SPG, as mentioned above, the highest proportion

* However, when radioactivities of liver and brain were compared, it was noted that uptake of radioactivity from 18:3 in the brain was proportionately higher than that from 18:2.

TABLE 3

Incorporation of radioactivity from carboxy-labelled fatty acids into brain lipids

| *Fatty acid administered* | *4 h after administration* | | | *24 h after administration* | | |
|---|---|---|---|---|---|---|
| | *Radioactivity administered/g body wt. μCi* | *Radioactivity of total lipids/g brain tissue c.p.m./g* | *% of given dose incorporated into lipids/g brain tissue* | *Radioactivity administered/g body wt. μCi* | *Radioactivity of total lipids/g brain tissue c.p.m./g* | *% of given dose incorporated into lipids/g brain tissue* |
| [1-$^{14}$C]acetic acid | 5 | 509980 | 4.59 | 3.1 | 75235 | 1.09 |
| [1-$^{14}$C]palmitic acid | 0.25 | 13275 | 2.39 | 0.25 | 11879 | 2.14 |
| [1-$^{14}$C]oleic acid | 0.25 | 13145 | 2.36 | 0.25 | 8570 | 1.54 |
| [1-$^{14}$C]linoleic acid | 0.16 | 5452 | 1.53 | 0.21 | 12714 | 2.7 |
| [1-$^{14}$C]linolenic acid | 0.16 | 4331 | 1.2 | 0.21 | 11008 | 2.5 |

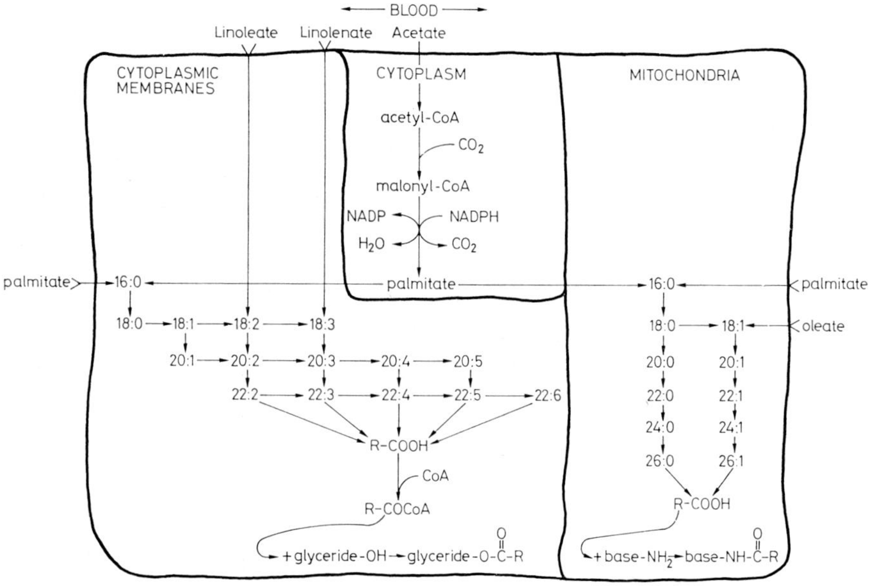


FIG. 2. Overall view of fatty acid derivation and metabolism in brain.
Horizontal arrows in the microsomal system do not imply inter-family conversions, which are not known to occur in animals. The figure represents conversions within an individual series, eg. in the *n*-9 series, 18:0 → 18:1 → 18:2; in the *n*-6 series, 18:2 → 18:3, etc.

appears in the CPG fraction with one interesting exception. In the case of linolenic acid (Dhopeshwarkar, Subramanian and Mead 1971*b*), a very high incorporation of activity into cerebroside occurs. Partial purification of this fraction reveals that the radioactivity is in the lower of the two cerebroside spots as separated by thin-layer chromatography. Since this is the spot usually considered to contain the hydroxy acids and since linolenate and its derivatives are not usually found in cerebrosides, this curious finding must be investigated further.

By whatever route the fatty acids have reached the brain, they are subjected to several different types of alteration in different locations, probably in different cells, before their final disposal. These reactions have been studied in a number of laboratories including this one and that of Radin (e.g. Hajra and Radin 1963).

In Fig. 2 are depicted some of the pathways open to the brain fatty acids. The mitochondrial elongation pathway (Boone and Wakil 1970), using acetyl-CoA, converts either palmitate or mono-unsaturated acids to form the very long-chain fatty acids of the sphingolipids. An example of the importance of this

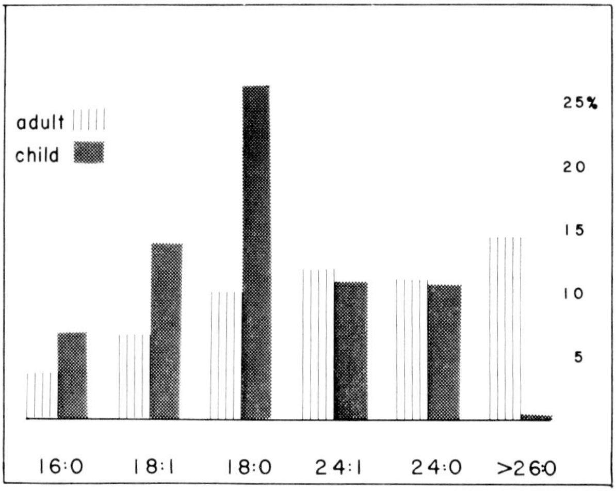


FIG. 3. Relative proportions of long- and very long-chain fatty acids in the cerebroside sulphate of adult and child brains.

system is shown in Fig. 3, in which the chain-lengths of fatty acids in the cerebroside sulphate from young and adult human brains are shown graphically. It is of interest, as stated above, that the product of this system appears to be found largely in amide link (i.e. sphingolipids).

The other major system, the microsomal elongation-desaturation system (Mead 1971), appears to be concerned largely with unsaturated and polyunsaturated acids usually obtained from dietary sources. This system uses malonyl-CoA for elongation and its products, long-chain polyunsaturated acids, seem to end up largely in ester linkage in seemingly more metabolically active phospholipids. Although it is not yet clear in which cell types these various reactions occur, a reasonable guess would be that the mitochondrial elongation system would surely be found in the oligodendrocytes, which must incorporate them into the myelin lipids. A culture of astrocytes, admittedly derived from an astrocytoma, was found to carry out the microsomal elongation-desaturation reactions with great rapidity, compared with other cells in culture (Mead and Haggerty 1971), and it is possible that the astrocytes are a site for this type of alteration.

Some of the fatty acids found in the brain lipids, particularly those in the sphingolipids of myelin, cannot be explained as the result of any of these processes. It was found in this laboratory that the long-chain odd and α-hydroxy-acids are a result of an α-oxidation or one-carbon chain-shortening process. This was first demonstrated in *in vivo* studies (Mead and Levis 1962, 1963) and was then investigated in a brain 'microsomal' fraction (Levis and

Mead 1964; MacDonald and Mead 1968). This system appears to be a mixed-function oxidase and requires only the 'microsomal' fraction, ferrous ion (which is partially contained in the particles) and the 110 000 **g** supernatant fraction, in which the active factor is ascorbic acid, which has the function of maintaining the iron in the +2 state. The reaction proceeds until the ascorbate is irreversibly oxidized and then ceases when the iron is oxidized to the +3 state. It can be renewed with additional ascorbate. Unfortunately, the complete mechanism has not yet been elucidated nor has the cellular location of the enzymes.

The conventional β-oxidation must also take place in the brain, since some of the enzymes involved have been found there (Vignais, Gallagher and Zabin 1958). However, the importance of this reaction in the brain is not at all certain.

Perhaps the most vital and intriguing questions are those concerning the functions of the various fatty acids in the general reactions of the brain. Presumably the polyunsaturated fatty acids serve the same function in the various cellular membranes in the brain as in other organs—control of the physical state of the non-polar portion of the membranes. The function of the very long-chain fatty acids of the myelin sphingolipids might be to add stability to the myelin membrane through their ability to form a stronger total of hydrophobic bonds (according to some authors, 'interdigitation'). However, recent freeze-etching studies appear to cast some doubt on the idea that the very long-chain acids extend completely through a lipid bilayer. Even more obscure are the functions of the products of the α-oxidation reaction. If the reaction is largely a degradative one, disposing of the very long-chain fatty acids, why then do the intermediate products appear in the myelin lipids? This can probably be explained in the case of the odd-chain fatty acids, since these may not be distinguishable from their even-chain homologues, but the hydroxy acids must impart some different properties to the sphingolipids of which they form an important part. Thus it might appear that an initially purely degradative process has been partially converted to the production of a uniquely useful product.

Finally, the question of the transport of the various lipids throughout the brain is an intriguing one. For example, the changes that occur in the fatty acids of the myelin lipids during maturation and aging must imply either that the pertinent enzymes have ready access to the inner myelin layers or that the fatty acids may be transported to the enzyme site or that certain of the enzymes are present in the myelin. It is not too difficult to visualize a steady state of 'vacant' positions on the myelin phospholipids, to be filled by available fatty acids from whatever source. It is possible that the passage of fatty acids into the brain, as discussed above, is a function of the number of 'vacant' positions rather than of a blood–brain barrier.

It is evident from this brief summary of our work and that of other laboratories that only a start has been made at answering the problem implicit in the title. A great deal of work remains to be done.

SUMMARY

Brain lipid fatty acids are derived in two ways—by synthesis within the brain and passage into the brain of fatty acids synthesized elsewhere in the body or obtained in the diet.

Synthesis within the brain is very rapid in the premyelination animal and falls off rapidly to a steady state in the adult. Even in the adult brain, however, fatty acid synthesis and incorporation into lipids is very rapid—less than 15 seconds following the intracarotid injection of labelled acetate.

Fatty acids, fed or injected intravenously, rapidly pass into the brain lipids. The blood–brain barrier appears to offer little impediment to the passage of free fatty acids and the controlling factors governing the rate of incorporation and fatty acid discrimination appear to be at the enzymic (transacylase) level.

Fatty acids thus derived are subjected to very rapid microsomal elongation and desaturation (probably in glial cells) and to elongation in mitochondria. Degradation by the α or β systems takes place but the location, mechanism and 'purpose' of these reactions are obscure.

ACKNOWLEDGEMENTS

These studies were supported in part by Contract AT(04-1) GEN-12 between the Atomic Energy Commission and the University of California and by United States Public Health Service research career award GM-K6-19, 177 from the Division of General Medical Sciences, National Institutes of Health, U.S.A.

# References

Abdel-Latif, A. A. and Abood, L. G. (1966) *J. Neurochem.* **13**, 1189-1196

Ansell, G. B. and Spanner, S. (1962) *Biochem. J.* **84**, 12P-13P

Ansell, G. B. and Spanner, S. (1968) *Biochem. J.* **110**, 201-206

Boone, S. C. and Wakil, S. J. (1970) *Biochemistry* **9**, 1470-1479

Davison, A. N. and Dobbing, J. (1959) *Biochem. J.* **73**, 701-706

Davison, A. N., Dobbing, J., Morgan, R. S., Wajda, M. and Wright, G. P. (1959) In *Biochemistry of Lipids* (Proc. 5th Int. Conf., Vienna), pp. 85-88. Pergamon Press, Oxford

Davson, H. (1967) *The Physiology of the Cerebrospinal Fluid*, pp. 82-119. Churchill, London
Dhopeshwarkar, G. A., Maier, R. and Mead, J. F. (1969) *Biochim. Biophys. Acta* **187**, 6-12
Dhopeshwarkar, G. A., Subramanian, C. and Mead, J. F. (1971*a*) *Biochim. Biophys. Acta* **248**, 41-47
Dhopeshwarkar, G. A., Subramanian, C. and Mead, J. F. (1971*b*) *Biochim. Biophys. Acta* **239**, 162-167
Dhopeshwarkar, G. A., Subramanian, C., McConnell, D. H. and Mead, J. F. (1972) *Biochim. Biophys. Acta* **255**, 572-579
Hajra, A. K. and Radin, N. S. (1963) *J. Lipid Res.* **4**, 1470-1479
Levis, G. M. and Mead, J. F. (1964) *J. Biol. Chem.* **239**, 77-80
MacDonald, R. C. and Mead, J. F. (1968) *Lipids* **3**, 275-283
Mead, J. F. (1971) In *Progress in the Chemistry of Fats and Other Lipids*, vol. 9, pp. 159-192, ed. R. T. Holman. Pergamon Press, Oxford
Mead, J. F. and Haggerty, D. F., Jr (1971) *Excerpta Medica Nutrition* **8**, 76-80
Mead, J. F. and Levis, G. M. (1962) *Biochem. Biophys. Res. Commun.* **9**, 231-234
Mead, J. F. and Levis, G. M. (1963) *J. Biol. Chem.* **238**, 1634-1636
Miyamoto, K., Stephanides, L. M. and Bernsohn, J. (1967) *J. Neurochem.* **14**, 227-237
Mohrhauer, H. and Holman, R. T. (1963) *J. Neurochem.* **10**, 523-530
Smith, M. E. (1968) *Biochim. Biophys. Acta* **164**, 285-293
Smith, M. E. and Eng, L. F. (1965) *J. Am. Oil Chem. Soc.* **42**, 1013-1018
Vignais, P. M., Gallagher, C. H. and Zabin, I. (1958) *J. Neurochem.* **2**, 283-287

# Discussion

*Young:* I've been getting quite interested in sex recently in relation to this field, and the fact that the essential fatty acid requirement of a male rat is so much higher than that of the female seems to be possibly of some significance. Have you, or other investigators, found a difference between the sexes, in animals or human beings, in any of this area? Dr Hugh Sinclair (1956, 1958) has painted a broad canvas, pointing out that the effects of smoking on carcinoma of the lung and on heart disease are more common in men than women, and suggests that this difference may relate to the greater male requirement for essential fatty acids. It might be worth noting any differences between the sexes in our discussions.

*Mead:* As you say, the essential fatty acids appear to have a very different quantitative effect in the male and female rat. Whether this extends to the brain I can't say, but we do know that the female either has greater stores of essential fatty acids or uses them more efficiently than does the male, because the female rat is fairly impervious to essential fatty acid deficiency whereas the male responds rapidly and we know that the female requires lower amounts of essential fatty acids than the male (e.g. Greenberg *et al.* 1950). We haven't investigated this in the brain. In our experiments we noted in each case the sex of the animal, but found no particular difference. In man, when we're considering nutrition in children and essential fatty acids appearing in the brain, sex may have an effect.

*Crawford:* A considerable amount of work has been done on sex differences and polyunsaturated fatty acids; the subject has been recently reviewed by R. L. Lyman (1968).

*Rossi:* Dr Mead, have you found any correlation between the quantity of labelled compounds that you injected and the incorporation in brain cells? Do you need to achieve certain gradients between blood and cells?

*Mead:* We haven't investigated this, because these were all tracer doses, so we were measuring not the effect of our injected fatty acid but reactions occurring continuously. In other words, our doses were small in comparison with the materials already there. As a matter of fact, we have done a few experiments along those lines, but the results have been so confusing that I would prefer not to discuss them at present.

*Ansell:* Dr Mead, you showed that if you injected dipalmitoyl phosphatidylcholine, very little of it was taken up by the brain. We have some indirect evidence that choline can be transported to the brain in lipid-bound form and I'd like to ask whether, since the plasma lecithin is all bound as lipoprotein, the dipalmitoyl phosphatidylcholine was complexed with protein before you injected it, or did you inject it as an emulsion?

*Mead:* We injected it as an emulsion, but it was complexed immediately, and was apparently readily available for lecithin:cholesterol acyltransferase and other enzymes, because 20% appeared in cholesterol ester, which is an apparently normal conversion.

*Crawford:* J. Hoelzl and H. P. Franck (1969) did experiments with doubly labelled lecithin and concluded that there was no blood–brain barrier for phospholipids. Most of the brain phospholipids will have a highly unsaturated long-chain fatty acid in the β-position, but you have used a phosphatidylcholine with a saturated acid in the β-position. This may not be acceptable to the lipoprotein complexes in the brain.

There may also be a question of degree: you are comparing the counts from phospholipid in the brain with the much higher counts obtained with free fatty acids, whereas Hoelzl was simply looking at phospholipids. Had he used free fatty acids as a standardization, he might have found they entered the brain faster than phospholipids. There are two variables: the degree of unsaturation in the phospholipid and the baseline for comparison.

*Mead:* This is something we have to do. However, I have seen no follow-up of the abstract describing this work (Hoelzl and Franck 1969). On closer examination, I'm loath to make the same conclusions as Dr Hoelzl did.

*Paoletti:* Have you studied diabetic animals? The level of free fatty acids in blood is increased, and the composition of this free fatty acid is quite different from that of fatty acids in the brain, so as a consequence, the brain phospholipid fatty acid would be changed in diabetic animals.

*Mead:* Why don't you do that experiment! If the free fatty acid is increased in such animals, I'm sure you would find more in the brain, because this is exactly what we have shown in our experiments.

*Dobbing:* I'm very puzzled by what is meant by 'the blood–brain barrier'. In the days before the availability of radioactive isotopes, Waelsch and others (see Schwerin, Bessman and Waelsch 1950) discovered that if you loaded the bloodstream with something like 40 times its normal amount of glutamate, this didn't alter the brain levels of that material in any way. When it became possible to label glutamate, it was discovered (Lajtha, Berl and Waelsch 1959) that the rapidity with which it exchanged with brain was so great that it wasn't possible to measure it. I submit that the first finding is an example of brain homeostasis, which is not a question of permeability at all, but of the control by the brain of its own composition. But as far as you know, Dr Mead, the fatty acids have this facility also? What you are measuring is exchange, not net flux, and I wonder whether the expression 'blood–brain barrier' ought not to be confined to flux, and that one shouldn't refer to exchange rates in this way.

*Mead:* This is exactly the conclusion I tried to make. We started off by assuming we were going to measure a barrier phenomenon, and we discovered that we hadn't. Our conclusion is that there is essentially no barrier in the true sense of the word, and that what we are measuring is an exchange. With acetate of course we are measuring synthesis as well, but with fatty acids we are measuring exchange and we are titrating what I would like to call 'vacant positions'. If there is a phospholipase operating in the brain, there will always be 'vacant positions', and these will be available for substitution by an incoming acyl (CoA). What we are measuring, then, is the availability of an exchangeable position rather than a barrier. This is a very rapid reaction but continues only so long as the supply of labelled fatty acids is not taken up by the liver and converted to less permeable compounds.

*von Muralt:* What part do you assign to the astrocytes in the 'blood–brain barrier'? Is it possible that astrocytes have an active transport system which might interfere with your flux measurements by selective transport of certain labelled compounds against the concentration gradient?

*Mead:* We have studied astrocytes *in vitro*, and they have an extremely active transport. As I mentioned, they take up fatty acids against a gradient and immediately convert them into other fatty acids. The blood–brain barrier may be concerned with astrocytes, and with other cell types, and with the permeability of the capillaries. This is a question for an anatomist.

*Bernsohn:* I think it is time that the term 'blood–brain barrier' is phased out, because I don't think it means anything in the *biochemical* sense. It's a relic of the old dye-injection experiments, and the term has persisted, but it seems obvious in the light of the results with labelled compounds that there is no such thing as a blood–brain barrier; even though many of these substances do so very slowly, they do enter the brain. This may not be true for macromolecules, because of the problem of membrane permeability and membrane pore size, but for the molecules we're discussing, the term 'blood–brain barrier' has outlived its usefulness.

*von Muralt:* However, there is a membrane barrier. The capillaries entering the brain are foreign structures and the brain maintains its basement membrane around every capillary.

*Bernsohn:* Electron micrographs (Peters, Palay and Webster 1970) showing that the astrocytic feet seem to interpose themselves between the capillary and the brain substance have lent credence to the idea of a physical barrier between the capillary and the brain, but in biochemical terms that concept is not valid. Even on a morphological basis, there are gaps in the astroglial end-feet which would therefore provide only a discontinuous barrier (Brightman 1967).

*Dobbing:* It's very heartening that Dr Bernsohn wants to demolish the blood–brain barrier. It's ten years since I had the temerity to write a review with the theme that the blood–brain barrier (Dobbing 1961) should be dropping out of our vocabulary, in this sense. Until you can show that there is a physical structure interposed between the blood and the brain which limits the rate of a metabolic process by limiting its rate of access to the brain, one has no right, in neurochemical terms, to speak of a blood–brain barrier. Every one of the instances which are quoted can be just as easily regarded as a reflection of brain metabolism rather than a limiting factor in it. Rather than state these questions in terms of a barrier, let us describe how fatty acid concentrations are changed, and how quickly.

*Ansell:* The classic examples of substances unable to pass through the blood–brain barrier are water-soluble quaternary ammonium compounds. Even so, Schuberth, Sparf and Sundwall (1969) have shown that in fact there must be a very active process which will take up water-soluble free choline into the brain.

*Crawford:* The converse to the difficulties of the water solubles is that ether enters the brain very rapidly!

*Dobbing:* The 'blood–brain barrier' becomes a nonsense with glucose and fructose. There can be very little physical difference between these two molecules, and yet one enters very rapidly and the other comparatively slowly. The explanation, if that's not too strong a term, surely is that the brain has a mechanism for dealing with glucose and deriving energy from it, which it doesn't have for fructose.

*Bovet:* Pharmacologically speaking I am not so sceptical about the blood–brain barrier. The concept is complicated and is not only based on the fate of injected dyes. Curare for example does not act on the brain unless it is directly injected into the ventricle. Then it acts very rapidly at cholinergic endings. There are also differences for serotonin and adrenaline.

*von Muralt:* How much of the total surface between the blood and the brain is made up of astrocytes?

*Menkes:* I understand that it consists almost entirely of astrocytes. I was brought up on Dr Dobbing's review (1961) and also feel that the word 'barrier' is inappropriate; perhaps one should use 'border'.

*Dobbing:* 'Blood–brain relationship' is quite a good term, because it implies function rather than obstruction, for a given substance.

# References


BRIGHTMAN, M. W. (1967) *Anat. Rec.* **157**, 219

DOBBING, J. (1961) *Physiol. Rev.* **41**, 130-188

GREENBERG, S. M., CALBERT, C. E., SAVAGE, E. E. and DEUEL, H. J. (1950) *J. Nutr.* **41**, 473-486

HOELZL, J. and FRANCK, H. P. (1969) *Abstracts 2nd International Meeting, International Society for Neurochemistry*, pp. 219-220, ed. R. Paoletti, R. Fumagalli and C. Galli. Tamburini Editore, Milan

LAJTHA, A., BERL, S. and WAELSCH, H. (1959) *J. Neurochem.* **3**, 322-332

LYMAN, R. L. (1968) In *Progress in the Chemistry of Fats and Other Lipids*, vol. 9, part 2, p. 193, ed. R. T. Holman. Pergamon Press, Oxford

PETERS, A., PALAY, S. L. and WEBSTER, H. DE F. (1970) *The Fine Structure of the Nervous System.* Harper and Row, New York

SCHUBERTH, J., SPARF, B. and SUNDWALL, A. (1969) *J. Neurochem.* **16**, 695-700

SCHWERIN, P., BESSMAN, S. P. and WAELSCH, H. (1950) *J. Biol. Chem.* **184**, 37-44

SINCLAIR, H. M. (1956) *Lancet* **1**, 381-383

SINCLAIR, H. M. (1958) *Proc. Nutr. Soc.* **17**, 28-37

# Biosynthesis of the myelin sheath

A. N. DAVISON*

*Department of Biochemistry, Charing Cross Hospital Medical School, London*

After the early embryogenesis of the mammalian nervous system and cellular multiplication, the growth of nerve cells and the deposition of myelin become of special importance, the latter accounting for much of the increase in dry weight during the late stages of development. Failure to form myelin (amyelination), faults in its structure (dysmyelination), or demyelination results in serious neurological disease, for the sheath provides an essential insulation for the propagation of nerve impulses along the axon. Apart from these clear-cut pathological effects, reduced deposition of myelin may serve as a permanent and useful indication of earlier stress to the brain during a vulnerable period of brain development (Davison and Dobbing 1966; Dobbing 1971). The detrimental effects of malnutrition and of amino acid or hormonal imbalance on the development of higher mental function are well established and in all these conditions some degree of amyelination has been demonstrated. Although it is likely that partial failure to synthesize other essential brain structures (e.g. nerve terminals) occurs at the same time, it remains possible that myelin may itself be associated in some way with the development of higher mental activity.

In man, myelin is most actively synthesized during the perinatal period and in the adult myelination is comparatively slow with relative metabolic stability of some components. It is therefore critical that the correct molecules are assembled into the membrane at the time of its most active synthesis. Of special interest in this respect is the finding of changes in the fatty acid esters of myelin in multiple sclerosis and the presence of phytanic acid in Refsum's syndrome. Deficits of sphingolipid long-chain fatty acids are found in the nervous system of mutant mice with neurological lesions, a subject to be

* *Present address:* Department of Neurochemistry, Institute of Neurology, Queen Square, London.

discussed by Dr Baumann (see pp. 91-100). Of even more general importance is the possibility that undernutrition and deficiencies in essential fatty acids may similarly lead to permanent molecular errors in brain membrane composition.

## THE MYELIN SHEATH

Myelin is an easily obtainable brain membrane and is therefore particularly valuable for study. Microscopic examination shows that the multi-lamellae of the myelin sheath are the most abundant membranes of the adult nervous system and are concentrated in the white matter and myelinated peripheral nerve tracts. This mass of lipid-rich myelin largely accounts for the marked difference in composition between the grey and white matter and between immature and adult brain. Such comparisons show that cholesterol, sphingolipids and certain phospholipids are concentrated in the myelin-rich areas of the nervous system. These complex lipids contain elongated chain structures such as sphingosine and the long-chain fatty acids of phospholipids and galactolipids. The presence of such extended molecules has led to the speculation that they would allow sufficient interaction to account for the high degree of metabolic stability associated with myelin (Vandenheuvel 1965; O'Brien 1967). Several different methods for the isolation of myelin by differential centrifugation and gradient density centrifugation have led to the availability of the membrane in relatively pure form (e.g. Autilio, Norton and Terry 1964; Cuzner, Davison and Gregson 1965; Woehneldt and Mandel 1970). In a typical separation, a brain mitochondrial pellet is layered over 0.66 M-sucrose solution and on centrifuging, a crude myelin preparation is isolated. The fraction floating at the interface contains myelin vesicles with trapped axoplasm and some microsomal contaminants. The axoplasm is released by suspending the crude myelin in ice-cold water and thus subjecting it to osmotic shock; the preparation is slowly centrifuged so that myelin sediments as a clear white pellet and microsomal and soluble contaminants remain in the supernatant. The procedure is repeated several times. There are disadvantages in using such an isolation procedure: (1) myelin is lost at each separation step; (2) repeated washing may remove loosely bound myelin components; and (3) some myelin components (e.g. basic protein and triphosphoinositide) may be degraded during centrifugation.

Analysis of separated myelin confirms the lipid composition of myelin as predicted by indirect means and shows that up to about 30% of the dry weight is protein. Besides proteolipid protein soluble in chloroform-methanol, a basic encephalitogenic protein and a third minor protein (Wolfgram 1966) seem to be present in central nervous system myelin, although Mehl (1971) has evidence to suggest that the last-mentioned protein is a contaminant of myelin. Small amounts of ganglioside (mainly $G_{M1}$) are present in mature myelin, but probably the most characteristic lipid component is cerebroside and its 3-sulphate ester (sulphatide). Phosphatidalethanolamine (ethanolamine plasmalogen) is the most abundant phospholipid; of the others, polyphosphoinositide is of special interest. Purified myelin has relatively little enzymic activity, but aminopeptidase and cathepsins present in myelin fractions may have an important physiological function. In contrast, the enzyme 2′:3′-cyclic nucleotide 3′-phosphohydrolase is concentrated in myelin and is a useful enzyme marker for myelin.

## CHANGES IN BRAIN LIPID COMPOSITION DURING DEVELOPMENT

During myelination the lipid content of both brain and nerve increases substantially. In the brain of the 6-day-old rat, before myelin has appeared, gangliosides, phosphatidylcholine, phosphatidylethanolamine and cholesterol are present in relatively high concentration. The phosphoglyceride fatty acids are predominantly saturated (for example, palmitic acid, 16:0, accounts for 55% of the lecithin fatty acid and stearic acid, 18:0, for 45% of the sphingomyelin fatty acid in the human; see Table 1). Immediately before myelination

TABLE 1

Unsubstituted fatty acid content of sphingomyelin from human myelin

| *Fatty acid* | *Percentage of total fatty acids* | |
| --- | --- | --- |
| | *10 months* | *35 years* |
| 16:0 | 9.0 | 5.4 |
| 18:0 | 62.8 | 33.6 |
| 18:1 | 2.3 | 0.4 |
| 24:1 | 10.0 | 40.0 |

Data after O'Brien and Sampson (1965). The most prominent fatty acid changes are recorded.

commences (at 10-12 days in the rat brain) the concentrations of sphingomyelin, triphosphoinositide, phosphatidic acid, ethanolamine plasmalogen, galactosyl diglyceride and sulphatide are less than 10% of those found in adult brain. Some sterol precursors (e.g. 24-dehydrocholesterol) are transiently incorporated into the myelin. Lipids tentatively identified as cholesterol esters and a sphingolipid (not cerebroside) accumulate in human premyelinating glial cells (Mickel and Gilles 1970). The cholesterol esters appear to be associated with the early myelin sheath (Adams and Davison 1959) but this phase of Marchi-positive sheaths is short-lived, for cholesterol esters are not normally present in adult myelin. It has previously been suggested that these cholesterol esters are possibly derived from the liver and incorporated into the brain via the plasma. However, the fatty acid spectrum of cholesterol esters of the developing chick brain is not identical with that of liver (Davison 1970). In the 21-day-old chick embryo, in brain, spinal cord and liver, the 16:0 cholesterol ester forms 16.5, 30.0 and 6.9% of the total sterol fatty acid ester. In the liver the most plentiful cholesterol fatty acid ester is 18:1, accounting for 62% of the total fatty acids, compared to 49.3% and 34.0% in brain and spinal cord of the chick. This suggests that cholesterol esters are synthesized within the brain. It could be, therefore, that cholesterol esters serve in some way as an intermediary in the intracellular transport of fatty acids at a time when lipogenesis is maximal, especially as cholesterol esterase activity correlates with the cholesterol ester concentration. Although Eto and Suzuki (1971) have been unable to find lecithin: cholesterol acyltransferase activity in young adult rat brain, it may be present in human foetal or infant nervous tissue. In their study they found an active cholesterol-esterifying enzyme, namely fatty acid: cholesterol acyltransferase. The enzyme catalysed the incorporation of [1-$^{14}$C]oleate into cholesterol esters with an activity of 40 μg of cholesterol esterified/hour per g young adult brain. Nearly half the activity was present in the crude mitochondrial fraction and none in purified myelin. The transferase in new-born rat brain was about 20% as active as in the adult. Two different cholesterol esterases were detected in the developing brain with activity which could be related to myelination. An esterase with a pH optimum of 6.6 was localized partially in the myelin and mainly in microsomes. In the chick sciatic nerve the cholesterol esterase activity is maximal for the first day after birth (Mezei, Newburgh and Hattori 1971). As myelin rings appear there is a steady increase in the amount of these lipids. Cholesterol, present early in relatively high concentration, increases less markedly in the rat brain during the period 12 to 330 days after birth. Cerebroside, but not sulphatide, is virtually absent from the brain until myelination commences, and then the initial rate of cerebroside accumulation is lower than that for other myelin lipids.

The overall picture, but not the timing, of such changes in lipid content of the developing central nervous system, is similar in all species so far examined. The same is true for specific areas of the nervous system. In the developing human peripheral nervous system, myelination is seen in the sciatic nerve at about 18 weeks menstrual age but traces of cerebroside only appear at about 20 weeks. The adult ratio of cerebroside is seen at not later than 32 weeks menstrual age (Table 2). During development there is a decrease in the proportion of phospholipid; in particular the lecithin content falls.

TABLE 2

Sciatic nerve lipids during development in man

| | *Menstrual age (weeks)* | | | *Adult* |
|---|---|---|---|---|
| | *14.8–17.7* | *20.6* | *24* | |
| Cholesterol (μmol/g wet wt.) | 7.68 ± 1.64 | 9.5 | 13.7 | 26.5 |
| Ratio of cholesterol (100): phospholipid : cerebroside | 100:138:0 | 100:142:4 | 100:110:12 | 100:124:30 |

(Unpublished data, A. N. Davison, S. Duckett and J. M. Oxberry.)

EARLY MYELIN

During the early stages of myelination, electron microscopy shows that the myelin lamellae are loosely wound around the axon (Caley and Maxwell 1968; Bass, Netsky and Young 1969; Peters and Vaughn 1970). At that time, 10-25 days postnatally in the rat brain, crude myelin isolated by centrifugation is deficient in cerebroside and basic protein (Cuzner and Davison 1968; Banik and Davison 1969; Agrawal *et al.* 1970; Einstein, Dalal and Csejkey 1970*a*, *b*; Dalal and Einstein 1969). It proved possible to separate this 'early' myelin into two fractions (see Norton 1971), one with a composition close to adult myelin and a second 'myelin-like' fraction which has a composition close to that of plasma membranes although the fraction contained the marker enzyme 2′:3′-cyclic nucleotide 3′-phosphohydrolase. Thus like plasma membranes and cytomembranes, the phospholipid fatty acids of the myelin-like fraction have shorter chains and are more saturated than those of mature myelin (Table 3). The myelin-like fraction contained relatively little cerebroside and had a higher phospholipid concentration. The yield of myelin-like material was greatest in the initial stages of the deposition of myelin and was relatively less in the mature brain.

Using [$^{14}$C]acetate for labelling lipids and [$^{14}$C]leucine for incorporation into proteins, we have not found any evidence of a precursor–product relationship (Agrawal *et al.* 1970). For this reason it was suggested that the myelin-like fraction is the loose myelin first formed directly in continuity with, and similar in composition to, the glial plasma membrane. According to this hypothesis,

TABLE 3

Phosphoglyceride fatty acids of myelin and microsomes of developing and adult rat brain

| Fatty acid | *Purified myelin* | | *'Myelin-like' fraction* | | *Microsomes* | |
|---|---|---|---|---|---|---|
| | *15 days* | *Adult* | *15 days* | *Adult* | *15 days* | *Adult* |
| 16:0 | 28.2 | 15.4 | 32.7 | 32.4 | 37.7 | 30.4 |
| 18:0 | 19.3 | 26.6 | 19.7 | 26.6 | 23 | 21.6 |
| 18:1 | 21.3 | 35.5 | 14.1 | 26.6 | 18.1 | 22.5 |
| 18:2 | 5.6 | 1.3 | 5.5 | — | 1.7 | 1.3 |
| 20:4 | 11.3 | 5.9 | 11.7 | 7.0 | 13.4 | 10.0 |

The fatty acids are expressed as a percentage of total fatty acids (Banik and Davison 1969).

compact mature myelin is formed at a later stage close to the axon and not in the glial cell body. New lamellae are synthesized with cerebroside as an important component; the basic protein may serve to cement together the membranes at the major dense line. Small quantities of antibody to basic protein can inhibit myelination in tissue culture, which indicates the importance of the protein in the synthesis of compact myelin. It is not known how this synthesis occurs nor is there any information about the site of formation of the basic protein. It has been suggested that the protein may be synthesized in the neuron and that the basic protein travelling down the axon could initiate myelination. There is evidence that cerebroside and sulphatide are synthesized in the endoplasmic reticulum and that at least the sulphatide galactolipid is transferred to newly forming myelin as a lipoprotein complex. Synthesis of the myelin unit would thus be confined to the membrane itself. Studies by Dobiasova and Radin (1968) on the incorporation of lipid *in vitro* into partially delipidated myelin preparations support the idea of self-assembly processes in the biogenesis of myelin.

## ABNORMALITIES OF MYELIN FORMATION

Schjeide, Lin and de Vellis (1968) X-irradiated the heads of 2-day-old rats with 700 R and found a reduction in yield of myelin up to 178 days after exposure. The myelin differed from normal myelin only in the proportion of total long-chain fatty acids; the 24:1 and 26:1 acids were lower than in controls. This points to the sensitivity of the chain-elongation system which seems to be affected in certain of the neurological mutants. In these diseases it appears that there may be an accumulation of the 'myelin-like' fraction. For example, in the myelin synthesis-deficient mouse described by Meier and McPike (1970) there may be a block in development leading to an accumulation of the myelin-like fraction. Thus the 'myelin' isolated from this condition is deficient in cerebroside, although it is not known whether or not the basic protein is also absent. Studies on Jimpy and Quaking mouse brain will be reviewed by Dr Baumann (pp. 91-100), and here too there may be an accumulation of the myelin-like material containing little galactolipid and less basic protein than normal myelin. In preliminary studies we have found no evidence of the myelin-like fraction in normal white matter in multiple sclerosis, but it would be interesting to look for the membrane in plaque areas.

## MYELIN METABOLISM

Previous experiments in which [4-$^{14}$C]cholesterol and various precursors were injected into developing animals led to the finding of the apparent persistence of radioactivity in the myelin lipids for remarkably extended periods. This work was interpreted as indicating the relative metabolic stability of myelin in comparison to other parts of the body. Consistent with this hypothesis is the demonstration that synthesis of fatty acids in the adult brain is slower than in developing brain and that labelled fatty acid is incorporated to a lesser extent into myelin than into any other subcellular fraction. The myelin proteolipid protein also appears to be metabolically relatively stable, with a half-life of about 100 days. However, at least part of the myelin sheath undergoes rapid exchange; for example, there is fast turnover of triphosphoinositide and also the basic encephalitogenic protein, possibly localized in the intraperiod line. Moreover, Smith and Eng (1965) have shown that certain phospholipids, such as lecithin, are metabolized more quickly than the sterols and galactolipids. Other evidence has made it necessary to reconsider the interpretation of radioactive experiments on brain lipids. Firstly, after injection of [$^{14}$C]acetate into young animals, radioactive cholesterol persisted not only in myelin but also unexpectedly in mitochondrial sterol, despite the fact that the mitochondrial membrane is known to undergo dynamic metabolism. Secondly, Rawlins and co-workers (1969) have found convincing radioautographic evidence for the re-utilization of [$^{14}$C]cholesterol in the sciatic nerve long after administration of the labelled sterol. These experiments suggested that recycling occurred between sterols in the Schwann cell cytoplasm and myelin. Thirdly, it has always been difficult to explain the degree of incorporation of isotopes into myelin lipid of the adult brain if, as was postulated, the lipids were metabolically stable. Further work has helped to explain these findings.

EXCHANGE OF MYELIN LIPID

If anti-cholesterolaemic drugs are injected into developing rats, large amounts of sterol precursors accumulate in the brain and myelin. When drugs such as AY9944 were injected together with [$^{14}$C]acetate into 4-day-old rats, 7-dehydrocholesterol in myelin was extensively labelled 17 days after injection; as the precursor disappeared, an equivalent of radioactive cholesterol was subsequently found in the myelin. This suggests a localized conversion of 7-dehydrocholesterol to the more saturated sterol. However, the 7-dehydrocholesterol reductase responsible for the conversion is present in brain microsomes and not in purified myelin (Banik and Davison 1971). These observations therefore suggest that in the developing rat brain 7-dehydrocholesterol can migrate from the myelin and become reduced by microsomal reductase and that the resultant cholesterol molecules can be re-incorporated into myelin. Myelin labelled with $^{14}$C-labelled lipid or with dehydrocholesterol was therefore incubated at 37°C for 30 minutes with a homogenate of whole rat brain or with isolated microsomes. After incubation, myelin and microsomes were re-isolated. Contamination was checked for by measurement of $^{14}$C-labelled protein and 2′:3′-cyclic nucleotide 3′-phosphohydrolase in the separate fractions. Labelled cholesterol and 7-dehydrocholesterol were found to undergo up to 10% exchange between myelin and microsomes. Phospholipid and cerebroside were also exchanged from one membrane to another.

Similar results were obtained when labelled microsomes were incubated with unlabelled myelin. Graham and Green (1967) have already demonstrated a 57% exchange of cholesterol from adult myelin with plasma lipoproteins after incubation at 37°C for 24 hours. It is also well established that cholesterol of erythrocyte stroma undergoes ready exchange with plasma sterols. In our experiments, exchange with whole-brain suspensions was faster than in myelin plus isolated microsomes. It has been demonstrated that a heat-labile supernatant factor, identified as a lipoprotein carrier (Wirtz and Zilversmit 1968; McMurray and Dawson 1969; Beattie 1969), is required for the exchange *in vitro* of phospholipid molecules between rat liver mitochondria and microsomes (Jungalwala and Dawson 1970). A similar protein carrier might be important in the exchange of cerebral lipid.

Dr M. Spohn has extended this work to adult rats. In her studies, [$^{14}$C]-acetate was injected into 16-day-old animals and the relative specific activities of cholesterol in cerebral subcellular fractions were measured. Ten minutes and 6 and 7 months after injection there was uniform specific activity of cholesterol in all fractions. In another series of experiments, adult rats were given intravenous injections of [4-$^{14}$C]cholesterol and killed at intervals. By 10 days afterwards the specific activity of cholesterol in myelin had increased to that of the sterol in all other fractions, a completely unexpected finding if adult myelin were inert. Similar results have been obtained in adult rats after labelling of 7-dehydrocholesterol.

Jungalwala and Dawson (1971) have examined the incorporation of [$^{32}$P]-phosphate, [U-$^{14}$C]glycerol and [2-$^{14}$C]ethanolamine into microsomes and a highly purified myelin fraction of adult rat brain. Initially, the specific activity of microsomal phospholipids was higher than that of myelin but by 20 days after intracerebral injection the reduced specific activities were similar. Labelling persisted when 10-day-old rats had been injected; this supports the previous concept that two metabolic pools exist in myelin, one a rapidly exchanging pool and the other a more persistent and slowly turning over part which can be significantly labelled only in the developing animal. This recent work indicates that the pool of exchangeable myelin lipid is larger and more accessible than had been previously assumed.

Exchange of myelin lipid will also depend on the binding of lipid to myelin protein. Braun and Radin (1969) have demonstrated a special interaction of sulphatide, phosphatidylserine and phosphatidylinositol with proteolipid protein which may be compared to the weaker binding of non-ionic lipids (cholesterol and cerebrosides). It has also been shown that polyphosphoinositides and lecithin readily combine with the myelin basic protein (Palmer and Dawson 1969). These myelin components are all known to turn over rapidly and may therefore be combined in some form in the myelin sheath. Despite the ready exchange of lipid within the nervous system it appears to be difficult to modify the brain lipids by altering whole-brain metabolism. Thus Dobbing (1968) found no changes in brain lipids of severely starved rats, and Galli, White and Paoletti (1970) found only minor changes in brain fatty acids during chronic deficiency of essential polyunsaturated fatty acids.

Rathbone (1965) fed 9 to 10-week-old rats diets containing sunflower-seed oil (high in linoleic acid, 18:2) and coconut oil (low in 18:2 and high in short-chain fatty acids) for periods up to 34 weeks. Small changes were seen in the fatty acid composition of the brain as a result of the prolonged dietary regime. In myelin the proportion of linoleic acid increased from 0.9% to 1.3% in the animals fed with sunflower-seed oil and dropped to 0.4% in those given supplements of coconut oil. There were therefore no very marked changes in fatty composition, and it seems that endogenous fatty acid synthesis or re-utilization of previously formed long-chain molecules predominates in the adult brain.

CONCLUSIONS AND SUMMARY

Changes in the lipid composition of the developing nervous system have been correlated with the important process of myelination. It is postulated that the basic encephalitogenic protein and cerebroside are critical components in the formation of compact myelin. Failure to form either results in accumulation of a 'myelin-like' fraction similar to that found in developing brain. Previous ideas about the metabolic stability of myelin are being modified. It now seems that proteolipid protein remains an essential and more permanent structure into which lipid molecules may readily exchange. The basic protein may serve to cement together the lipoprotein myelin lamellae at the major dense line. Despite the flux between membrane lipids within the brain, the metabolism of sterols, fatty acids and many other lipids is slow, for the nervous system seems to conserve such molecules for re-utilization in membrane structures. Such a conclusion emphasizes the critical importance of normal development of the central nervous system, especially with regard to the synthesis of structural protein and the formation of complex lipid molecules.

## References

ADAMS, C. W. M. and DAVISON, A. N. (1959) *J. Neurochem.* **4**, 282-289

AGRAWAL, H. C., BANIK, N. L., BONE, A. H., DAVISON, A. N., MITCHELL, R. F. and SPOHN, M. (1970) *Biochem. J.* **120**, 635-642

AUTILIO, L. A., NORTON, W. T. and TERRY, R. D. (1964) *J. Neurochem.* **11**, 17-27

BANIK, N. L. and DAVISON, A. N. (1969) *Biochem. J.* **115**, 1051-1062

BANIK, N. L. and DAVISON, A. N. (1971) *Biochem. J.* **122**, 751-758

BASS, N. H., NETSKY, M. G. and YOUNG, E. (1969) *Neurology* **19**, 405-414

BEATTIE, D. A. S. (1969) *J. Membrane Biol.* **1**, 383-401

BRAUN, P. E. and RADIN, N. S. (1969) *Biochemistry* **8**, 4310-4318

CALEY, D. W. and MAXWELL, D. S. (1968) *J. Comp. Neurol.* **133**, 45-70

CUZNER, M. L. and DAVISON, A. N. (1968) *Biochem. J.* **106**, 29-34

CUZNER, M. L., DAVISON, A. N. and GREGSON, N. A. (1965) *J. Neurochem.* **12**, 469-481

DALAL, K. B. and EINSTEIN, E. R. (1969) *Brain Res.* **16**, 441-451

DAVISON, A. N. (1970) In *Handbook of Neurochemistry*, vol. 3, pp. 547-560, ed. A. Lajtha. Plenum Press, New York

DAVISON, A. N. and DOBBING, J. (1966) *Br. Med. Bull.* **22**, 40-44

DOBBING, J. (1968) In *Malnutrition, Learning and Behaviour*, pp. 181-202, ed. N. S. Scrimshaw and J. E. Gordon. M.I.T. Press, Cambridge, Mass.

DOBBING, J. (1971) In *Chemistry and Brain Development*, pp. 399-412, ed. R. Paoletti and A. N. Davison. Plenum Press, New York

DOBIASOVA, M. and RADIN, N. S. (1968) *Lipids* **3**, 1

EINSTEIN, E. R., DALAL, K. B. and CSEJKEY, J. (1970*a*) *J. Neurol. Sci.* **11**, 109-121

EINSTEIN, E. R., DALAL, K. B. and CSEJKEY, J. (1970*b*) *Brain Res.* **18**, 35-49

ETO, Y. and SUZUKI, K. (1971) *Proc. 3rd International Meeting, International Society for Neurochemistry, Budapest*, p. 374

GALLI, C., WHITE, H. B., Jr and PAOLETTI, R. (1970) *J. Neurochem.* **17**, 347-355
GRAHAM, J. H. and GREEN, C. (1967) *Biochem. J.* **103**, 16C
JUNGALWALA, F. B. and DAWSON, R. M. C. (1970) *Biochem. J.* **117**, 481-490
JUNGALWALA, F. B. and DAWSON, R. M. C. (1971) *Biochem. J.* **123**, 683-693
MCMURRAY, W. C. and DAWSON, R. M. C. (1969) *Biochem. J.* **112**, 91-108
MEHL, E. (1971) *Proc. 3rd International Meeting, International Society for Neurochemistry, Budapest*, p. 414
MEIER, H. and MCPIKE, A. D. (1970) *Exp. Brain Res.* **10**, 512-525
MEZEI, C., NEWBURGH, R. W. and HATTORI, T. (1971) J. *Neurochem.* **18**, 463-468
MICKEL, H. S. and GILLES, F. H. (1970) *Brain* **93**, 337-346
NORTON, W. T. (1971) In *Chemistry and Brain Development*, pp. 327-337, ed. R. Paoletti and A. N. Davison. Plenum Press, New York
PETERS, A. and VAUGHN, J. E. (1970) In *Myelination*, pp. 3-79, ed. A. N. Davison and A. Peters. Thomas, Springfield, Ill.
PALMER, F. B. and DAWSON, R. M. C. (1969) *Biochem. J.* **111**, 637-646
O'BRIEN, J. S. (1967) *J. Theor. Biol.* **15**, 307-324.
O'BRIEN, J. S. and SAMPSON, E. L. (1965) *J. Lipid Res.* **6**, 545-551
RATHBONE, L. (1965) *Biochem. J.* **97**, 620-628
RAWLINS, F. A., HEDLEY-WHYTE, E. T., VILLEGAS, G. and UZMAN, B. G. (1969) *Abstracts 2nd International Meeting, International Society for Neurochemistry, Milan*, p. 334, ed. R. Paoletti, R. Fumagalli and C. Galli. Tamburini Editore, Milan
SCHJEIDE, O. A., LIN, R. I. and DE VELLIS, J. (1968) *Radiat. Res.* **33**, 107-128
SMITH, M. E. and ENG, L. F. (1965) *J. Am. Oil Chem. Soc.* **42**, 1013-1018
VANDENHEUVEL, F. A. (1965) *Ann. N.Y. Acad. Sci.* **122**, 57-76
WIRTZ, K. W. A. and ZILVERSMIT, P. B. (1968) *J. Biol. Chem.* **243**, 3596-3602
WOLFGRAM, F. (1966) *J. Neurochem.* **13**, 461-470
WOEHNELDT, T. V. and MANDEL, P. (1970) *FEBS Lett.* **9**, 209-212

# Discussion

*Chapman:* You suggested that from a mere inspection of molecular models it was fairly obvious that the mitochondrial membrane was less stable than the myelin membrane. Could you explain what you mean by stable in this situation?

*Davison:* I mean both metabolically stable *in vivo*, and physically stable in a physical-chemical sense. Thus, the closely packed myelin lamellae prevent easy exchange with cytoplasm and the parallel lipid chains, as in myelin, are stabilized by Van der Waals forces and similar interactions, as you described; whereas in the mitochondrial membrane, where the whole structure is more open, the fatty acid chains are shorter and have much less opportunity for these types of interactions to occur.

*Chapman:* If the mitochondrial membrane is essentially a lipid bilayer like the myelin membrane I can understand, in terms of the difference in saturation of the fatty acids, that a difference of water permeability can be expected. I can also envisage that it may be more difficult for some of the lipids of the myelin membrane to 'leave the structure'. I think 'stability' has to be defined rather carefully. Both myelin and mitochondrial membranes could be equally unstable if the appropriate enzymes were present.

*Davison:* One of the features of myelin is the absence of enzymes that would break it down.

*Chapman:* You found that there is an exchange of lipids from myelin. Is there an equal exchange of all the different lipid classes or is it primarily lecithin?

*Davison:* It seems that all classes of lipids exchange, including galactolipid, but cholesterol and lecithin exchange relatively rapidly.

*Mead:* Dr O'Brien was delighted when I told him that I had found fatty acids up to 36 carbons in length in the cerebrosides of myelin, because he has always talked about 'interdigitation'; he refers to a situation in which the chain of the fatty acid goes completely through the myelin membrane, and it can be estimated that if the chain were in the extended form this would be possible. He thinks of the long-chain fatty acids as a 'stitching'. This is stability in a different sense, perhaps. One would suspect that there would be no cleavage plane in such a membrane. However, freeze-etching experiments indicate that myelin cleaves very much as any other membrane and that apparently the fatty acid chains do not go through it. So is it possible that these long-chain fatty acids are concentrated in certain areas, separated by areas of concentration of the shorter-chain fatty acids where myelin has different properties, and that myelin is not at all homogeneous? In the freeze-etching experiments we may be looking at a part that is cleaved readily, rather than one in which the fatty acids pass through. Or is it possible that the fatty acid chains never pass through the membrane but are simply held together, by Van der Waals or other forces, throughout their length but not *through* the myelin membrane?

*Davison:* What proportion of these exceptional fatty acids do you find?

*Mead:* In the old human brain it is a significant proportion; fatty acids above $C_{26}$ are about 4% of the total fatty acids of cerebroside but as high as 25% of the total in ceramide and cerebroside sulphate.

*Davison:* That is not negligible. However, it seems that chain elongation goes on throughout development and that perhaps the increased proportion of long-chain fatty acid in myelin lipids may be correlated with greater metabolic stability of the adult myelin sheath. Where shorter fatty acid chains are present in developing myelin there will be more opportunity for exchange than in the adult. There is some justification for this idea, because it takes much longer to introduce 7-dehydrocholesterol into the adult rat myelin sheath, by giving anti-cholesterolaemic drugs, than it does when the drugs are given to young rats. On the question of homogeneity of myelin in relation to chain length and the $C_{36}$ acids, these very long chains could only be accommodated if they were bent round to fit in laterally rather than in a radial direction.

*Svennerholm:* Dr Mead kindly sent me his manuscript on the very long-chain fatty acids of brain cerebrosides. Since we (Svennerholm and Ställberg-Stenhagen 1968) had not been able to detect any fatty acid with a chain length longer than $C_{28}$, we decided to hydrolyse a large amount of cerebrosides and sulphatides from human brain and separate the fatty acids by the counter-current distribution technique. With this method no loss of very long-chain fatty acids occurs. We found no fatty acids with more than 28 carbon atoms; the $C_{28}$ acids constituted approximately 1% and were mainly mono-unsaturated. The main fatty acids were $C_{24}$ acids (55%). $C_{26}$ acids constituted 10% or a little more. The age changes described by Professor Davison agree with those found by us (Svennerholm and Ställberg-Stenhagen 1968) for human brains.

*Mead:* We found the very long-chain fatty acids by gas-liquid chromatography on very efficient capillary columns. You need something like 10 000 theoretical plates to see them as anything more than a slight change in the base-line.

*Svennerholm:* The counter-current technique in combination with mass spectrometry is a more reliable method for identifying a fatty acid.

*Mead:* Roger Kornberg (Kornberg and McConnell 1971), using an artificial lipid vesicle preparation, showed extremely rapid sideways movement of phospholipids, as well as a slow inner to outer movement in the vesicle. This would mean, if it can be applied to something like a natural membrane such as myelin, that the enzyme can remain in one position and the lipids can move sideways to it. This might also explain the high mobility of phospholipids within the myelin membrane, provided there is some enzyme close by, perhaps within the myelin–protein structure itself.

*Davison:* I would say that lecithin in the myelin must be in equilibrium with lecithin in the cytoplasm, and that the catabolic enzymes are in the cytoplasm, not in the myelin. The major hydrolytic enzymes in myelin are the protein-degrading enzyme, neutral cathepsin, and an aminopeptidase.

*Mead:* Myelin has a good sialidase also.

*Chapman:* How does the lipid leave the myelin membrane? Does it leave it as a lipoprotein, or does it leave it as lipid?

*Davison:* All these lipid exchanges have been shown, as far as I know, to require a lipoprotein carrier or intermediate. During the next few years we shall probably hear much more about the nature and specificity of this carrier which allows movement of the lipid from one membrane to another.

*Chapman:* You mentioned that there is a time sequence of lipids being inserted into the membranes. Do you envisage that the membranes are formed and particular lipids such as the cerebrosides are then incorporated into the membrane at a later stage of brain development?

*Davison:* We have studied the turnover of the early, loose myelin, and have found that the turnover rates for both lipids and proteins were similar to those of the compact myelin. If this membrane is synthesized in the glial cell body, transferred to the glial plasma membrane and then progresses round the axon, we would have expected to find transference of radioactivity from early to compact myelin. There is no evidence of a precursor–product relationship between the hypothetical loose (myelin-like) membrane and the inner compact myelin. We are hoping to show that the first step in myelination consists of the formation of loose winding of the glial plasma membrane, followed by synthesis of compact myelin close to the axon. The key factors for formation of compact myelin are basic protein, possibly cementing together the lipoprotein membrane units, and cerebroside, whose important role in the formation of the myelin membrane has not been delineated.

*Chapman:* So when the cerebroside content increases with age, is that due to the fact that you are creating more membrane containing cerebroside? It is not that you already have existing membranes into which cerebrosides are inserted?

*Davison:* Our work supports the first hypothesis, that completely new membrane is synthesized close to the axon containing increasing proportions of galactocerebroside.

*von Muralt:* The myelin sheaths of peripheral nerve have clefts—the so-called clefts of Schmidt-Lantermann—which might facilitate the exchange of lipids.

*Chapman:* There's no doubt that diffusion of lipid molecules along a phospholipid bilayer can take place. On the other hand, when cholesterol is present in the membrane, this must limit to some extent the possibility of diffusion of phospholipid occurring. Of course if the cholesterol moves out from the membrane the diffusion rate could increase.

*Davison:* Diffusion within myelin must be slower than it is in other biological membranes. Our earlier idea was that myelin was very stable, with a half-life of about 100 days. We now think that exchange occurs in the adult, so that one lipid molecule might have a half-life of about a month.

*Ansell:* On the subject of the so-called metabolic stability in myelin, the very elegant early experiments of Professor Davison and his colleagues certainly convinced us that myelin was stable and we did experiments which showed, for example, that the optic chiasma also behaved in this metabolically stable way (Ansell and Spanner 1961). It was only when we and others started to do intracerebral injections that we saw intensive labelling of myelin (Ansell and Spanner 1967; Horrocks 1969). This method uses a pulse of label as opposed to a continuous supply of labelled material to the brain. As far as I know, no one has ever really compared these two types of injections in the same series of animals.

If myelin becomes labelled but doesn't contain the enzymic equipment to label its own phospholipids, it must be receiving these phospholipids (and other lipids) from somewhere else. Recent experiments of Dawson and Jungalwala (1971) suggest that the primary source of these materials is the endoplasmic reticulum, which they isolate as a microsomal fraction. But as far as I know, and the same point is made by Dawson and Jungalwala (1971), the transfer of phospholipids synthesized in the microsomal fraction to myelin *in vitro* has not been demonstrated, whereas it is possible for phospholipids to be transferred from liver microsomes to mitochondrial membranes (McMurray and Dawson 1969). This seems to me to be a crucial point. How does the transfer of phospholipid from the endoplasmic reticulum occur and which endoplasmic reticulum is involved? Is it the endoplasmic reticulum of the glial cell or some other cell?

*Davison:* We know that a protein is involved in the transport of sulphatide to myelin. In our experiments with 7-dehydrocholesterol we showed enhanced exchange of sterol only when whole homogenate was used, but Dr Dawson's results were with phospholipids and our experience agrees with his when using isolated microsomes and myelin.

*Herschkowitz:* You showed that an age-dependent increase in cerebroside takes place in myelin fractions. Could you show that for other subcellular fractions too, or was that unique to the myelin fractions?

*Davison:* No; changes in cerebroside, phospholipid and ganglioside concentrations are largely restricted to myelin, and not found in mitochondria or endoplasmic reticulum.

*Menkes:* Did you analyse your myelin-like material for fatty acid composition? What was the fatty acid composition of the cerebrosides?

*Davison:* There is virtually no cerebroside in the myelin-like material—only 2%, which wasn't enough to analyse. We looked at phosphoglyceride fatty acids; during development relatively short-chain fatty acids predominate and in the myelin-like fraction the fatty acid spectrum is similar to that of other plasma membranes.

*Menkes:* Like Dr Mead, I believe fatty acid metabolism in myelin is not homogeneous. Evidence in support of this comes from a patient with diffuse sclerosis. Myelin derived from this patient has a reduced amount of cerebroside, plasmalogens and phosphatidylethanolamine. The loss of cerebrosides is almost exclusively due to the reduction of cerebrosides containing long-chain fatty acids. This abnormality was not due to contamination of myelin by white matter, because it was less marked in the surrounding white matter than in purified myelin. I think that with demyelination there is a preferential loss of material containing long-chain fatty acids which anatomically may be located in the outer layers of the myelin (Eviatar and Menkes 1972).

*Davison:* That is very interesting, because it raises one of the very practical questions posed in this symposium, of whether or not chain elongation is critical for normal, healthy brain membranes. Relevant to this basic theme is Dr Baumann's work on chain elongation in relation to the inborn errors of metabolism.

*Svennerholm:* Dr Menkes spoke about diffuse sclerosis. We have isolated myelin from brains with multiple sclerosis (Alling, Vanier and Svennerholm 1971). In the purified myelin we found no change in the composition of cerebrosides and sulphatides.

*Crawford:* One thing disturbs me about this kind of technique: if you isolate myelin and develop a very sophisticated technique for purifying it, by definition you have isolated purified myelin which from a diseased person and a healthy person, again by definition, will be closely similar. The analogy is with kwashiorkor: if you isolate cytochrome *c* from children who have died from kwashiorkor and from normal children you find no difference in the amino acid composition or possibly the sequence of amino acids. This point tends to be overlooked by those who analyse various fractions after very detailed purifications in disease states.

*Davison:* That criticism also applies to studies of neurological diseases in which only small proportions of myelin can be isolated. It is not surprising to find, say, only 2% of apparently normal myelin in one of these very severe diseases. Purified myelin must be regarded as an operational term; such procedures with repeated washing and centrifugation may not be truly representative of the myelin *in vivo* and the abnormal myelin may be lost in the supernatant. However, if the yields of myelin in a diseased and a non-diseased individual are comparable, any chemical differences detected are of more significance.

*Baumann:* What are the different percentages of the myelin-like fraction and of adult myelin at the very early stages of myelin development?

*Davison:* In the rat brain at 10 days, about 70 or 75% of myelin that one isolates by floating down, as we described, would be 'myelin-like' material. In the 15-day-old rat brain, something like 40% would be. In the adult about 5% is myelin-like; it stays constant relative to the increase in the purified myelin, so the absolute amount is the same, but the proportion between the two differs. That's another reason why I think there is no direct precursor–product relationship between the two.

*Baumann:* Did you look at the ganglioside pattern? Suzuki, Poduslo and Norton (1967) have shown that it evolves with age.

*Davison:* The ganglioside pattern or lipid *N*-acetylneuraminic acid content of the myelin-like fraction was higher than that of purified myelin. This high content of *N*-acetylneuraminic acid present in the myelin-like fraction may in some way be related to a galactolipid-rich cell coat thought to be present in the glial cell plasma membrane (Lehninger 1968). As Suzuki showed, the actual proportion of different gangliosides (a useful marker of change of lipid composition) does alter systematically in myelin with age.

*Winick:* There is an analogy between myelination and DNA synthesis, in that both are used as markers for growth. One reason is their stability, allowing one to measure quantitatively the addition of either myelin or DNA in a developing brain. With DNA we find that those *qualitative* changes that occur for example with malnutrition in the developing brain, one area being differently affected from another, are in fact probably quantitative rather than qualitative changes, due to differing rates of DNA synthesis at the time of malnutrition. I wonder if the same is true for myelination? Is there evidence that with malnutrition the quantity of *normal* myelin is altered in particular areas of the brain, as a result of an effect on the rate of myelination in those areas, or is this a qualitative change as well, in the *kind* of myelin being deposited, secondary to alterations in nutrition?

*Davison:* In terms of the proportions of lipids there's no evidence that the actual quality of the myelin alters in malnutrition. We have looked in some diseases for the presence of the 'myelin-like' fraction, which might be evidence of more primitive myelin, but have not found it. There are some inborn errors of metabolism where this does occur, such as the Jimpy mouse, and there are undoubtedly some human diseases where amyelination occurs and where abnormal types of myelin are produced. Metachromatic leucodystrophy, where the ratio of sulphatide to cerebroside alters, is another example. In Krabbe's disease the reverse occurs—there is possibly a decrease in sulphatide concentration. I don't think there are other examples, *due* to malnutrition; just the quantity of myelin produced is less.

*Winick:* So it's fair to say at the present time that with the models of malnutrition studied, there is a quantitative decrease in the amount of myelin, and where this occurs depends on the rate of myelination of the particular area?

*Davison:* Yes, and since myelination occurs at maximal rate in man during the perinatal period, if stress continues for more than a few months it would have a permanent effect: this is the thesis being investigated.

*Dobbing:* It's fair to say that investigations of the long-term effects of growth restriction at this time have been very crudely tackled and it needs good lipid neurochemists to look into it. For example, the work as far as I know is practically all concerned with the analysis of whole-brain lipid extracts. I don't think anyone has looked specifically at 'pure myelin' in adults previously undernourished during the perinatal period. Would you say that the lipid composition of the other brain membranes was so different from myelin that all we may be showing in a whole-brain lipid extract of a previously malnourished animal is that this brain is deficient in membrane?

*Davison:* Yes, definitely. I began my paper with the point that it is convenient to look at myelin but there are other, perhaps more critical parts of the nervous system structure which are affected at the same time, and I quite agree with you.

*Dobbing:* A permanent effect on mitochondria, in fact, might be functionally more significant for the things we are ultimately concerned with than a few laminae less on the myelin sheath?

*Davison:* Multiplication of organelles such as mitochondria can apparently occur quite readily. I would have thought that this is not true for synaptic connections where a permanent reduction in their number may present an even more serious problem, and if true, could be an explanation of effects on the physiological functions of the brain. Since gangliosides are localized in neurons and their synapses, ganglioside concentrations have been examined in undernutrition (Bass 1971) and in hypothyroidism, and slight alterations found (Balázs *et al.* 1969), but gangliosides are not specific markers of synaptic endings. It would be valuable to study brains from undernourished subjects by subcellular fractionation with biochemical analysis, for example estimation of the protein distribution in different fractions. Unfortunately most such studies reported in the literature have been on deep-frozen brain which from a cytological point of view has been maltreated. It would be best, if such material becomes available, to use fresh brain, kept at 0°C. In my opinion, even 24 hours after death a lot of useful work could be done.

## References


ALLING, C., VANIER, M. T. and SVENNERHOLM, L. (1971) *Brain Res.* **35**, 325

ANSELL, G. B. and SPANNER, S. (1961) *Biochem. J.* **79**, 176-184

ANSELL, G. B. and SPANNER, S. (1967) *J. Neurochem.* **14**, 873-885

BALÁZS, R., BROOKSBANK, B. W. L., DAVISON, A. N., EAYRS, J. T. and WILSON, D. A. (1969) *Brain Res.* **15**, 219-232

BASS, N. H. (1971) In *Chemistry and Brain Development*, pp. 413-424, ed. R. Paoletti and A. N. Davison. Plenum Press, New York

DAWSON, R. M. C. and JUNGALWALA, F. B. (1971) *Biochem. J.* **123**, 683-693

EVIATAR, L. and MENKES, J. H. (1972 )In preparation

HORROCKS, L. A. (1969) *J. Neurochem.* **16**, 13-18

KORNBERG, R. D. and MCCONNELL, H. M. (1971) *Biochemistry* **10**, 1111-1120

LEHNINGER, A. L. (1968) *Proc. Natl. Acad. Sci. U.S.A.* **60**, 1069-1080

MCMURRAY, W. C. and DAWSON, R. M. C. (1969) *Biochem. J.* **112**, 91-108

SUZUKI, K., PODUSLO, S. E. and NORTON, W. T. (1967) *Biochim. Biophys. Acta* **144**, 375-381

SVENNERHOLM, L. and STÄLLBERG-STENHAGEN, S. (1968) *J. Lipid Res.* **9**, 215-225

# Genetic disorders of myelination

N. A. BAUMANN, J. M. BOURRE, C. JACQUE and S. POLLET

*Laboratoire de Neurochimie, Hôpital de la Salpêtrière, Paris*

Myelination is an important part of brain development. Its timing is evidently specified in the genetic code, since it always occurs at a particular time in a given species. At this critical period, numerous factors interact so that the process, which has this once-and-for-all opportunity, develops normally. If the right conditions are not present, myelination is impaired (Dobbing 1970). Thus, undernutrition can lead to a reduction in the extent of myelination, which nevertheless still occurs at its normal time. To understand this effect, information is required on the sequential histological events leading to myelination, their biochemical correlates, and also the metabolic and hormonal influences on this process and its genetic control.

Animal experiments provide the only available method of experimental investigation, and in mice, where myelination occurs after birth, it is possible to follow its development. In addition, there are two myelin-deficient mutants in mice (Sidman, Dickie and Appel 1964), presumably blocked at specific steps of myelination. These mutants enable morphological and biochemical investigations to be made under strictly controlled conditions of genetic background, rearing, housing and food. The two myelin-deficient mutant mice, Quaking and Jimpy, manifest symptoms at the time of myelination, around the 10th or 12th day after birth. Although they have the same apparent phenotype, characterized by the abnormal gait, tremor and seizures, they have different genotypes. The Quaking mutation is an autosomal recessive; the Jimpy mutation is an X-linked recessive mutation. This implies that genes located on at least two chromosomes are involved in the formation of myelin.

We have been working for several years on the Quaking mutation. Among the myelin-deficient mutants, Quaking mice are the only ones with a normal lifespan; they live for at least a year. It is therefore probable that the genetic defect primarily involves the myelin membrane.

Myelination is a sequential event, and a correlation between histological and biochemical data should be fruitful for understanding this process. Berger (1970, 1971) at La Salpêtrière has made histological and ultrastructural studies in correlation with our work. The axonal diameter, which may play a role in initiating and controlling the degree of myelination (Friede and Samorajski 1967), appears to be identical in Quaking and normal mice. Glial cells multiply more than normally before the onset of myelination; some are multivesiculated. Oligodendroglial cells lie in rows among myelinating fibres, constituting a myelinating glia, but the processes they extend around the axons contain dense round lipid inclusions and vacuoles, and numerous cytoplasmic loops. The oligodendrocytes of Quaking mice are therefore qualitatively abnormal; consequently, the number of myelin lamellae is considerably reduced and their compaction does not occur. Wisniewski and Morrell (1971) have also described this arrest in the growth and maturation of myelin and its possible relationship to oligodendrocyte metabolism. In Jimpy mice (Farkas *et al.* 1970), the multiplication of glial cells is deficient and there is a lack of myelinating glia, indicating a block at an earlier step in the sequential events leading to myelin development.

In attempting to establish the metabolic block in the Quaking mutant, we began by studying the lipid components of the brain in Quaking mice compared to normal control littermates. We found a considerable decrease in myelin lipids, including plasmalogens, cholesterol, cerebrosides and proteolipids (Baumann *et al.* 1967, 1968). We extended the analysis to see whether the reduction was uniform or whether a particular group was reduced within each lipid class. Plasmalogens were as usual essentially located in the ethanolamine phosphoglycerides in Quaking mice, and dimethylacetal analysis showed no difference between control and mutant mice.

The various diacyl phosphoglycerides were present in Quaking mice and no abnormal fatty acid pattern was detected in phosphatidylserine (Jacque, Harpin and Baumann 1969), phosphatidylethanolamine and phosphatidylcholine. Quantitative data on phospholipid content obtained by Hogan and Joseph (1971) and by Dawson and Clarke (1971) are in agreement with our results. Cholesterol esters were not present in the mutant. The only qualitative difference was a disappearance of the major group of galactolipids, those containing long-chain fatty acids (Jacque, Harpin and Baumann 1969), which normally constitute 80% of these brain lipids. Sphingomyelins containing long-chain fatty acids were also reduced. The deficiency was essentially in non-hydroxylated long-chain fatty acids, both saturated and mono-unsaturated. Sphingolipids containing long-chain acids are essential and specific components of myelin (O'Brien 1965; Menkes, Philippart and Concone 1966; Svennerholm and Ställberg-Stenhagen 1968).

These results suggested that the paucity of myelin in the mutants is caused by this lack of long-chain fatty acids necessary to myelin sphingolipids, perhaps as a result of a block at a particular stage of myelin formation at which these fatty acids normally appear. According to Vandenheuvel (1963) and O'Brien (1965), the long-chain fatty acids are necessary for the formation and stability of myelin. We therefore isolated cerebrosides from control and mutant mice at various ages to try to detect a block at a particular stage of maturation in the evolution of the fatty acid composition of these compounds in the mutant. In relation to this, it was interesting to find that in adult Quaking mice, the cerebrosides, although lacking long-chain fatty acids, were present at 35% of their normal amount, expressed in micromoles per brain (Baumann *et al.* 1967). Pilz and Mehl (1966) and Norton and Autilio (1966) pointed out that 34% of total brain galactolipids are found in structures other than myelin in white matter. It was also found that the adult concentration of galactolipids in the brain of Quaking mice was close to the amount found in control littermates at early stages of myelination, and that galactolipid concentration did not rise significantly in the myelination period (Table 1). Nevertheless, there was a

TABLE 1

Concentration of galactolipids (μmol/g wet weight) in brains of mutant and normal mice during the myelination period

| *Days postnatally* | *Control mice* | *Quaking mice* | *Jimpy mice** |
|---|---|---|---|
| 10 | 1.38 | — | |
| 12 | 2.95 | 1.4 | |
| 15 | 4.30 | 1.6 | |
| 20 | 6.7 | 2.1 | 0.15 (19 days) |
| 25 | 9.6 | 2.5 | 0.14 (26 days) |

* Data of Nussbaum, Neskovic and Mandel (1969).

constant although very slight increase of galactolipids throughout myelination. On the other hand, the normal rise of $C_{24}$ fatty acids, correlated with myelination between 15 and 20 days, was not found in the total brain lipid extract of Quaking mice (Fig. 1). The percentage of long-chain non-hydroxylated fatty acids in the cerebrosides of adult Quaking mice was closer to that observed in cerebrosides of 8-day-old controls than that in normal adults (Table 2). This is evidence in favour of a block at the step at which long-chain fatty acids appear in sphingolipids necessary to myelin.

In Jimpy mice, Nussbaum, Neskovic and Mandel (1969) found only traces of cerebrosides (Table 1). Recent studies by Nussbaum, Neskovic and Mandel

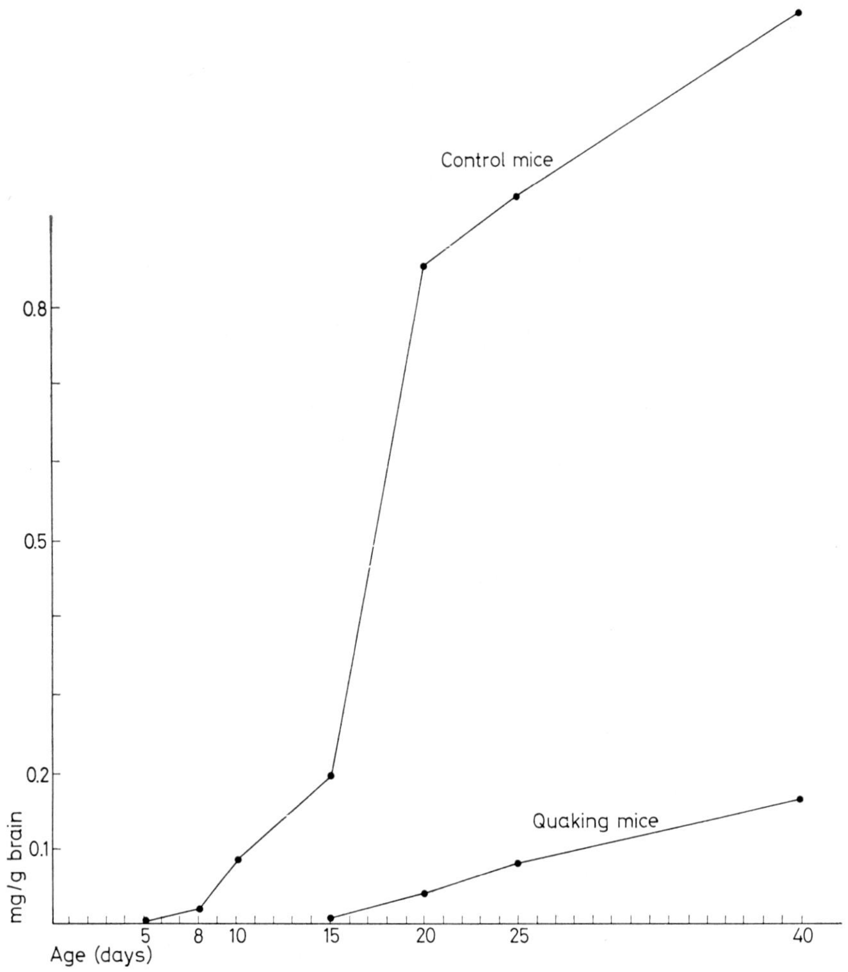


FIG. 1. Content of $C_{24}$ non-hydroxylated fatty acids in brain lipids in control and Quaking mice as a function of age.

(1971) and by Hogan and Joseph (1971) have shown that the very small amount of cerebrosides, sulphatides and sphingomyelins present is essentially made up of medium-chain length fatty acids in this mutant. It is noteworthy that long-chain hydroxylated fatty acids are less affected than non-hydroxylated fatty acids in both mutants.

The data of Norton, Poduslo and Suzuki (1967), Eng and Noble (1968) and Horrocks (1968) indicated that the composition of myelin varies with age. It was therefore interesting to see whether the defect in long-chain myelin sphingo-

TABLE 2

Percentage composition of long-chain non-hydroxylated fatty acids in the cerebrosides of control and mutant mice

| | Normal mice | | | | Mutant mice | |
|---|---|---|---|---|---|---|
| *Fatty acids* | *1 day* | *9 days* | *12 days* | *Adults* | *Quaking adults* | *Jimpy* 18 days* |
| 16:0 + 16:1 | 18.1 | 9.8 | 3.1 | 3.4 | 21.2 | 27.6 |
| 18:0 + 18:1 | 67.8 | 35.7 | 25.4 | 10.8 | 51.0 | 41.5 |
| 20:0 + 20:1 | 1.9 | — | 2.9 | — | — | 3.2 |
| 22:0 + 22:1 | 2.1 | 11.6 | 23.4 | 5.1 | 4.2 | 9.30 |
| 24:0 + 24:1 | 10.1** | 31.5 | 37.8 | 81.0 | 23.4 | 13.6 |
| Ratio of long-chain (19–24) to short-chain acids | 0.16 | | 2.25 | 6.06 | 0.38 | 0.30 |

* Data of Nussbaum, Neskovic and Mandel (1971).
** Plus α-hydroxylated fatty acids.

lipids meant a block in myelin maturation itself and at what stage. Myelin was isolated (Baumann, Harpin and Bourre 1970) according to Norton, Poduslo and Suzuki (1967) and its constituents were analysed. We found (Table 3), as did others, that it is essentially the ratio of galactolipids to phospholipids which increases with age and not the ratio of cholesterol to phospholipids. In adult Quaking mice the ratio of galactolipids to phospholipids is less than that found in the myelin of 12-day-old normal littermates. The fatty acids of the cerebrosides were analysed. We found no major differences in the long-chain fatty acid content of myelin from 12-day-old controls and adult controls. The long-chain non-hydroxylated fatty acids were considerably reduced in Quaking mice; the proportion of long-chain hydroxylated fatty acids was tremendously increased, which remains puzzling. In Jimpy mice, Nussbaum, Neskovic and Mandel (1971) also found a diminution in the long-chain fatty acid content of myelin cerebrosides. Hydroxylated fatty acids were not analysed. These data imply that the formation and compaction of myelin is impaired by the absence of these complex lipids.

TABLE 3

Lipid composition of myelin from Quaking mice and 12-day-old and adult normal littermates (lipids expressed as μmol/100 mg myelin)

| | *12-day-old controls* | *Adult controls* | *Quaking adults* |
|---|---|---|---|
| Cholesterol | 46.0 | 42.4 | 47.9 |
| Phospholipids | 49.6 | 50.0 | 51.6 |
| Galactolipids | 23.9 | 28.9 | 14.4 |

Cuzner and Davison (1968) have shown that 'early myelin' can be separated into an adult type of myelin and a myelin-like fraction thought to be derived from the oligodendroglial plasma membrane. We have also shown that even before myelination, at the 7th day after birth in mice, a detectable amount of membranes sediments in the myelin fraction on discontinuous sucrose gradients. In Quaking mice, it may well be that the difference in composition reflects mostly the presence of the oligodendroglial cell plasma membrane. This will be hard to confirm, as pure preparations of this cell fraction have not been obtained. Nevertheless, other modifications have been shown to occur in the myelin of mutants that are also seen in preparations of early myelin. The ganglioside content in Quaking mice is close to that observed by Suzuki, Poduslo and Norton (1967) in the myelin fraction of the maturing brain of the rat and, in our hands, to that observed at 12 days in mice, although the importance of gangliosides other than $G_{M1}$ seems even greater. In isolated myelin, we have also found a modification of the protein pattern. Although the basic protein was slightly diminished, the main modification was in the proteolipid pattern (Jacque *et al.* 1971; Greenfield, Norton and Morell 1971).

Comparison with the evolution of myelin in controls as a function of age is illuminating. According to Uzman and Rumley (1958) and others, myelination involves to a great extent the reorientation of existing lipids, already present in the cells, cell processes and cell membranes of brain, which thereby acquire the properties by which myelin is defined and recognized, and they attribute a key role to cerebrosides (and one would now say to cerebrosides containing long-chain fatty acids). It is now clear that these are the only lipids which are represented only in trace amounts in the Quaking mice.

When the different mutants are compared, the lack of oligodendroglial cells in Jimpy mice can be correlated with the lack of cerebrosides, and the qualitative defects observed in the oligodendroglial cells in Quaking mice can be correlated with a loss of metabolic differentiation, shown by the failure of long-chain fatty acids to appear in cerebrosides.

There is much experimental evidence to indicate a defect in long-chain fatty acid biosynthesis in Quaking mice. In this mutant, we had found (Baumann *et al.* 1968) that the amount of $C_{18}$ acids was normal although that of $C_{24}$ was considerably reduced. As the synthetase synthesizes essentially palmitic acid ($C_{16}$) (Pollet, Bourre and Baumann 1969) and as Kishimoto, Davies and Radin (1965) have pointed out that the turnover is the same for $C_{16}$ and $C_{18}$, we postulated that there are at least two systems for fatty acid elongation, one synthesizing $C_{18}$, the other synthesizing $C_{24}$ acids. In rats, X-ray irradiation data obtained by Schjeide, San-Lin and de Vellis (1968), which indicated a specific block in the formation of long-chain fatty acids and therefore of

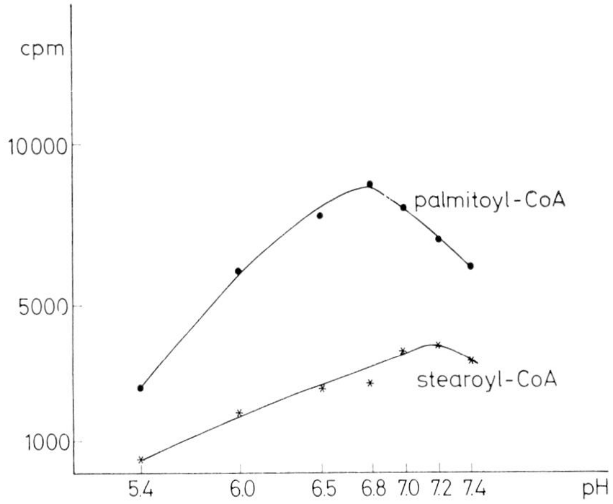


FIG. 2. Elongation of palmitoyl-CoA and stearoyl-CoA by brain m. rosomal preparations, in relation to the pH of the incubation medium.

myelin when the brain was irradiated at 2 days of age, also support this hypothesis. A difference in pH optimum has been shown for palmitoyl-CoA and stearoyl-CoA as substrates (Fig. 2) in long-chain fatty acid biosynthesis by microsomes (Bourre *et al.* 1970). In the presence of stearoyl-CoA, the amount of long-chain fatty acids is considerably reduced in Quaking mice (Table 4; Bourre *et al.* 1971), which indicates a defect in this second system (Pollet *et al.* 1971). There is clearly a specific defect in the biosynthesis of long-chain fatty acids in these mutants.

TABLE 4

Percentages of elongation products in fatty acid biosynthesis by microsomes from normal and Quaking mice

| | | *Product chain length* | | | | |
|---|---|---|---|---|---|---|
| | | *16* | *18* | *18–OH+20* | *20–OH+22* | *24* |
| Palmitoyl-CoA + | Control | 6 | 77 | 5 | 7 | 5 |
| [14C]malonyl-CoA | Quaking | 9.5 | 86.5 | 2.5 | 1.5 | — |
| [14C]Palmitoyl-CoA | Control | — | 95 | 3 | 0.5 | 1.5 |
| + malonyl-CoA | Quaking | — | 97 | 2 | 0.7 | 0.3 |
| Stearoyl-CoA + | Control | 23 | 34 | 20 | 11 | 12 |
| [14C]malonyl-CoA | Quaking | 46.3 | 50 | 3 | 0.7 | trace |
| [14C[Stearoyl-CoA | Control | — | — | 78.5 | 10.5 | 11 |
| + malonyl-CoA | Quaking | — | — | 99 | 0.8 | 0.2 |

The enzyme UDPgalactose:sphingosine galactosyltransferase has been shown to be diminished in Quaking mice (Costantino-Ceccarini and Morell 1971). This may be a consequence of the lack of one of its major substrates, ceramides containing long-chain fatty acids, since long-chain fatty acids are lacking. Neskovic, Nussbaum and Mandel (1970) showed a reduction in the concentration of psychosine, which is not a precursor of cerebroside biosynthesis, according to Morell, Ceccarini and Radin (1970). This reduction may be due, as they suggest, to a lack of specificity of the transferase. If the reduction of the transferase is a result of the lack of substrate, a lack of synthesis of long-chain non-hydroxylated fatty acid-containing ceramides should also be observed. The enzyme necessary for the synthesis of stearoyl ceramides is present in normal amount in Quaking mice (Costantino-Ceccarini and Morell 1971; P. Girard and N. A. Baumann, unpublished results, 1971). The existence of a second system specific for ceramides containing long-chain fatty acids is not excluded; it could also explain the specific lack of long-chain sphingomyelins. Substrate specificity for ceramide formation may be determined by the length of the fatty acid as well as the nature of the sphingosine base, since the amount of sphingosine compared to dihydrosphingosine evolves in parallel with the lengthening of the fatty acids in the maturing brain cerebrosides (Isaacson and Moscatelli 1970).

The peripheral nervous system is histologically normal in Quaking mice. It contains normal amounts of cerebrosides (Herschkowitz, Vassella and Bischoff 1971). Nevertheless, there is a 50% diminution of sphingolipids containing long-chain fatty acids (Kishimoto 1971). In the kidney there is no difference between controls and Quaking mice in the content of long-chain sphingomyelins (Kishimoto 1971) and cerebrosides. A structural gene mutation modifying the activity of an enzyme always manifests itself in all organs where the enzyme is necessary. Unless several enzymic systems are involved in the synthesis of long-chain fatty acids, these results suggest that there is a controller gene specific to the central nervous system, and different for oligodendrocytes and for Schwann cells. Regulatory mechanisms are necessary to explain the reduction in 2′:3′-cyclic nucleotide 3′-phosphohydrolase (Kurihara, Nussbaum and Mandel 1970) observed in both mutants.

Quaking mice also have a defect in reproduction. The females are less fertile than normal and the males are aspermatogenic. Although genetic studies have been made at the Jackson laboratory, no dissociation of the effects on the central nervous system and on the reproductive organs has been observed, so the existence of a pleiotropic controller gene cannot be excluded.

In conclusion, we are still far from understanding the sequential events leading to myelin formation, but nevertheless the biosynthesis of cerebrosides and sulphatides and especially of galactolipids (and sphingomyelins) containing long-chain fatty acids seems to play a crucial role. Although the hormonal controls are not well known, the thyroid hormone plays a role in myelin metabolism and seems to be involved at some stage in the biosynthesis of these compounds (Walravens and Chase 1969; Balasz *et al.* 1969).

SUMMARY

Mutations in mice which block specific steps in myelination can give clues to the sequential timing of the histological and biochemical events leading to the elaboration of this very special membrane and to its genetic control. The Quaking mutation is recessive autosomal, and the Jimpy mutation is X-linked. Histological studies point to specific modifications of the oligodendroglial cells in these mutations.

The content of cerebroside and sulphatide is negligible in the Jimpy mutation, which correlates with a very early histological impairment of myelin formation. Cerebrosides and sulphatides are formed in the Quaking mouse, although they are deficient in long-chain fatty acids with 24 carbon atoms, as are sphingomyelins.

Several arguments are in favour of control steps being involved rather than inborn errors of metabolism related to enzymic defects, as several enzymes of cerebroside and sulphatide metabolism are affected and as there are no general consequences on similar pathways in other organs.

In Quaking mice, the appearance of long-chain non-hydroxylated fatty acids in myelin sphingolipids is impaired; comparison with normal myelin at different ages suggests that this may be one of the latest steps in myelin formation. In relation to this fact a special function must be attributed to a long-chain fatty acid-specific synthetase, and perhaps also to long-chain-specific enzymes for fatty acid fixation on myelin sphingolipid precursors. Myelin membrane proteolipids are also diminished in Quaking mice. The exact significance of this fact remains unclear.

# References

Balasz, R., Brooksbank, B. W. L., Davison, A. N., Eayrs, J. T. and Wilson, D. A. (1969) *Brain Res.* **15**, 219-232

Baumann, N., Jacque, C., Pollet, S. and Harpin, M. L. (1967) *C. R. Hebd. Séances Acad. Sci., Sér. D*, **264**, 2953-2956

BAUMANN, N. A., JACQUE, C. M., POLLET, S. A. and HARPIN, M. L. (1968) *Eur. J. Biochem.* **4**, 340-344.

BAUMANN, N. A., HARPIN, M. L. and BOURRE, J. M. (1970) *Nature* (*Lond.*) **227**, 960-961

BERGER, B. (1970) In *Les mutants pathologiques chez l'animal, leur intérêt pour la recherche biomédicale*, pp. 91-98, ed. M. Sabourdy. Centre National de la Recherche Scientifique, Paris

BERGER, B. (1971) *Brain Res.* **25**, 35-53

BOURRE, J. M., POLLET, S., DUBOIS, G. and BAUMANN, N. (1970) *C.R. Hebd. Séances Acad. Sci., Sér. D* **271**, 1221-1223

BOURRE, J. M., POLLET, S., DAUDU, O. and BAUMANN, N. (1971) *C.R. Hebd. Séances Acad. Sci., Sér. D* **273**, 1534-1537

COSTANTINO-CECCARINI, E. and MORELL, P. (1971) *Brain Res.* **29**, 75-84

CUZNER, M. L. and DAVISON, A. N. (1968) *Biochem. J.* **106**, 29-34

DAWSON, R. M. C. and CLARKE, N. (1971) *J. Neurochem.* **18**, 1313-1316

DOBBING, J. (1970) *Am. J. Dis. Child.* **120**, 411-415

ENG, L. F. and NOBLE, E. P. (1968) *Lipids* **3**, 157-162

FARKAS, E., ZAHND, J. P., NUSSBAUM, J. L. and MANDEL, P. (1970) In *Les mutants pathologiques chez l'animal, leur intérêt pour la recherche biomédicale*, pp. 21-26, ed. M. Sabourdy. Centre National de La Recherche Scientifique, Paris

FRIEDE, R. L. and SAMORAJSKI, T. (1967) *J. Comp. Neurol.* **130**, 223-232

GREENFIELD, S., NORTON, W. T. and MORELL, P. (1971) *J. Neurochem.* **18**, 2119-2128

HERSCHKOWITZ, N., VASSELLA, F. and BISCHOFF, A. (1971) *J. Neurochem.* **18**, 1361-1363

HOGAN, E. L. and JOSEPH, K. C. (1971) *J. Neurochem.* **18**, 1209-1214

HORROCKS, L. A. (1968) *J. Neurochem.* **15**, 483-488

ISAACSON, E. and MOSCATELLI, E. A. (1970) *J. Neurochem.* **17**, 365-371

JACQUE, C. M., HARPIN, M. L. and BAUMANN, N. A. (1969) *Eur. J. Biochem.* **11**, 218-224

JACQUE, C., LOUIS, CH., BOURRE, J. M. and BAUMANN, N. A. (1971) *Abstracts 3rd International Meeting, International Society for Neurochemistry, Budapest*, p. 83

KISHIMOTO, Y. (1971) *J. Neurochem.* **18**, 1365-1368

KISHIMOTO, Y., DAVIES, E. W. and RADIN, N. S. (1965) *J. Lipid Res.* **6**, 515-531

KURIHARA, T., NUSSBAUM, J. L. and MANDEL, P. (1970) *J. Neurochem.* **17**, 993-997

MENKES, J. H., PHILIPPART, M. and CONCONE, M. C. (1966) *J. Lipid Res.* **7**, 479-486

MORELL, P., CECCARINI, E. C. and RADIN, N. S. (1970) *Arch. Biochem. Biophys.* **141**, 738-748

NESKOVIC, N., NUSSBAUM, J. L. and MANDEL, P. (1970) *Brain Res.* **21**, 39-53

NORTON, W. T. and AUTILIO, L. A. (1966) *J. Neurochem.* **13**, 213-222

NORTON, W. T., PODUSLO, S. E. and SUZUKI, K. (1967) *Abstracts 1st International Meeting, International Society for Neurochemistry, Strasbourg*, p. 61

NUSSBAUM, J. L., NESKOVIC, N. and MANDEL, P. (1969) *J. Neurochem.* **16**, 927-934

NUSSBAUM, J. L., NESKOVIC, N. and MANDEL, P. (1971) *J. Neurochem.* **18**, 1529-1543

O'BRIEN, J. S. (1965) *Science* **147**, 1099-1107

PILZ, H. and MEHL, E. (1966) *Hoppe-Seyler's Z. Physiol. Chem.* **346**, 306-309

POLLET, S., BOURRE, J. M. and BAUMANN, N. (1969) *C.R. Hebd. Séances Acad. Sci., Sér. D* **268**, 2146-2149

POLLET, S., BOURRE, J. M., DAUDU, O. and BAUMANN, N. (1971) *C.R. Hebd. Séances Acad. Sci., Sér. D* **273**, 1426-1429

SCHJEIDE, O. A., SAN-LIN, R. E. and DE VELLIS, D. (1968) *Radiat. Res.* **33**, 107-128

SIDMAN, R. L., DICKIE, M. M. and APPEL, S. H. (1964) *Science* **144**, 309-310

SUZUKI, K., PODUSLO, S. E. and NORTON, W. T. (1967) *Biochim. Biophys. Acta* **144**, 375-381

SVENNERHOLM, L. and STÄLLBERG-STENHAGEN, S. (1968) *J. Lipid Res.* **9**, 215-225

VANDENHEUVEL, F. A. (1963) *J. Am. Oil Chem. Soc.* **40**, 455-472

WALRAVENS, P. and CHASE, H. P. (1969) *J. Neurochem.* **16**, 1477-1484

WISNIEWSKI, H. and MORELL, P. (1971) *Brain Res.* **29**, 63-73

UZMAN, L. L. and RUMLEY, M. K. (1958) *J. Neurochem.* **3**, 170-184

## Discussion

*Mead:* In confirmation of your idea that there are two systems that elongate fatty acids: the cytoplasmic (or soluble) palmitate-synthesizing system is capable of synthesizing stearate, and Norman Radin and I now agree that this does take place in the brain to some extent, so it is possible that this system could be operating normally in the mutants but that the mitochondrial system, which produces further elongation, might be deficient. I am at a loss to explain the normality of the α-hydroxy acids, which, I believe, must be formed from the long-chain unsubstituted acids.

*Baumann:* Is it possible that a small amount of long-chain fatty acids is being formed and that from then on the system that makes long-chain α-hydroxylated fatty acids is more active than the one forming ceramides containing long-chain non-hydroxylated fatty acids? That might be one explanation.

On the question of the microsomal long-chain fatty acid synthesis, you seemed to be saying that long-chain non-hydroxylated fatty acids are only made in mitochondria; is that from Dr Boone's data (1969) or have you other data?

*Mead:* Boone and Wakil (1970) have shown that brain mitochondria are perfectly capable of making $C_{24}$ out of $C_{18}$, and that the co-factors are the familiar ones for that particular system, but I don't think he has said that this is the *only* system that makes long-chain fatty acids.

*Baumann:* We found, like Dr Menkes, that there are a lot of long-chain fatty acids in microsomes.

*Menkes:* I think there are three chain-elongating systems in the brain: the soluble system, which tends to make palmitic acid and a little stearic acid; a mitochondrial system, which does what Dr Boone has shown, namely elongate fatty acids, both saturated and unsaturated; and a microsomal system. In liver, this microsomal system elongates polyunsaturated fatty acids preferentially, but in brain, particularly in the *developing* brain—that is, at the time of maximum myelination—the microsomal system has a marked predilection for the elongation of saturated fatty acids. In the presence of thyroid hormone, chain elongation of saturated fatty acids is preferentially stimulated (Grippo and Menkes 1971). So that when you, Dr Baumann, say that the microsomal chain elongation is lost, I think this explains why you continue to get the formation of hydroxy fatty acids. Perhaps the mitochondrial chain elongation system is still able to function and produce long-chain fatty acids, even though this may occur at a slow rate.

*Baumann:* In fact, when one looks at the $C_{24}$ fatty acid pattern in the brains of mice as a function of age there seems to be at first a low rate of synthesis and then suddenly a boost between the 15th and the 18th day, as if a second system were coming into action.

*Davison:* Could you feed the mutant mice with long-chain fatty acids?

*Baumann:* We have obtained labelled lignoceric acid that we would like to feed to the mice. The only problem is the form in which it should be given.

*Mead:* Lignoceric acid is almost impossible to handle in aqueous systems. It doesn't complex with albumin. One way of dealing with it is to form a micellar solution. If you dissolve the acid in a small amount of monoglyceride, add bile acid solution (we use taurocholate), and then sonicate it, you get a clear micellar solution that is stable for quite a while.

*Davison:* If you formed a long-chain fatty acid ester would it not go to the brain and there be hydrolysed?

*Mead:* I don't think it would go to the brain. We haven't attempted this because of the difficulty. We haven't tried getting lignoceric acid into the brain except by direct injection. One could inject the micelle directly into the brain and take the chance that the bile acid or other emulsifying agent might be toxic to the brain.

*Svennerholm:* It would be better to use nervonic acid, because it is more soluble.

*Rossi:* Dr Baumann, what is the condition of the heterozygote parents of the affected mice? Does heterozygosis affect the genetic expression (functional, morphological or chemical)?

*Baumann:* Heterozygotes have not been studied yet, as they cannot be distinguished from normal homozygotes in litters containing Quaking mice. It is not possible to breed from Quaking individuals, as the females are not very fertile and the males are sterile.

*Chapman:* Have you shown that the myelin of the Quaking mouse does not exhibit its normal function as a myelin membrane?

*Baumann:* The mice have tremors and seizures, which suggests a defect in nervous conduction, but it's harder to detect this in the central nervous system than in the peripheral nervous system, and the studies have not been done.

*Chapman:* Is the turnover rate for this myelin different from that of normal myelin?

*Baumann:* We have not studied this.

*von Muralt:* Do you find differences in the conduction velocity or in reflex actions of these mice? If myelination is abnormal, you should get abnormal electrophysiological behaviour of the peripheral nerves, too—or is the defect in myelin restricted to the central nervous system?

*Herschkowitz:* The current view is that the disorder is limited to the central nervous system.

*Chapman:* This is the point I was trying to reach. I wonder whether the difference between the presence of $C_{18}$ and $C_{24}$ fatty acids in the membrane would make a major difference in the electrical resistivity or conductivity of myelin.

*Bovet:* What is the sensitivity of the mutant strains for convulsive drugs or for electroshock?

*Baumann:* For electroshock, I don't know, but they convulse spontaneously.

*Herschkowitz:* In connection with the clinical appearance and defects of myelin, I would like to add a note of caution. In the Jimpy mouse it is thought to be exclusively a myelination defect of the oligodendrocytes. However, we checked the neurons, which we separated by two methods: those of Norton and Poduslo (1970) and of Johnson and Sellinger (1971). *In vitro* and *in vivo* experiments have shown that sulphatide synthesis is significantly diminished. Neuronal metabolism is therefore also affected in the Jimpy mice (although the neurons appear normal when seen by electron microscopy). We haven't looked at the Quaking mice.

*Svennerholm:* We have studied the lipid composition of neurons and glial cells from rabbit cerebral cortex (Hamberger and Svennerholm 1971). The plasma membranes of the two cell types were isolated by gradient centrifugation on ficoll-sucrose. The same concentrations of cerebrosides and sulphatides were found in the neuronal plasma membrane as in the glial cell membrane. These results would explain the finding of a disturbed glycolipid metabolism in the neurons as well as in the glial cells, because the plasma membranes of the two cell types contain the same components.

*Davison:* Dr Baumann pointed out the proteolipid protein band and the basic protein band, but there were also several protein bands higher up on the gel-electrophoresis pattern. These were presumably the so-called Wolfgram proteins, but there's now some doubt whether these proteins are myelin components. The other thing that struck me, in relation to the concept of myelin-like material, was that if this material did accumulate in these inborn errors, I would have expected to see much less basic protein, but a normal amount of proteolipid protein, whereas you find a membrane which in many ways fits the bill of the myelin-like membrane, which appears in the brain just at the beginning of myelination, but differs in certain respects in its composition. It is similar in having a lack of cerebrosides, but it has a basic protein (see also Greenfield, Norton and Morell 1971). In addition, these authors isolated a pellet containing no basic protein which resembles our myelin-like fraction.

*von Muralt:* When we discuss myelination, it should be clear about what we are talking. The term 'myelin membrane' is not correct. In the brain, the oligodendroglial membrane and in peripheral nerve, the Schwann cell membrane surrounds the myelin, which is a sort of filling substance inside the membrane. The axon also has a membrane of its own which is covered by the innermost layer of the Schwann cell membrane in peripheral nerves. In myelinated nerves, the axonal membrane is inexcitable in the internode, where it is covered by the Schwann cell membrane, and it is only excitable at the nodes, where there is no myelination, giving the saltatory transmission of the impulse from one node to the next one. In so-called 'non-myelinated' fibres there is a small amount of myelin present, but the Schwann cell usually surrounds several axons. Brain function is based on the electrical excitation of nerve cell membranes, axonal elements and dendrites. The glial apparatus, containing myelin, is responsible for the electrical insulation of these elements from each other. At the present time, it seems impossible to extrapolate data obtained from deficiencies of myelin to explain the behaviour of the neuronal apparatus.

*Bernsohn:* I believe that the oligodendroglial membrane has quite a different lipid composition from the myelin itself, both qualitatively and quantitatively. It's therefore difficult to visualize myelin as a simple extrusion of the oligodendroglial membrane. Does the plasma membrane ultimately turn out to be myelin? Is there an extrusion of myelin material between the inner and outer membrane layers, or is there an elaboration of some new substance from the oligodendroglial cell? How does this myelin then wrap around the axon? Does the glial cell migrate, or does the axon turn? In our attempt to explain this process we seem to avoid some inherent problems posed by the explanation.

*Davison:* I think there may be a winding by promulgation of the Schwann cell or glial membrane loosely around the axon, but the site of subsequent membrane synthesis is completely unknown. We have not explored the possibility that membrane protein and complex lipid are synthesized in the nerve cell and transported down the axon. Perhaps the basic protein is formed in the neuronal perikaryon; alternatively myelin may be synthesized much closer to the axon, through participation of glial (or Schwann) cell cytoplasm. In the diagrams of myelinating nerve on the theory of Alan Peters and J. E. Vaughn (1970) and the diagram by Hirano and Dembitzer (1967), for example, there is always trapped glial cytoplasm close to the axon and this glial cytoplasm contains ribosomes and smooth endoplasmic reticulum. Synthesis of myelin close to the axon has the advantage that macromolecules do not have to go through the long drawn-out process of transport from the neuron via the axon or from the glial perikaryon via the tortuous glial process.

*Dobbing*: Does the myelin shunt radially from there once it's formed, or does it have to shear right round the axon?

*Davison:* I think it could be a radial movement, but this is of course only speculation.

*von Muralt:* Seddon, Medawar and Smith (1943) studied the regeneration of nerves after war injuries and found that regeneration is a repetition of the embryonic development (see also Shawe 1955). First there is axonal outgrowth towards the periphery. When this outgrowth is completed and a signal for myelination is given, the Schwann cells build up around the axon, at first with a small internodal distance. As regeneration goes on, myelination becomes important, the size of the Schwann cells increases and their number falls. At the same time, the internodal length increases, together with the conduction velocity, until it becomes almost normal.

*Davison:* Webster (1971) has shown that even within one internode supplied by one Schwann cell, the number of lamellae is not constant throughout the length, again suggesting that there is some kind of local synthesis so that myelination is patchy and you can't think of the whole sheath wrapping round in continuity.

# References

Boone, S. C. (1969) *Abstracts 2nd International Meeting, International Society for Neurochemistry*, p. 98, ed. R. Paoletti, R. Fumagalli and C. Galli. Tamburini Editore, Milan

Boone, S. C. and Wakil, S. J. (1970) *Biochemistry* **9**, 1470-1479

Greenfield, S., Norton, W. T. and Morell, P. (1971) *J. Neurochem.* **18**, 2119-2128

Grippo, J. and Menkes, J. H. (1971) *Pediatr. Res.* **5**, 466

Hamberger, A. and Svennerholm, L. (1971) *J. Neurochem.* **18**, 1821-1829

Hirano, A. and Dembitzer, H. M. (1967) *J. Cell Biol.* **34**, 555-567

Johnson, D. E. and Sellinger, O. Z. (1971) *J. Neurochem.* **18**, 1445

Norton, W. T. and Poduslo, S. E. (1970) *Science* **167**, 1144-1146

Peters, A. and Vaughn, J. E. (1970) In *Myelination*, pp. 3-79, ed. A. N. Davison and A. Peters. Thomas, Springfield, Ill.

Seddon, H. J., Medawar, P. B. and Smith, H. J. (1943) *J. Physiol. (Lond.)* **102**, 191

Shawe, G. D. H. (1955) *Br. J. Surg.* **42**, 474-488

Webster, H. de F. (1971) *Neurosci. Res. Program Bull.* **9** (4), 470-477

# Critical periods in brain development

N. HERSCHKOWITZ and E. ROSSI

*Department of Neurochemistry, Universitäts-Kinderklinik, Bern*

The development of the brain is the result of highly complex interactions between the genome and a multitude of exogenous factors. It is the purpose of this symposium to explore the ways in which one of these exogenous factors, nutrition, in particular the lipids, can influence the growth and differentiation of the nervous system.

An important problem with which we have to deal is the question of whether there are certain periods during brain development at which alterations of metabolism (due to exogenous factors) are particularly likely to cause a definite change in the course of future brain development. As a contribution toward the understanding of this complex problem, the following three subjects will be discussed:

1. Development of the brain at the cellular level.

2. Genetic mechanisms involved in development.

3. Exogenous regulation of genetic expression.

## BRAIN DEVELOPMENT

The growth and maturation of an organ at the cellular level comprises four stages: (1) proliferation; (2) migration; (3) differentiation; and (4) death. This sequence of events is observed in all parts of the brain; however, the timing differs from one cell type to another and from region to region. This results in an extremely complex pattern of development when the brain is regarded as a whole.

*Proliferation*

The formation of the brain in, for example, the mouse begins around the 6th gestational day, at about the time when implantation occurs in the uterus. Proliferation of cells from the ventricular zone of the primitive brain begins around the 11th day and proceeds very rapidly, producing an enormous number of cells in a few days. Slight changes in the cell cycle affect the rate of mitosis and will have a great effect on the final cell number. The number of neurons depends, however, not only on the number and rate of mitoses but also on the rate of cell death. Retrograde flow of metabolites from the periphery may influence the rate of cell degeneration. Malnutrition during early pregnancy can reduce the number of cells formed, as measured by the DNA content of the brain. It is not yet clear whether this is due to a decrease in cell formation, increased cell death, or both. However, this is an example of how nutrition can alter brain development from the very beginning.

*Migration*

After an unknown number of mitoses, some cells start to migrate out from the ventricular zone and form layers of homogeneous cells. De Long (1970) has recently shown that migration is a self-organizing process guided by the membrane characteristics of the cells themselves. If cells from the hippocampus and isocortex of mouse embryos at 18½ days of gestation are dissociated and allowed to reaggregate in liquid cell cultures, two main features can be observed:
1. Different cell types separate from each other, and cluster together. This process is equivalent to the cell migration observed *in vivo* and may be due to specific surface conditions which produce group-specific affinities.
2. Within the homogeneous cell population the cells align in parallel to each other, they show a basal-apical orientation, they form layers of approximately constant thickness and they orient in asymmetrical curves which are comparable to the *in vivo* layers. This self-orientation may be due to specific asymmetrical patches on the surface of the membranes which differentiate the side of the cell from the ends.

The capacity for self-organization is strictly limited to a short period during embryonic development. If brains were taken from mice younger or older than 18½ days of gestational age, the formation and organization of layers was not observed *in vitro*. The appearance of these time-dependent membrane characteristics is part of cellular differentiation and is genetically regulated. The example of the mutant Reeler mouse, in which neurons are formed at a normal rate but no migration takes place, underscores the metabolic control of cellular migration (De Long and Sidman 1970).

## *Differentiation*

During or following migration a second type of differentiation takes place: the formation of cell-specific structures. Neurons grow axons and dendrites and form synaptic interconnections. There seem to be two main populations of dendrites, one under exclusive genetic control and the other regulated by external stimulation (Jacobson 1969). Glial cells differentiate into astroglia and oligodendroglia. The oligodendrocytes develop and differentiate their plasma membrane into myelin sheaths.

Short-axoned microneurons have been observed to proliferate postnatally in the rat and kitten, in the rat until about the 16th postnatal day. This is in contrast to the macroneurons, where there is no postnatal proliferation. The significance and function of microneurons has not yet been established. Altman (1967) has suggested that they may play a role in the storage of memory.

The correlation of biochemical events with cellular development and brain functions is not yet understood. The following example illustrates the situation in a very simplified form (Fig. 1). In the rat, galactocerebroside sulphotransferase activity increases around the 8th postnatal day (McKhann and Ho 1967). How does this increase in activity correlate with the observed increase in the amount of sulphatide in whole brain (Wells and Dittmer 1967)? How well does the increase in sulphatide reflect the formation of myelin, which

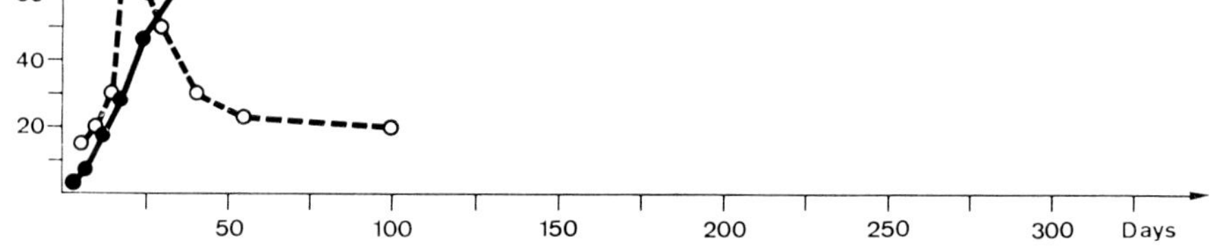


FIG. 1. Sulphatide content and galactocerebroside sulphotransferase activity in the developing rat brain.

can be observed at that time, and what is the role of sulphatide in the myelin membrane? Finally, what is the significance of myelin in motor and 'psychological' function? This chain of events has to be kept in mind when studying the effects of undernutrition on brain development.

In this paper, we deal mainly with the regulation of enzymic activity.

## GENETIC REGULATION OF BRAIN DEVELOPMENT

Genetic expression is related to the structure of the genome. The work of Callan (1967), Britten and Kohne (1968) and others has shown that in higher organisms some DNA base sequences can be repeated serially, up to many thousand times. One terminal unit can serve as a 'master' gene followed by 'slave' genes, which are more or less congruent to the master gene, but not involved in recombinational events.

Paigen (1971) for convenience divides the genes into four classes:

1. Structural genes, which code for the amino acid sequences of enzyme proteins and determine their catalytic functions as expressed by substrate specificity, physical stability, pH optimum and susceptibility to regulatory effectors.
2. Regulatory genes, which control enzyme activity and enzyme turnover. The presence of these genes has not been proved in mammals.
3. Architectural genes, which control the intracellular sites of enzymes.
4. Temporal genes, which control the timing of the activation and de-activation of structural, architectural and regulatory genes at specific stages during development.

Temporal genes are of special interest in development. The mutation in the Jimpy mouse (an X-linked recessive mutation causing leucodystrophy) may be an indication of their presence. The Jimpy male shows normal development until about the 11th postnatal day, when excessive tremor appears. Around the 20th day, tonic seizures occur and the animals die before the age of 30 days. Histologically there is almost no myelin in the central nervous system but normal myelin is found in the peripheral nervous system (Sidman, Dickie and Appel 1964). There are no major indications of demyelination. Biochemically there is a significant decrease of myelin lipids, particularly the glycolipids, cerebroside and sulphatide (Galli and Galli 1968; Nussbaum, Neskovic and Mandel 1969; Hogan, Joseph and Schmidt 1970).

Neskovic, Nussbaum and Mandel (1969) found decreased activity of UDP galactose:sphingosine galactosyltransferase in Jimpy brain, but the $K_m$ values for UDP-galactose were normal. Decreased synthesis of cerebroside in Jimpy brain was found by Galli, Kneebone and Paoletti (1969).

A deficiency of long-chain fatty acids of cerebrosides, sulphatides and ceramides was found by Joseph and Hogan (1971), which was more pronounced than in the Quaking mouse (Baumann, Harpin and Bourre 1970). In the Jimpy brain we found decreased sulphatide synthesis *in vivo* and *in vitro* (Herschkowitz, Vassella and Bischoff 1971). When homogenates of normal and Jimpy brains were mixed, no inhibition of galactocerebroside sulphotransferase activity was seen.

In normal mice the synthesis of sulphatide increases sharply around the 8th postnatal day, reaching a maximum at the 20th day. In the Jimpy mouse the increase of enzyme activity starts at the same time but reaches only 15% of the activity shown by normal mice. The remaining enzyme activity, however, shows normal heat inactivation, pH optimum and $K_m$ values for galactocerebroside and 3′-phosphoadenosine 5′-phosphosulphate. These results indicate the presence of an enzyme protein with a normal structure.

The fact that at least two enzymes (UDP galactose: sphingosine galactosyltransferase and galactocerebroside sulphotransferase) do not show the age-dependent activity increase in the Jimpy mutant but may be of normal protein structure, could be explained by the mutation of a temporal gene. However, a structural gene mutation in the X-chromosome which affects an energy-requiring step necessary for activation of the different enzymes, could also be responsible for the observed multiple enzyme deficiency.

TABLE 1

Regulation of genetic expression

| *Localization* | *Mechanism* |
|---|---|
| Gene | Activation, amplification, suppression |
| m-RNA | Turnover, transport |
| t-RNA | Turnover, amino acid binding |
| Ribosomes | Turnover |
| Polysomes | Aggregation, disaggregation |
| Protein synthesis | Initiation, elongation, termination |
| Protein structure | Turnover, structural changes |

## REGULATION OF GENETIC EXPRESSION

There are three different ways in which enzyme activity can be regulated:

1. By changing the concentration of the enzyme protein.

2. By altering the structure of the enzyme protein.
3. By changing the availability of substrates and removal of end products.

Some possible mechanisms of the control of enzyme activity at the molecular level are shown in Table 1. Some of these will be discussed.

*Control at the transcriptional level*

Production of messenger RNA starts in mammalian cells simultaneously with the first cleavages of the fertilized egg. Cytoplasmic factors are involved in this activation. When the nucleus from an amphibian ectodermal cell which is synthesizing RNA is removed and implanted into an egg from which the inactive nucleus has been removed, RNA synthesis will stop. It starts again in the descendants of the transplanted nucleus at the normal time for that cell. It is possible that these cytoplasmic factors may be influenced by exogenous factors which thereby affect gene activation. In mammals, the very close metabolic relationship of the egg with its surroundings may enhance this possibility. The egg is already exposed to the secretions of the maternal oviduct and the embryo, later, to the circulation and metabolism of the uterus.

In addition to gene activation there are mechanisms of specific gene suppression which may play a role in development. For instance, only 5% of the DNA of the mammalian hepatocyte is transcribed. Histones, together with other factors such as acidic proteins, are involved in this suppression. Of importance is the finding of Langan (1969) that cyclic 3′:5′-adenosine monophosphate stimulates phosphorylation of histones in nuclear preparations from rat liver. Again, it is possible that exogenous factors can act on these mechanisms. Gene amplification has not yet been shown in mammals. If it exists, it could be an important means of providing higher rates of enzyme synthesis. The presence of repeated sequences of DNA in higher organisms makes this a very possible hypothesis.

*Control at the post-transcriptional level*

In contrast to bacterial m-RNA, mammalian messenger RNA seems to be quite stable, which makes a regulation of specific protein synthesis possible by means of factors which either selectively stabilize messenger RNA or change the rate of translation.

Working with rat hepatoma cells in culture, Tomkins and co-workers (1969) studied the effect of dexamethasone phosphate on the activity of tyrosine aminotransferase. When the hormone was added to the culture medium, the activity of the enzyme increased rapidly and after 12 hours reached a new steady state, which was five to 15 times higher than the basal activity. By immunoprecipitation of the enzyme protein, it could be shown that the observed increase in activity was due to an actual increase in the protein concentration. The increased incorporation of amino acids into the enzyme protein indicated an increased synthesis of protein and not a decreased degradation. The synthesis of other proteins was not affected. When the synthesis and inducibility of tyrosine aminotransferase were studied in synchronized cell cultures, it became evident that the enzyme can be synthesized during the whole cell cycle, but that no induction is possible during the post-DNA-synthetic phase, mitosis and the beginning of the presynthetic period. A model of post-transcriptional control has been proposed, based on this work (Gelehrter 1971) (see Fig. 2).

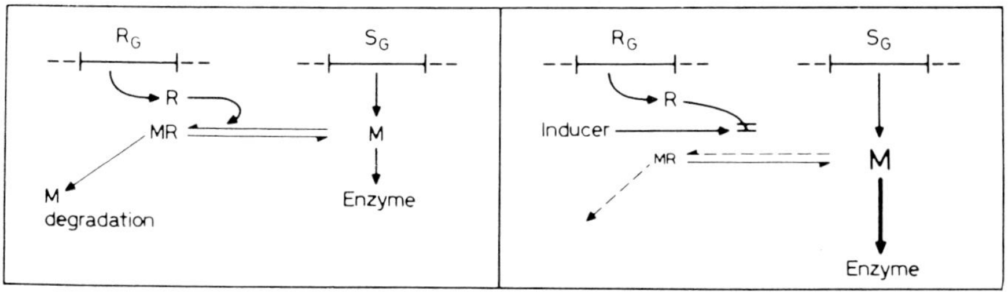


FIG. 2. Schematic model for the induction of tyrosine aminotransferase in rat hepatoma cells. (From Gelehrter 1971, with permission.)

In this model, tyrosine aminotransferase is coded in the gene, $S_G$, which is transcribed during the inducible phase into messenger, M. A regulatory gene $R_G$ produces a repressor, probably a protein R, at a constant rate. The repressor reacts in the cytoplasm reversibly with the tyrosine aminotransferase message, forming a complex, MR. This complex is not translated and the messenger is degraded at a constant rate. The role of the inducer (in this case the hormone) would then be to inhibit the formation of the MR complex; more M is therefore formed and more enzyme synthesized. Future work will determine whether this hypothesis is true and how widely it can be generalized. An example of the depression of enzyme synthesis has been studied by Jost, Khairallah and Pitot (1968). Rats which had previously fasted for a short period received glucocorticoid hormone, which produced a rapid increase of threonine dehydratase activity in the liver. Glucose administration inhibited this increase in activity. Studies of incorporation of amino acids into the enzyme protein and of immunoprecipitation have shown that the synthesis of the enzyme was decreased, probably at the translational level.

Transfer RNA is another control site for protein synthesis and degradation. Cortisone, for example, can stimulate synthesis of transfer RNA (Kenney, Wicks and Greenman 1965).

The omission of tryptophan from an amino acid mixture decreases protein synthesis *in vitro* (Sidranski *et al.* 1968). The role of tryptophan is interesting in this context. The administration of tryptophan-free amino acid mixtures may cause a breakdown of polysomes in the liver, and the addition of tryptophan restores the normal pattern (Wenner, Bell and Munro 1966). It should be mentioned that actinomycin D may cause polysomal disaggregation. This would make the use of actinomycin D inhibition questionable as an indication of the requirement for *de novo* RNA synthesis in induction (Soeiro and Amos 1966).

In many instances it has been observed that changes in nutrition alter the activity of enzymes. The mechanisms by which these alterations occur are, however, not known. Thus the biosynthesis of cholesterol in the liver is almost completely prevented when the cholesterol content in the food exceeds 0.5 %, in man and in rat (Siperstein and Fagan 1964). The exact mechanism of this inhibition is unknown. Work along the lines discussed will help to clarify such questions.

The previously discussed examples, illustrating the varied interaction between genome and nutrition, and the following observation, raise a general question. Mutant bacteria which lack the ability to synthesize histidine multiply better than the wild-type bacteria when histidine is added to the medium. As the enzyme for histidine synthesis does not have to be synthesized, more DNA, RNA and protein is available for replication (Zamenhof and Eichhorn 1967). Is it, therefore, possible that dependence upon nutrition becomes an important selective advantage in evolution, thereby making nutrition of primary significance in regulating genetic expression?

## SUMMARY AND CONCLUSION

1. Normal brain development depends on an exact sequence of integrated biological events: cell proliferation, migration, differentiation and death.
2. Metabolic reactions are the basic mechanisms regulating the cellular events. They are primarily determined by the genome. However, exogenous factors can interfere at any time at many sites of regulation and alter the selective genetic expression.
3. If such an alteration occurs at a period when the affected metabolic reaction is rate-limiting—'critical'—for the formation of a structure, brain development can be changed in a definite way.

4. During the whole period of brain development, theoretically rate-limiting metabolic events can be altered by exogenous factors, especially nutrition. Therefore, the entire developmental period may be 'critical' for the final outcome of the mature brain.
5. Assuming that alterations of brain development have a *functional* significance, the study of the effect of nutrition on brain development will then serve *two* purposes:
   (*a*) The prevention of possible harmful effects on brain function.
   (*b*) The optimizing of conditions which may improve brain function.

ACKNOWLEDGEMENT

This work has been supported by grant no. 3.145.69 from the Swiss National Foundation.

# References

ALTMAN, J. (1967) In *The Neurosciences: A Study Program*, pp. 723-743, ed. G. C. Quarton, T. Melnechuk and F. O. Schmitt. Rockefeller University Press, New York
BAUMANN, N. A., HARPIN, M. L. and BOURRE, J. M. (1970) *Nature* (*Lond.*) **227**, 960-961
BRITTEN, R. J. and KOHNE, D. E. (1968) *Science* **161**, 529-540
CALLAN, H. G. (1967) *J. Cell Sci.* **2**, 1-7
DE LONG, G. R. (1970) *Dev. Biol.* **22**, 563-583
DE LONG, G. R. and SIDMAN, R. (1970) *Dev. Biol.* **22**, 584-600
GALLI, C. and GALLI, R. C. (1968) *Nature* (*Lond.*) **220**, 165-166
GALLI, C., KNEEBONE, G. M. and PAOLETTI, R. (1969) *Life Sci.* **8**, 911-918
GELEHRTER, T. D. (1971) In *Enzyme Synthesis and Degradation in Mammalian Systems*, pp. 165-199, ed. M. Rechcigl, Jr. Karger, Basel
HERSCHKOWITZ, N., VASSELLA, F. and BISCHOFF, A. (1971) *J. Neurochem.* **18**, 1361-1363
HOGAN, E. L., JOSEPH, K. C. and SCHMIDT, G. (1970) *J. Neurochem.* **17**, 75-83
JACOBSON, M. (1969) *Science* **163**, 543-547
JOSEPH, K. C. and HOGAN, E. L. (1971) *J. Neurochem.* **18**, 1639-1645
JOST, J. P., KHAIRALLAH, E. H. and PITOT, H. C. (1968) *J. Biol. Chem.* **243**, 3057-3066
KENNEY, F. T., WICKS, W. D. and GREENMAN, D. C. (1965) *J. Cell. & Comp. Physiol.* **66**, 125-136
LANGAN, T. A. (1969) *J. Biol. Chem.* **244**, 5763
MCKHANN, G. M. and HO, W. (1967) *J. Neurochem.* **14**, 717-724
NESKOVIC, N. M., NUSSBAUM, J. L. and MANDEL, P. (1969) *FEBS Lett.* **3**, 199-201
NUSSBAUM, J. L., NESKOVIC, N. and MANDEL, P. (1969) *J. Neurochem.* **18**, 927-934
PAIGEN, K. (1971) In *Enzyme Synthesis and Degradation in Mammalian Systems*, pp. 1-46, ed. M. Rechcigl, Jr. Karger, Basel
SIDMAN, R. L., DICKIE, M. M. and APPEL, S. H. (1964) *Science* **144**, 309-311
SIDRANSKI, H., SARMA, D. S. R., BONGIORNO, M. and VERMEY, E. (1968) *J. Biol. Chem.* **243**, 1123-1132
SIPERSTEIN, M. D. and FAGAN, V. M. (1964) *Adv. Enzyme Regul.* **2**, 249-264

Soeiro, R. and Amos, H. (1966) *Biochim. Biophys. Acta* **129**, 406-409
Tomkins, G. M., Gelehrter, T. D., Martin, D. G. D., Samuels, H. H. and Thompson, E. B. (1969) *Science* **166**, 1474-1480
Wells, M. A. and Dittmer, J. C. (1967) *Biochemistry* **6**, 3169-3175
Wenner, W. H., Bell, J. and Munro, H. N. (1966) *Biochem. J.* **101**, 417-427
Zamenhof, S. and Eichhorn, H. H. (1967) *Nature* (*Lond.*) **216**, 456

# Discussion

*Aebi:* What is the exact molecular basis for the apparent enzyme deficiency condition in Jimpy mice? Some time ago I had trouble myself in distinguishing between a structural gene mutation and a regulator gene mutation in acatalasaemia (Aebi 1967; Aebi and Suter 1971). From this experience I think that even though you have already measured a number of parameters, such as $K_m$, pH optimum, and heat stability, you should still leave it open whether the defect in Jimpy mice is due to a structural gene mutation or not. In principle, there are two possible consequences to which an altered structure may lead: it is either an unstable enzyme variant, or a variant of low specific activity. In order to decide this, it might be of interest to establish the half-life of your enzyme variant compared to that of the normal enzyme and measure the specific activity of the purified variant and see whether it differs from that of the normal.

*Herschkowitz:* We have begun to purify the enzyme, galactocerebroside sulphotransferase, and will estimate the specific activity and, if possible, determine the amino acid sequence.

*Davison:* If it were a structural gene mutation, would you not expect there to be just one enzymic fault? But from Dr Baumann's paper it would seem that the chain-elongation system is also impaired, which suggests that at least two structural genes are involved, if in fact they are structural genes. And are not other enzyme proteins affected?

*Herschkowitz:* At least four enzymes show decreased activity. It is conceivable that a mutation in one structural gene is responsible for the fact that the activity of these enzymes does not increase around the 8th postnatal day.

*Menkes:* The finding of lower enzyme activity is not so surprising. I wonder what would be found if you expressed enzyme activity per number of glial cells available. Dr Baumann mentioned that there is a marked failure in the multiplication of glial cells in Jimpy mice, so if you express enzyme activity per cell, it might be perfectly normal.

*Herschkowitz:* We have checked the synthesis of [$^{35}$S]sulphatide in neurons isolated from Jimpy brain by the method of Norton and Poduslo (1970).

Sulphatide synthesis in Jimpy neurons (when calculated per cell protein) *in vivo* and *in vitro* is only about 20% of that found in normal neurons. This means that neurons are able to synthesize sulphatide and that this ability is reduced in the Jimpy mutant. Unfortunately, glial cells cannot be isolated with the same degree of purity as neurons, which makes it impossible to repeat this experiment with glial cells. From the neuron experiment, however, we can conclude that sulphatide synthesis is decreased not only by a possible reduction of cell number but also by a decrease in enzymic activity per cell. Since the increase in sulphatide synthesis around the 8th postnatal day is a step in the normal development of the cell, the question remains open of how the mutation affects this development.

*Bernsohn:* Has anyone tried enzyme replacement experiments? What would happen if you administered the galactosyl transferase to these Jimpy mice or Quaking mice? Since you are talking about young mice under 30 days of age, the possibility that enzymes may get into the brain after intraperitoneal or intravenous administration is fairly strong. It would be interesting to see whether this modified the natural course of the disease.

*Herschkowitz:* We have not tried to substitute galactocerebroside sulphotransferase, a microsomal enzyme, in Jimpy mice. However, we successfully replaced a lysosomal enzyme, arylsulphatase A (cerebroside sulphatase) in fibroblasts of patients with metachromatic leucodystrophy. These fibroblasts lack the enzyme which degrades sulphatide. If a preparation of enriched arylsulphatase A is added to the medium in which the cells grow, the fibroblasts take up the enzyme by pinocytosis and become capable of degrading the lipid. As far as I know it is not possible to replace microsomal enzymes, but there might be a possibility of inducing the enzyme activity. This has not yet been tried.

*Hollingsworth:* When you were speaking of nutritional effects, Dr Herschkowitz, did you mean a specific lack of tryptophan or some other amino acid in the diet or a specific lack of a vitamin or a fatty acid? People have been discussing the elongation of fatty acid chains, presumably by enzyme activity. Evidently the elongation of certain fatty acid chains requires the presence of pyridoxine (vitamin $B_6$). What really do you mean by the nutritional factors you are talking about?

*Herschkowitz:* In my paper I was using mostly models which show general principles and I was not thinking in terms of specific nutritional defects, apart from tryptophan. I wanted to suggest that in general, environmental factors of nutrition could interfere in one of these ways with these mechanisms.

*Mead:* There has been a continuous controversy about the role of pyridoxine in the chain elongation of essential fatty acids since Witten and Holman (1952) and others found that skin symptoms in deficiencies of both factors are similar and respond partially to administration of either. There has since been considerable argument for and against such a role, but most of the evidence seems to support only an indirect action of pyridoxine, possibly concerned with the formation of the enzymes involved. As a matter of fact, Stoffel (1963) has reported that pyridoxal phosphate actually inhibits fatty acid elongation *in vitro*.

*Winick:* On the specificity of tryptophan, Munro used tryptophan as a limiting amino acid as measured by the disaggregation of polysomes, but he feels that this can be done *in vitro* by limiting almost any amino acid and that tryptophan happens to be the usual limiting amino acid in proteins as they are supplied (see Munro 1964-1970). This too may be a more general phenomenon and may involve the limiting of any amino acid or in fact a protein deprivation, rather than a specific reaction to tryptophan.

*Aebi:* Dr Herschkowitz mentioned cholesterol biosynthesis as an example of end-product inhibition in enzyme regulation. He stated that synthesis of cholesterol stops in rat and man when cholesterol exceeds 0.5% in the diet. I am not sure whether this is true for man. As you know, this problem is of considerable practical relevance regarding the recommendations to be given to the public about lipid intake.

*Mead:* In the rat, as you say, dietary cholesterol regulates cholesterol synthesis in the liver, but in man it is much more complicated and the synthesis of cholesterol in the liver does not respond to dietary cholesterol. I think this is partly because in man, the enterohepatic circulation provides enough cholesterol to inhibit its own synthesis in the liver, and a dietary increase of cholesterol provides little more, so we don't really know how cholesterol synthesis is regulated in man.

*Crawford:* What sort of man are you talking about? We have studied the El Molo in Africa who have blood cholesterol concentrations averaging about 96 mg% in the 16-25 year age group and 139 mg% for the adult middle-aged group. This is quite different from the value in age-matched Europeans, which was 215 mg% (Crawford, Crawford and Hansen 1971).

*Mead:* If you isolate the cholesterol-synthesizing enzymes from a man, whatever his colour, the system responds to cholesterol in the same way as does the cholesterol synthetase from rat liver. So in man we are dealing with a different type of regulatory mechanism, probably at a different level.

*Crawford:* I agree that the enzymic equipment is similar, regardless of race or creed, but there are major differences among people living on contrasting food structures: you can find groups with plasma cholesterols of less than 100 mg% as adults. Has anyone looked at people who normally have low blood cholesterol concentrations and established whether cholesterol synthesis is shut off by exogenous cholesterol?

*Mead:* Cholesterol absorption is regulated by dietary cholesterol in man, which is apparently not true in the rat.

*Paoletti:* The inhibition of cholesterol biosynthesis in liver by dietary cholesterol is present at least in the Masai, because, apparently, they absorb more cholesterol than Caucasian populations. This may be enough to suppress the biosynthesis of cholesterol for many hours during the day. What is more relevant to this meeting is that the synthesis of cholesterol in brain is not affected by dietary cholesterol, or even by diet. In starvation, brain cholesterol biosynthesis still goes on in young animals while liver cholesterol biosynthesis is completely stopped. The brain is quite independent of caloric intake in this respect.

*Dobbing:* The brain is a place where there are enormous quantities of cholesterol which are almost entirely synthesized there, although the whole molecule will enter the brain, but under ordinary circumstances this is a very small proportion of the amount accumulated (Dobbing 1963). In the rat, plasma cholesterol levels in the first 3 weeks are three times those in the adult rat. It seems to me very unlikely, and I'm glad to have Dr Paoletti confirm this, that alterations of dietary cholesterol or even plasma cholesterol would alter this state of affairs.

*Paoletti:* Brain tumours, by contrast, are sensitive to dietary conditions, and during starvation a growing brain is still able to make cholesterol but cholesterol synthesis in brain tumours is greatly reduced. This is of practical interest, because brain tumours do not utilize plasma cholesterol; the rate of growth of brain tumours depends directly on the amount of cholesterol synthesized in the tumour cells. Any dietary or pharmacological means of reducing cholesterol biosynthesis in brain tumours also reduces the rate of growth of the tumour. This is a different condition from many peripheral tumours.

## References

AEBI, H. (1967) In *Proc. 3rd International Congress of Human Genetics*, pp. 189-205, ed. J. F. Crow and J. V. Neel. The Johns Hopkins Press, Baltimore

AEBI, H. and SUTER, H. (1971) *Advances in Human Genetics*, pp. 143-199, ed. H. Harris and K. Hirschhorn. Plenum Press, New York and London

CRAWFORD, M. A., CRAWFORD, S. M. and HANSEN, I. B. (1971) *Biochem. J.* **122**, 11P

DOBBING, J. (1963) *J. Neurochem.* **10**, 739-742

MUNRO, H. N. (1964-1970) *Mammalian Protein Metabolism*, vol. 1-4, ed. H. N. Munro and J. B. Allison. Academic Press, New York

NORTON, W. T. and PODUSLO, S. E. (1970) *Science* **167**, 1144-1146

STOFFEL, W. (1963) *Z. Physiol. Chem.* **333**, 71-88

WITTEN, P. W. and HOLMAN, R. T. (1952) *Arch. Biochem.* **41**, 266-273

# Effects of essential fatty acid deficiency on the central nervous system in the growing rat

R. PAOLETTI and C. GALLI

*Institute of Pharmacology and Pharmacognosy, University of Milan*

Deficiency in essential fatty acids (EFA) initiated before birth and continued up to one year induces extensive modifications in rat brain. The brain weight is decreased, total lipid and phospholipid concentrations are diminished and the fatty acid composition of the phospholipids, especially ethanolamine phosphoglyceride (EPG), which is a major, highly unsaturated phospholipid constituent of brain membranes, is considerably modified (Galli, White and Paoletti 1970; White, Galli and Paoletti 1971).

Previous investigations in this laboratory have shown that substitution of a control diet for the deficient diet, after different periods of deficiency, induces a rebound of the levels of the *n*–6 fatty acids, so that values for 20:4, 22:4 and 22:5 exceed the corresponding amounts in the control animals. Concomitantly, the *n*–9 acids decrease below the control level, whereas *n*–3 fatty acids remain or return to normal. The overadjustment in the n–6 and *n*–9 families continues even after a prolonged recovery period on the control diet (White, Galli and Paoletti 1971).

In the present study the phospholipids of brain subcellular fractions such as myelin, mitochondria, microsomes and synaptosomes, which differ in their fatty acid composition (Cotman *et al.* 1969; Sun and Horrocks 1970), have been analysed after purification from brains of normal and EFA-deficient rats.

In particular, the fatty acid compositions of EPG in myelin, mitochondrial, microsomal and synaptosomal fractions have been determined both in normal rats and in rats kept from birth up to a period of 140 days on an EFA-deficient diet.

MATERIALS AND METHODS

Pregnant rats of the Sprague-Dawley strain were fed *ad libitum* with either a fat-free diet, or the same diet with 2% corn oil added, starting approximately one week before delivery (Aaes-Jørgensen and Holman 1958).

The basic percentage composition of the two diets was: sucrose 70, alpha-cellulose 4, vitamin-free casein 20, vitamin mix 1, salt mix 4, choline chloride 1. The relative contents of essential fatty acids in the two diets were 0.84% linoleate and 0.004% linolenate in the control diet and 0.023% and 0.001%, respectively in the deficient diet.

The fatty acid composition of the milk of the lactating rats kept on the deficient diet was considerably modified from that of the controls. Linoleic acid decreased from 14.2% to 4.2% after 5 days of lactation and from 9.3% to 1.3% after 10 days. These results indicate that the EFA intake of the suckling deficient rats was considerably decreased.

Groups of control and deficient rats were sacrificed at 3, 10, 30, 60, 90, 180 and 365 days after birth. Four additional groups of rats on a combination dietary programme (initial period on the deficient diet, D, followed by a period on the control diet, C) were also studied (groups 10D + 20C, 30D + 30C, 10D + 50C, 90D + 90C).

Body and brain weights were measured and brains from all groups were pooled for lipid analysis, with the exception of the 60-day-old control and deficient animals, which were examined individually.

The lipids were extracted (Rouser *et al.* 1966), ethanolamine phosphoglyceride was isolated by thin-layer chromatography (White, Galli and Paoletti 1971) and fatty acid methyl esters were prepared, purified from aldehydes and analysed by gas-liquid chromatography (Galli, White and Paoletti 1970). By this procedure total fatty acids, deriving from both the monoacyl (plasmalogen) and the diacyl forms of EPG, were analysed. Fatty acids were identified by the use of reference compounds and by a combination of gas chromatography and mass spectrometry (model LKB 9000).

Further groups of control and deficient animals were sacrificed at 140 days and used for the preparation of subcellular fractions. The brains were divided longitudinally, one half being used for subfractionation and the other for total lipid extraction.

Myelin was prepared by the method of Smith (1968). Microsomal and mitochondrial fractions were prepared according to Sun and Horrocks (1970). Synaptosomal fractions were prepared as the $P_2B_2$ fraction according to Whittaker, Michaelson and Kirkland (1964). The purity of the fractions was checked by electron microscopy.

## RESULTS AND DISCUSSION

### *Effect of EFA deficiency and refeeding on brain growth*

The effects of the different diets on brain and body weights in developing rats are shown in Tables 1 and 2. Brain weights up to the age of 6 months are always lower in the deficient animals than in the controls (White, Galli and Paoletti 1971) (Table 1).

TABLE 1

Body and brain weights of growing rats fed control diets (C), EFA-deficient diets (D) and EFA-deficient diets followed by control diets

| | | *Body weight* | | *Brain weight* | |
|---|---|---|---|---|---|
| *Group* | *Number in group* | *Observed g* | *% difference from control* | *Observed mg* | *% difference from control* |
| 10C | 11 | 21 ± 0.4* | | 955 ± 14 | |
| 10D | 9 | 18 ± 0.4° | −14 | 858 ± 8° | −10 |
| 30C | 4 | 46 ± 1.0 | | 1388 ± 7 | |
| 30D | 4 | 45 ± 1.6 | − 2 | 1346 ± 30 | − 3 |
| 10D + 20C | 4 | 56 ± 1.0° | +22 | 1477 ± 19† | + 6 |
| 60C | 6 | 177 ± 9 | | 1702 ± 35 | |
| 60D | 5 | 108 ± 6° | −39 | 1655 ± 21 | − 3 |
| 10D + 50C | 7 | 147 ± 8† | −17 | 1680 ± 12 | − 1 |
| 30D + 30C | 3 | 180 ± 13 | + 2 | 1642 ± 54 | − 4 |
| 90C | 4 | 375 ± 8 | | 1911 ± 46 | |
| 90D | 3 | 128 ± 1° | −66 | 1517 ± 39· | −21 |
| 180C | 2 | 400 ± 4 | | 1838 ± 1 | |
| 180D | 2 | 214 ± 6· | −46 | 1726 ± 56 | − 6 |
| 90D + 90C | 2 | 385 ± 7 | − 4 | 1955 ± 18 † | + 6 |

* Values are means ± S.E.M.
Values indicated as follows are significantly different from control values at the *P* levels shown: °, $P < 0.001$; ·, $P < 0.01$; †, $P < 0.05$.

In animals made EFA deficient for 30 and 90 days respectively and then kept on the control diet for equal periods of time, brain and body size show a complete rehabilitation. Table 2 shows that EFA deficiency modifies the normal brain weight/body weight percentage ratio in a reversible way.

TABLE 2

Brain weight as percentage of body weight

| *Treatment* | *% brain weight* | |
|---|---|---|
| 10 C | 4.61 | ± 0.12 |
| 10 D | 4.68 | ± 0.08 |
| 30 C | 3.01 | ± 0.08 |
| 30 D | 2.99 | ± 0.16 |
| 10 D + 20 C | 2.66 | ± 0.08• |
| 60 C | 0.97 | ± 0.04 |
| 60 D | 1.56 | ± 0.11° |
| 10 D + 50 C | 1.17 | ± 0.07† |
| 30 D + 30 C | 0.92 | ± 0.05 |
| 90 C | 0.51 | ± 0.02 |
| 90 D | 1.18 | ± 0.03° |
| 180 C | 0.45 | ± 0.01 |
| 180 D | 0.81 | ± 0.07† |
| 90 D + 90 C | 0.50 | ± 0.03 |

Significance levels in respect of controls: °, $P < 0.001$; •, $P < 0.02$; †, $P < 0.05$.

The fatty acid composition of brain phospholipids, and especially of ethanolamine phosphoglyceride, a lipid class particularly affected by essential fatty acid deficiency (Galli, White and Paoletti 1970), is progressively modified at various periods of deficiency (3 days to one year after birth), as shown in Table 3. The three major fatty acid families of oleate (*n*–9), linoleate (*n*–6) and linolenate (*n*–3) show different changes. In normal development, *n*–9 acids

TABLE 3

Ethanolamine phosphoglyceride fatty acid families in brain as molar percentages of total fatty acids in control (C) and EFA-deficient (D) rats

| *Days* | *(n–9) acids* | | *(n–6) acids* | | *(n–3) acids* | | *Unsaturation index* | |
|---|---|---|---|---|---|---|---|---|
| | *C* | *D* | *C* | *D* | *C* | *D* | *C* | *D* |
| 3 | 11.2 | 11.8 | 30.8 | 29.2 | 14.8 | 16.5 | 233 | 238 |
| 10 | 11.8 | 10.6 | 30.2 | 27.9 | 14.7 | 16.3 | 225 | 225 |
| 30 | 23.5 | 29.4 | 28.2 | 24.1 | 12.9 | 14.0 | 218 | 223 |
| 60 | 32.1 | 38.8 | 24.3 | 21.0 | 10.3 | 9.7 | 201 | 191 |
| 90 | 34.8 | 41.8 | 24.7 | 19.5 | 10.2 | 12.2 | 201 | 201 |
| 180 | 41.1 | 52.4 | 19.6 | 14.4 | 13.7 | 7.2 | 202 | 181 |
| 365 | 38.4 | 49.0 | 17.3 | 11.8 | 9.8 | 5.3 | 167 | 163 |

(mostly monoenes with 18 and 20 carbon atoms) increase continually, whereas *n*–6 (mostly 20:4, 22:4 and 22:5) are reduced to about two-thirds after 12 months and *n*–3 acids (mostly 22:6) do not change significantly up to 6 months and decrease later on. In EFA-deficient animals, *n*–9 acids increase after 20 days, and, in contrast *n*–6 decrease after 10 days, compared to control values; *n*–3 fatty acids are affected only after 6 months.

It is of interest that the modification in the fatty acid composition of EPG continues long after the peak of brain growth and lipid deposition, which occurs at the age of 15 days in the rat (Dobbing 1971).

The unsaturation index, which represents the average number of double bonds per fatty acid molecule (White, Galli and Paoletti 1971), remains unchanged in the deficient group, however, indicating that the phospholipid molecule maintains a constant level of unsaturation of its fatty acids, regardless of the amount of essential fatty acids in the diet.

The modifications observed in the *n*–9 and *n*–6 fatty acid families consist mainly of a rise of *n*–9 trienes (20:3 and 22:3) and a reduction of *n*–6 tetraenes (20:4 and 22:4), resulting in an increase of the triene/tetraene ratio, which is considered to be a biochemical index of EFA deficiency (Holman 1960). This ratio increases almost linearly up to the age of 12 months in the deficient rats, indicating that replacement of fatty acids in the brain is practically independent of the deposition of new lipids (Table 4).

TABLE 4

Triene/tetraene ratios in brain ethanolamine phosphoglycerides at various ages in control and EFA-deficient rats

| | *Days of age* | | | | | | |
|---|---|---|---|---|---|---|---|
| | *3* | *10* | *30* | *60* | *90* | *180* | *365* |
| Control rats | 0.063 | 0.054 | 0.073 | 0.079 | 0.070 | 0.068 | 0.041 |
| EFA-deficient rats | 0.083 | 0.083 | 0.216 | 0.381 | 0.590 | 1.370 | 1.960 |

## *Reversal of EFA deficiency in growing rats*

When the control diet is fed to rats previously kept deficient for various periods of time, there is a reduction of the *n*–9 and an elevation of the *n*–6 fatty acids, in comparison to control values (White, Galli and Paoletti 1971). Tetraenes, especially, are consistently higher in the deficient rats put on a control diet (D + C) than in the controls (C) of the same age group, as shown in Table 5. This is termed the ‘rebound’ phenomenon.

TABLE 5

Dietary influence on fatty acids of the *n*–9, *n*–6 and *n*–3 families in ethanolamine phosphoglycerides (molar percentages) of brains of male rats

| | *Age of rats and dietary treatment* | | | | | | | | | |
|---|---|---|---|---|---|---|---|---|---|---|
| | *30 days* | | | *60 days* | | | | *180 days* | | |
| | *30 C* | *10 D + 20 C* | *30 D* | *60 C* | *10 D + 50 C* | *30 D + 30 C* | *60 D* | *180 C* | *90 D + 90 C* | *180 D* |
| | (*4*)* | (*4*) | (*4*) | (*6*) | (*7*) | (*3*) | (*5*) | (*2*) | (*2*) | (*2*) |
| *n–9 family* | | | | | | | | | | |
| 18:1 | 19.2 | 16.7 | 23.0 | 26.6 | 25.1 | 23.7 | 27.7 | 32.2 | 25.9 | 32.0 |
| 20:1 | 3.1 | 2.5 | 3.5 | 4.5 | 4.5 | 4.6 | 5.1 | 8.1 | 6.2 | 7.8 |
| 20:2 | 0.5 | 0.5 | 0.6 | 0.4 | 0.5 | 0.6 | 0.8 | 0.3 | 0.4 | 0.9 |
| 20:3 | 0.5 | 0.4 | 1.2 | 0.3 | 0.4 | 0.8 | 3.7 | 0.3 | 0.6 | 8.6 |
| 22:3 | 0.2 | 0.2 | 1.1 | 0.3 | 0.3 | 0.5 | 1.5 | 0.2 | 0.8 | 3.1 |
| Total | 23.5 | 20.3 | 29.4 | 32.1 | 30.8 | 30.2 | 38.8 | 41.1 | 33.9 | 52.4 |
| *n–6 family* | | | | | | | | | | |
| 18:2 | 0.5 | 0.5 | 0.2 | 0.4 | 0.4 | 0.3 | 0.2 | 0.6 | 0.4 | 0.1 |
| 20:2 | 0.5 | 0.4 | 0.4 | 0.4 | 0.3 | 0.3 | 0.2 | 0.3 | 0.2 | — |
| 20:3 | 0.9 | 1.0 | 0.9 | 0.7 | 0.7 | 0.5 | 1.7 | 0.7 | 0.3 | 0.6 |
| 20:4 | 14.6 | 15.2 | 12.5 | 12.0 | 12.8 | 12.8 | 10.2 | 10.9 | 12.2 | 6.8 |
| 22:3 | 0.3 | 0.3 | 0.8 | 0.3 | 0.2 | 0.2 | 0.3 | — | 0.1 | 0.3 |
| 22:4 | 7.6 | 8.7 | 5.6 | 7.2 | 7.3 | 6.8 | 5.0 | 6.4 | 7.2 | 3.1 |
| 22:5 | 3.0 | 3.4 | 2.4 | 2.6 | 4.4 | 4.2 | 2.8 | 0.4 | 2.7 | 3.5 |
| 24:4 | 0.8 | 1.0 | 1.3 | 0.7 | 0.7 | 0.7 | 0.6 | 0.3 | 0.7 | 0.02 |
| Total | 28.2 | 30.5 | 24.1 | 24.3 | 26.8 | 25.8 | 21.0 | 19.6 | 23.8 | 14.42 |
| *n–3 family* | | | | | | | | | | |
| 22:5 | 0.3 | 0.5 | 1.4 | 0.4 | 0.3 | 0.4 | 0.2 | 0.3 | 0.6 | 0.02 |
| 22:6 | 12.6 | 14.8 | 12.6 | 9.9 | 10.2 | 10.2 | 9.5 | 13.4 | 13.8 | 7.2 |
| Total | 12.9 | 15.3 | 14.0 | 10.3 | 10.5 | 10.6 | 9.7 | 13.7 | 14.4 | 7.2 |

* Number of animals in group.
10 D + 20 C = 10 days on deficient diet + 20 days on control diet.
10 D + 50 C = 10 days on deficient diet + 50 days on control diet.
30 D + 30 C = 30 days on deficient diet + 30 days on control diet.
90 D + 90 C = 90 days on deficient diet + 90 days on control diet.

## *EFA deficiency and myelin fatty acids*

The fatty acid composition of ethanolamine phosphoglyceride isolated from myelin obtained from 180-day-old control rats, deficient rats, and deficient rats subsequently put on a control diet (90D + 90C), reveals changes similar to those observed in the whole brain (Table 6). Tetraenes are sharply reduced in the group of rats made deficient for 6 months, whereas trienes are considerably

TABLE 6

Fatty acid distribution (molar percentage) of ethanolamine phosphoglyceride in myelin of 180-day-old male rats

| | *Dietary treatment* | | |
|---|---|---|---|
| *Fatty acids* | *Control diet for 6 months* | *Deficient diet for 3 months + control diet for 3 months* | *Deficient diet for 6 months* |
| Saturates | 14.2 | 14.7 | 14.5 |
| Monoenes | 65.1 | 64.7 | 61.5 |
| Polyenes | 20.7 | 20.5 | 24.0 |
| Dienes | 1.8 | 1.9 | 1.8 |
| Trienes | 2.3 | 3.9 | 12.2 |
| Tetraenes | 12.9 | 11.9 | 6.8 |
| Pentaenes | 0.5 | 1.0 | 1.6 |
| Hexaenes | 3.2 | 1.8 | 1.6 |
| *n*–9 acids | 64.9 | 67.0 | 72.7 |
| *n*–6 acids | 16.4 | 14.8 | 9.7 |
| *n*–3 acids | 3.4 | 1.9 | 1.8 |
| Unsaturation index | 149 | 144 | 147 |
| Triene/tetraene ratio | 0.18 | 0.33 | 1.79 |

elevated. In the D + C group, these changes are practically reversed, except for trienes and pentaenes remaining slightly higher, and hexaenes slightly lower than in control myelin. The rebound phenomenon of *n*–6 acids does not appear in myelin EPG fatty acids, suggesting a relatively slower turnover in a more stable structure. The considerable reduction of trienes and elevation of tetraenes in myelin EPG in the 90D + 90C group, however, indicates that the turnover of myelin lipids or the exchange of their fatty acids continues even in the adult brain.

It is also interesting to note that the triene/tetraene ratio is higher in myelin (1.79) than in the whole brain (1.37) of the same animals.

## *Effects of EFA deficiency on brain subcellular fractions*

Table 7 shows the molar percentages of ethanolamine phosphoglyceride fatty acids in brain subcellular fractions of 140-day-old control and deficient rats. The results are the averages of at least two analyses on each of two preparations of the subcellular fractions.

The normal fatty acid composition of myelin, mitochondria and microsomes is found to be rather similar to that reported by Sun and Horrocks (1970) for the corresponding fractions isolated from normal mouse brain. Myelin has distinctly higher levels of monoenes and lower levels of saturates, tetraenes and

TABLE 7

Fatty acid composition (molar percentage) of ethanolamine phosphoglyceride in brain subcellular fractions in 140-day-old control (C) and deficient (D) rats

| | *Synaptosomes* | | *Mitochondria* | | *Microsomes* | | *Myelin* | |
|---|---|---|---|---|---|---|---|---|
| | *C* | *D* | *C* | *D* | *C* | *D* | *C* | *D* |
| Saturates | 35.3 | 31.2 | 38.1 | 39.3 | 29.8 | 32.2 | 18.4 | 17.2 |
| Monoenes | 9.0 | 8.4 | 10.2 | 11.2 | 16.4 | 13.9 | 56.5 | 54.7 |
| Dienes | 0.3 | 0.4 | 0.3 | 0.2 | trace | 0.4 | 1.5 | 2.0 |
| Trienes | trace | 12.6 | 0.3 | 10.2 | trace | 11.0 | 2.2 | 13.2 |
| Tetraenes | 24.7 | 17.4 | 22.3 | 13.5 | 22.8 | 14.2 | 15.6 | 6.9 |
| Pentaenes | 6.8 | 6.4 | 8.5 | 6.0 | 9.7 | 7.1 | 2.5 | 2.4 |
| Hexaenes | 24.0 | 23.3 | 19.9 | 19.4 | 21.9 | 21.2 | 3.1 | 2.8 |
| Polyenes | 55.8 | 60.1 | 51.3 | 49.3 | 54.4 | 53.9 | 24.9 | 27.3 |

hexaenes (mainly 22:6 (*n*–3)), whereas in mitochondria, microsomes and synaptosomes, saturates, tetraenes and hexaenes (especially in synaptosomes) predominate. The values for the EFA-deficient rats show changes similar to those previously described for the whole brain, mainly consisting of a rise in *n*–9 trienes (20:3 and 22:3) and a decrease in *n*–6 tetraenes, whereas hexaenes are practically unaffected. It is of interest that the rise in trienes in myelin during EFA deficiency is greater than that in other fractions.

Calculation of the product/precursor ratios for acids of the *n*–6 family, derived from arachidonate (A = 22:4/20:4 and B = 22:5/22:4), provides an index of the prevalence of elongation (A) or desaturation (B) within the family. In myelin the ratio favours elongation, as shown in Table 8, whereas in the other fractions desaturation is higher. In the deficient rats, the 22:4/20:4 ratio is decreased while the 22:5/22:4 is increased in all fractions, suggesting a shift towards more unsaturated members of the *n*–6 series in structural phospholipids of subcellular membranes in EFA deficiency.

A shift towards more elongated members of the same family in myelin is also supported by the higher 22:3/20:3 ratio in this fraction than in the other subcellular components (Table 8).

The ratios of trienes to tetraenes in the various subcellular fractions of control and deficient rats are shown in Table 9. Myelin EPG in EFA-deficient animals has a triene/tetraene ratio which is more than twice that observed in the mitochondrial and microsomal fractions, indicating that the fatty acid composition of myelin lipids is more deeply modified than that of other structures, in contrast to the widely accepted concept that myelin has a greater metabolic stability than other types of membranes. These results suggest a progressive accumulation of trienes in myelin, by way of continuous exchange of the non-polar residues of the lipid components within the myelin sheath.

TABLE 8

Product: precursor ratios for fatty acids of the $n$–6 and $n$–9 families in ethanolamine phosphoglyceride from brain subcellular fractions of control (C) and deficient (D) rats

| *Ratio* | | *Whole brain* | | *Synaptosomal fraction* | | *Mitochondrial fraction* | | *Microsomal fraction* | | *Myelin fraction* | |
|---|---|---|---|---|---|---|---|---|---|---|---|
| | | *C* | *D* | *C* | *D* | *C* | *D* | *C* | *D* | *C* | *D* |
| ($n$–6) | 22:4/20:4 | 0.466 | 0.341 | 0.383 | 0.282 | 0.303 | 0.193 | 0.490 | 0.347 | 0.709 | 0.680 |
| ($n$–6) | 22:5/22:4 | 0.554 | 1.627 | 0.986 | 1.611 | 1.642 | 2.400 | 1.322 | 1.790 | 0.271 | 0.469 |
| ($n$–9) | 22:3/20:3 | — | 0.33 | — | 0.20 | — | 0.19 | — | 0.25 | — | 0.52 |

TABLE 9

Triene: tetraene ratio in ethanolamine phosphoglyceride in whole brain and subcellular fractions from control (C) and deficient (D) rats

| *Whole brain* | | *Synaptosomal fraction* | | *Mitochondrial fraction* | | *Microsomal fraction* | | *Myelin fraction* | |
|---|---|---|---|---|---|---|---|---|---|
| *C* | *D* | *C* | *D* | *C* | *D* | *C* | *D* | *C* | *D* |
| 0.053 | 1.264 | 0.083 | 0.724 | 0.016 | 0.752 | — | 0.778 | 0.132 | 1.920 |

*EFA deficiency and behavioural changes*

The same groups of rats kept for 90 days on an EFA-deficient diet have been tested behaviourally, together with control animals of the same strain (C. Galli and R. Oberosler, unpublished data). The rats have been tested for conditioned-avoidance responses (Cicala and Corey 1965) in a shuttle-box apparatus. The performance of the EFA-deficient rats was lower than that of the control rats, the difference being highly significant after the third, fourth and fifth session of a 5-day training programme (Fig. 1). This difference may be accounted for by

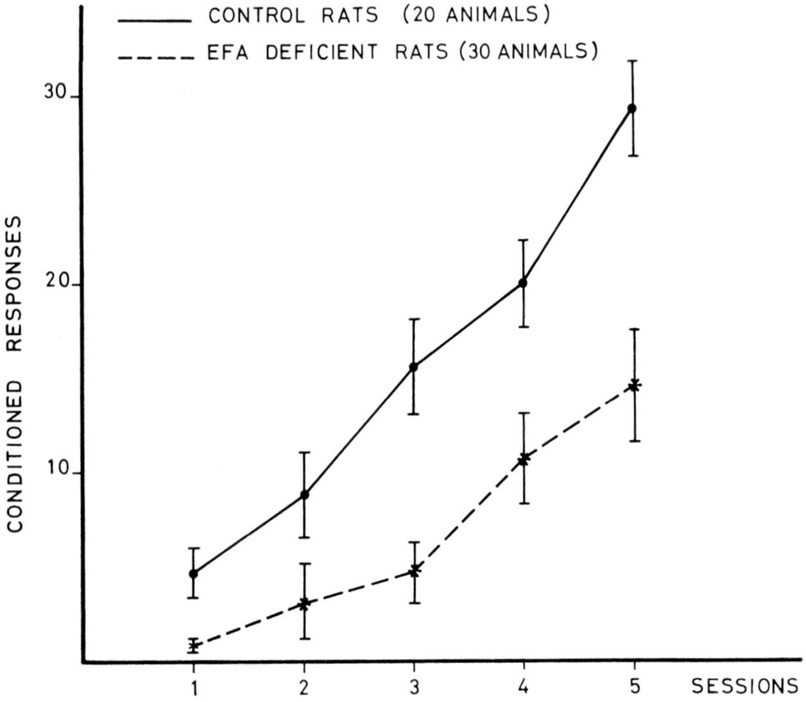


FIG. 1. Conditioned-avoidance responses of control and EFA-deficient rats tested in a shuttle-box apparatus.

the larger number of deficient animals unable to respond to the avoidance test in comparison to the control rats (Fig. 2).

These results, confirmed in many independent experiments, suggest a correlation between changes in dietary and brain lipid composition and one behavioural parameter at least. Investigations on the significance and reversibility of this behavioural change are in progress.

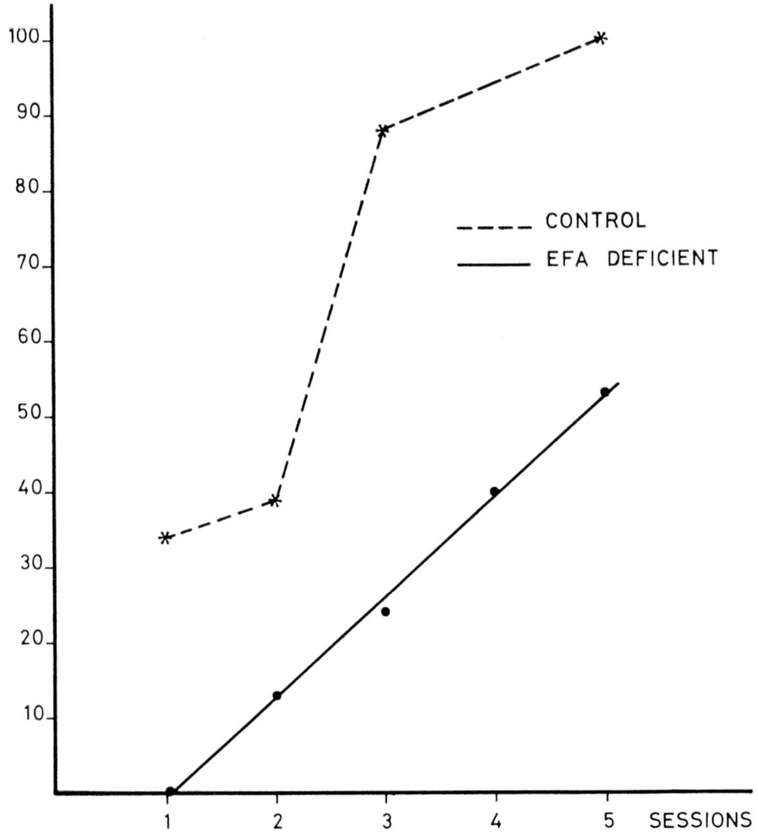


FIG. 2. Percentages of EFA-deficient and control rats which became conditioned in the avoidance-response test. The total number of trials was 50.

SUMMARY

Groups of rats were kept during the last week of pregnancy on a diet deficient in essential fatty acids (EFA), and their offspring were maintained on the same diet for various periods of time after weaning.

The deficient rats were examined for the fatty acid composition of phospholipid of total brain and of brain fractions (myelin, synaptosomes, mitochondria and microsomes) and changes were evaluated during the EFA deficiency and in the periods of recovery on a control diet.

During the period of growth, the EFA-deficient rats were able to recover completely if they were returned to the control diet.

The behaviour of normal and EFA-deficient rats has also been compared. The EFA-deficient rats show impairment of performance in a specific behavioural test.

ACKNOWLEDGEMENTS

The technical assistance of Mrs Dora Di Girolamo and the suggestions of the experimental psychologist Dr Rolando Oberosler are gratefully acknowledged.
The investigations have been supported in part by the Consiglio Nazionale delle Ricerche, Rome.

## References

AAES-JØRGENSEN, E. and HOLMAN, R. T. (1958) *J. Nutr.* **65**, 633-641
CICALA, G. A. and COREY, J. R. (1965) *Exp. Psychol.* **70**, 436-7
COTMAN, C., BLANK, M. L., MOEHL, A. and SNYDER, F. (1969) *Biochemistry* **8**, 4606-4612
DOBBING, J. (1971) In *Chemistry and Brain Development*, pp. 399-412, ed. R. Paoletti and A. N. Davison. Plenum Press, New York
GALLI, C., WHITE, H. B., JR and PAOLETTI, R. (1970) *J. Neurochem.* **17**, 347-355
HOLMAN, R. T. (1960) *J. Nutr.* **70**, 405-410
ROUSER, G., KRITCHEVSKY, G., GALLI, C., YAMAMOTO, A. and KNUDSON, A. G., JR (1966) In *Inborn Disorders of Sphingolipid Metabolism*, pp. 303-316, ed. S. M. Aronson and B. W. Volk. Pergamon Press, Oxford
SMITH, M. E. (1968) *Biochim. Biophys. Acta* **164**, 285-293
SUN, G. Y. and HORROCKS, L. A. (1970) *Lipids* **5**, 1006-1012
WHITE, H. B., JR, GALLI, C. and PAOLETTI, R. (1971) *J. Neurochem.* **18**, 869-882
WHITTAKER, V. P., MICHAELSON, I. A. and KIRKLAND, R. J. (1964) *Biochem. J.* **90**, 293-303

## Discussion

*Davison:* How many animals were studied in the measurements of fatty acid changes in whole brain and the different subcellular fractions, including myelin?

*Paoletti:* The groups varied in number from two (one-year-old rats) to eleven animals; there were usually six animals in each group. We studied both individual animals and pooled brains (four in each group) for the preparation of subcellular fractions. The studies on the distribution of fatty acids were made on individual animals at one age (60 days) and on pooled brains for the other age groups.

*Ansell:* Did you distinguish between the two major ethanolamine phospho glycerides, the diacyl and the plasmalogen forms?

*Paoletti:* This distinction was not made in this study.

*Lloyd*: Have you information on changes in lipids in tissues other than brain? Presumably there is considerable deficiency of essential fatty acids in other tissues; is it possible to make the assumption that if changes are detected in blood, or adipose tissue, or the red cell membrane, similar changes will be found in brain? If so, we can get a good deal of information in the early weeks and months of life on children in whom deficiency of essential fatty acids may occur and can be demonstrated in blood and red cell membranes. This brings me to a further question: do we really have evidence for the 'essentiality' of these fatty acids in the human infant?

*Paoletti:* In rat liver, plasma and adipose tissue the changes are much more profound than in brain at the same age. If the deficient diet is given to rats older than 30 days, the brain is only slightly affected, while the fatty acid composition in peripheral tissue is greatly changed.

We have no direct experience of human deficiency. However, studies in our laboratory have revealed that a chemical marker may be used to follow brain maturation; this is the ratio between desmosterol and cholesterol. Desmosterol (24-dehydrocholesterol) is a constant component of foetal and growing animal and human brains until myelin is completely deposited. In newborn human brain, desmosterol represents 1-2% of total brain sterols and practically disappears later on (Fumagalli and Paoletti 1963).

*von Muralt:* What happens in a deficiency of essential fatty acids in man?

*Lloyd:* I think it is still very difficult to find evidence for a clear-cut role for essential fatty acids in man. We have had the opportunity over the past 11 years to study a small group of children in whom severe essential fatty acid deficiency (as judged by blood, red cell membrane and adipose tissue studies) has been present from birth (Barnard, Fosbrooke and Lloyd 1970). These are children with the rare condition of abetalipoproteinaemia, in whom not only is there malabsorption of fat due to failure of chylomicron formation, but also gross depletion of the plasma lipoprotein transport system (Farquhar and Ways 1966). Part of the symptomatic treatment of this disorder is to control steatorrhoea by further reduction of the fat intake. Thus there is continuing deficiency in the intake and absorption of the essential fatty acids. Other deficiencies are, of course, also present, for example, of vitamins A and E. We have attempted to keep the vitamin A and E status of the children constant by giving large supplements, but we have not given additional essential fatty acids to any of the seven children in infancy, and only two of the seven have received small amounts of corn oil in later childhood. None of the children has shown any of the symptoms or signs ascribed to essential fatty acid deficiency in early childhood; their physical growth is satisfactory, and only one child shows evidence of intellectual retardation. Mental subnormality is not a feature of abetalipoproteinaemia. It is known, however, that towards the end of the first decade and during adolescence, individuals with this disorder develop an unusual ataxic neuropathy and a pigmentary retinopathy. Only one pathological study of nervous tissue has been described (Sobrevilla, Goodman and Kane 1964) which did suggest a demyelinating process, but no chemical studies have been reported.

*Paoletti:* One difference between children and our rats is that, at birth, children already have a depot of essential fatty acids in adipose tissue, while the rats have not, because the deficient diet has been given to the pregnant rats during the last part of pregnancy and continued during lactation.

*Lloyd:* These infants in fact have little adipose depot fat.

*Crawford:* But the child is born with about a 3-month supply of phospholipids in the liver, which it gets from the mother. It theoretically could survive on that, without considering other stores in muscle or depot fats. Lipid deficiency is concerned with long-term factors. Deficient animals can appear healthy from outside, but things may go wrong inside, and take effect later. The same may be true with your children. Our rat pups born from deficient mothers look healthy, but they die (see pp. 154, 277). In any event, we will not find out about the relevance of the lipids until we study them.

*Paoletti:* If the deficient diet is given to the offspring and not to the pregnant rats, as we did in earlier experiments, there is much less change in the brain. This indicates that the amount of essential fatty acids present in the newborn tissues, if they are not depleted before birth, is sufficient to provide the essential fatty acids supply for the brain.

*Winick:* On the possible non-specificity of this reaction, are your rats pair-fed? In other words, do you know that the experimental rats are eating as much of the fatty acid-deficient diet as the controls?

*Paoletti:* After weaning, the amount consumed is similar; this is shown by the curve of body growth which, in many groups of deficient rats, is not considerably changed. Up to the age of 21 days, during the lactation period, we don't know how much milk is taken.

*Winick:* So it is conceivable that during the first 21 days you have more than a fatty acid deficiency; that you may have a deficiency in the amount of milk consumed?

*Paoletti:* I tend to exclude this, because when we have measured the amount of milk present in the stomach of the newborn rats, it was not considerably different in the two groups, so I think lactation has been fairly normal. This is confirmed by the similar body weight in normal and EFA-deficient offspring at the end of lactation (Table 1, p. 123).

*Houtsmuller:* In rats, we find that with the same food consumption, growth is less on the essential fatty acid-deficient diet. That means that the caloric efficiency is lower. This has also been observed in man. Skin lesions occur in infants with too low a linoleic acid intake, as shown by Hansen and co-workers (1963) and by Warwick and co-workers (1959), and they have cured it by giving only linoleic acid.

*Crawford:* Some of the evidence on frank EFA deficiency in children has recently been reviewed (Soderhjelm, Wiese and Holman 1970).

*Mead:* Dr Houtsmuller has practically answered Dr Lloyd's question, but I could add a surprising observation made by Dr Holman, who has found essential fatty acid deficiency in an adult human, namely his mother, who, as she became elderly, went on a special diet and began suffering from essential fatty acid deficiency symptoms including severe dermatitis and loss of appetite. When he included essential fatty acid in her diet she recovered. This is the opposite end of the scale from the one of interest in this symposium, but Dr Holman has since found that elderly people have a tendency to suffer from this disease when they are on special diets.

Now, what is the cellular effect of essential fatty acid deficiency? We have lately been concerned mainly with cells in culture, because we think the whole animal is too complex to study this deficiency. In deficient cultured normal cells we have found a decrease of oxidative phosphorylation and a decrease in respiratory control, changes in transport into and out of the cell, and a decrease in growth rate. There may be other changes also, but these might all depend on a deficient membrane function (mitochondrial and plasma membrane), and possibly would be reflected in the symptoms we see in the whole animal.

*Paoletti:* The decrease in body weight in some of our deficient rats and in many other experiments is probably related to changes in endocrine and sympathetic nervous system functions which are modulated by prostaglandins—cyclized derivatives of essential fatty acids. Some of the symptoms of fatty acid deficiency are the symptoms of hyperthyroidism, and again I think this may be explained by a reduced formation of prostaglandins.

*Svennerholm:* I recently had the opportunity of seeing a 3-month-old Indian girl at the medical service of the Children's Hospital in Göteborg. She had essential fatty acid deficiency and presented the clinical picture of this deficiency described by Hansen and co-workers (1958). She had 13% eicosatrienoic acid (20:3(*n*–9)) in plasma lecithin and the linoleic acid was reduced to 8%. She was treated with intravenous infusion of Intralipid, in which linoleic acid constitutes 50% of the fatty acids. She recovered completely within 10 days on the ordinary hospital diet fortified with the linoleic acid infusion. From birth until first seen at the hospital she had been fed with diluted cow's milk, but nothing else. We have seen similar but milder subclinical forms in Finnish infants fed diluted cow's milk only.

*Lloyd:* While I am prepared to accept the individual instances of deficiency that are well documented, I remain sceptical about the overall concept; we certainly do not have the kind of evidence for a clear-cut deficiency state that we have, for example, for vitamin A deficiency or vitamin D deficiency. I think we need to examine the possibility of other factors operating in these individual case reports. There does seem to be a considerable difference in the experience of paediatricians in relation to so-called 'essential fatty acid deficiency' in infant human nutrition, and we clearly need a great deal more information.

*Svennerholm:* I don't fully understand this viewpoint. Professor Paoletti has described animal studies in which the animals were fed an almost completely linoleic acid-free diet. In these animals a pure form of essential fatty acid deficiency could be produced. We can never expect to get such unequivocal evidence for a pure essential fatty acid deficiency in human infants, but it appears warranted to classify a clinical syndrome in an infant as essential fatty acid deficiency if the biochemical tests show the same biochemical changes as in animals with a 'pure' deficiency. Do you mean that we should give infants a diet without any essential fatty acids in order to obtain more experience on fatty acid deficiency in human infant nutrition?

*Lloyd:* That is impossible.

*Hollingsworth:* In your experiments, Professor Paoletti, I take it that the dietary deficiency extended beyond linoleic acid to the other essential fatty acids?

*Paoletti:* The rats used in our experiments received a diet containing only trace doses of lipids and therefore, it was deficient in all the essential acids, including linolenic and arachidonic acids.

*Crawford:* What about the levels of arachidonic acid in the milk of the deficient mothers? You have analysed the milk of the pregnant rats and found that linoleic acid is low in the milk of those on the deficient diet. What about arachidonic and docosahexaenoic acids? One often finds that while linoleic and linolenic acids fall, lipids may still be quite rich in the long-chain polyunsaturated fatty acids (20:4 to 22:6).

*Paoletti:* The concentration of arachidonic acid in milk was measured and was decreased to 50-60% of the control levels. We have not measured docosahexaenoic acid.

*Aebi:* Is the type and intensity of manifestation of deficiency symptoms in your rats affected when different amounts of saturated fatty acids are given?

*Paoletti:* Not in very young rats. However, behavioural changes and chemical changes in phospholipid composition were more pronounced when the deficient diet was supplemented with saturated fat. In adult rats, published data indicate that saturated fats increase the symptoms of EFA deficiency (Evans and Lepkovsky 1932; Deuel *et al.* 1951; Aaes-Jørgensen and Holmer 1969).

*Aebi:* In Switzerland, the official figure for the dietary requirement for essential fatty acids is 4 to 7 g/day (for adults). This is likely to be a guess and should probably be revised. What would be your recommendation?

*Paoletti:* I think that 0.7 or 0.8% by weight of the unsaturated fatty acids might be sufficient. This was the amount present in the control diet used.

*Rossi:* Have you studied carbohydrate metabolism in these experiments? Clinically there is a special kind of hypoglycaemic state with a high level of free fatty acid, which is leucine-sensitive. In many cases there is no excretion of catecholamines. In these children the brain becomes atrophic and the head circumference is often smaller than normal, which suggests a relationship between carbohydrate metabolism and brain development (see Cochrane *et al.* 1956; Rossi, Zuppinger and Joss 1969).

*Paoletti:* I wonder if some of these effects may be related to changes in secretion of the growth hormone. Changes in blood glucose considerably affect the output of growth hormone. On the other hand, there is evidence that while the brain grows almost to its maximal size even in the absence of growth hormone, the skull growth requires growth hormone. So, if during the critical periods the release of growth hormone is modified, an altered relation between brain growth and skull growth may be seen (Goodman and Gilman 1970; see also p. 25).

*Davison:* Did you examine other things besides lipids in the milk of the deficient rats, such as the quality of the protein? Just conceivably, the effect of the deficiency was a lowering of the concentration of essential amino acids.

*Paoletti:* We measured only the fatty acid composition, because it is rather difficult to collect the milk. Better studies of the composition of the milk of essential fatty acid-deficient mothers should be made, using another species.

*Chapman:* You showed that the fatty acids of phosphatidylethanolamine were particularly affected in the myelin membranes. Have you shown that myelin function was grossly affected?

*Paoletti:* No, we have done no experiments in this area.

*Chapman:* There could be compensating effects occurring or it may even be that these particular changes in fatty acid composition may not have a dramatic effect on the myelin function.

*Paoletti:* I would emphasize that the unsaturation index remains the same in myelin phospholipids of the deficient rats.

*Hollingsworth:* Within that constant unsaturation index, you show big changes in the tetraene/triene ratio. Does this have any influence on the structure of the myelin?

*Paoletti:* We asked Dr F. Clementi to make some electron microscopic studies on myelin, and the myelin preparation looked normal.

*Houtsmuller:* Caldwell and Churchill (1966) fed pregnant rats a diet free of fatty acids. Directly after birth, all rats were put on a standard diet. The authors then tested the behaviour of the offspring at 50 days of age. They found exactly the same results as you had: decreased learning ability and also a lower capability to retain the learned information. In your experiments, if you return these animals to their normal diet, what is their performance on behavioural testing? Is the effect of the deficiency irreversible?

*Paoletti:* We have not enough data on this yet.

*Dobbing:* I think Professor Paoletti has added a whole new set of phenomena to our thinking in this matter of early undernutrition, brain development and behaviour. What is fascinating is that if you take the brain weight and body weight data and the changes in ratio (Tables 1 and 2, pp. 123 and 124), which are not altered until later than 30 days, in spite of the fact that the diet has been modified during gestation and lactation, he is producing the kind of picture which you could mimic in gross terms by not underfeeding *until* around 30 days, in which conditions the body weight would not only be affected much more than the brain, to give brain/body weight ratios comparable to those found, but you would also have the phenomenon of complete 'catch-up' of the body, which you also found. It would be interesting to know whether, if you began the reduction of dietary fatty acid after weaning, the same sort of results would be found, not only with body weight (I am convinced that this could be found), but with the compositional and behavioural changes as well.

*Paoletti:* This has not been done. We plan to substitute the deficient diet for the normal diet during lactation. The behaviour should then be followed for one year after the diet has been changed to see if behaviour can be reversed.

*Dobbing:* I would like more opportunity to study the behavioural data, because you are testing animals during the course of a period of growth restriction as adults, from which there is possible catch-up. If one does similar kinds of tests on recovered animals, previously undernourished in our sense, during the subsequent period, one gets the opposite answer. The rats which refrain on the second test from going into the shock compartment of the shuttle-box—that is, those which appear to have learned more successfully to avoid this shock—are the previously undernourished animals (Smart and Dobbing 1971). The possible explanation is that the previously undernourished animals are more fearful. This can be demonstrated in other ways:

they freeze on a stimulus; they freeze when they are put in the shuttle-box itself, and on handling. Here again, I'd simply like to add a word of caution, that these behavioural experiments are extremely difficult to interpret in terms which are meaningful for our own species.

*Paoletti:* I agree about the limitations of the behavioural studies. Other factors may affect them, such as the simple change of room humidity. This may affect the behaviour of the deficient rats much more than that of the normal rats. This condition can easily be controlled, but many variables cannot.

*Klein:* Can you tell us something more about the behaviour of the control and experimental animals in free situations, apart from your structured learning test?

*Paoletti:* In optimum conditions or when the room temperature and humidity are controlled, the gross behaviour is not different. As soon as the humidity is reduced, the deficient rats tend to 'freeze' more than the control rats. For this reason it is very difficult to establish the best conditions for investigating the behaviour of these animals.

*Houtsmuller:* In answer to Dr Dobbing, the rats from Churchill and Caldwell's experiment must have been normal during almost their complete lifespan with respect to body weight and other criteria that are usually studied, such as skin permeability. Nevertheless, their behaviour was different at 50 days of age.

*Dobbing:* I remain profoundly worried about the interpretation of animal experiments. Even those which are meticulously described in the published literature are extremely difficult to interpret unless you actually were there; factors like humidity may not appear in the published report, and there are many other artifacts of the behaviourists' experimental set-up which profoundly affect the interpretation even of apparently clear-cut examples. I would personally like to reserve judgement.

*Paoletti:* Probably the only large number of behavioural studies on humans kept on a diet with multiple deficiencies, including essential fatty acid deficiency, are those made at the Psychiatric Clinic in Glowno, Poland, on children who were in concentration camps during the war for the first 3 years of life. They have now reached the age of 27 to 29 years. The diet for children was reasonably balanced for calories, but apparently not for polyunsaturated fatty acids. These children during their growth and development have complete physical recovery, and the I.Q. level seems to be normal, but memory and social adjustment were affected (Rydzynski 1971).

*Dobbing:* These particular children may have been nutritionally deficient in some way in the concentration camps, but this circumstance of their environment must have been the least of their worries; there are so many other features of that environment which would produce the same answer.

# References

AAES-JØRGENSEN, E. and HOLMER, G. (1969) *Lipids* **4**, 501-506

BARNARD, G. B., FOSBROOKE, A. S. and LLOYD, J. K. (1970) *Clin. Chim. Acta* **28**, 417-422

CALDWELL, D. F. and CHURCHILL, J. A. (1966) *Psychol. Rep.* **19**, 99-102

COCHRANE, W. A., PAYNE, W. W., SIMPKISS, M. J. and WOOLF, L. J. (1956) *J. Clin. Invest.* **35**, 411

DEUEL, H. J., GREENBERG, S. M., ANISFELD, L. and MELNICK, D. (1951) *J. Nutr.* **45**, 535

EVANS, H. M. and LEPKOVSKY, S. (1932) *J. Biol. Chem.* **96**, 157

FARQUHAR, J. and WAYS, P. (1966) In *Metabolic Basis of Inherited Disease*, pp. 509-522, ed. J. B. Stanbury, J. B. Wyngaarden and D. S. Fredrickson. McGraw-Hill, New York

FUMAGALLI, R. and PAOLETTI, R. (1963) *Life Sci.* **2**, 291-296

GOODMAN, L. S. and GILMAN, A. (1970) *The Pharmacological Basis of Therapeutics*, 4th edn, p. 1516. Macmillan, London and Toronto

HANSEN, A. E., HAGGARD, M. E., BOELSCHE, A. N., ADAM, D. J. D. and WIESE, H. F. (1958) *J. Nutr.* **66**, 565-576

HANSEN, A. E., WIESE, H. F., BOELSCHE, A. N., HAGGARD, M. E., ADAM, D. J. D. and DAVIS, H. (1963) *Pediatrics* **31** (suppl. 1, pt. 2), 171-192

ROSSI, E., ZUPPINGER, K. and JOSS, E. (1969) *Monatsschr. Kinderheilkd.* **117**, 225-229

RYDZYNSKI, Z. (1971) In *Chemistry and Brain Development*, p. 437, ed. R. Paoletti and A. N. Davison. Plenum Press, New York

SOBREVILLA, L. A., GOODMAN, M. L. and KANE, C. A. (1964) *Am. J. Med.* **37**, 821-828

SODERHJELM, L., WIESE, H. F. and HOLMAN, R. T. (1970) In *Progress in the Chemistry of Fats and Other Lipids*, vol. 9, part 4, p. 555, ed. R. T. Holman. Pergamon Press, Oxford

SMART, J. L. and DOBBING, J. (1971) *Dev. Psychobiol.* in press.

WARWICK, W. J., HOLMAN, R. T., QUIE, P. G. and GOOD, R. A. (1959) *Am. J. Dis. Child.* **98**, 317-329

[For further discussion of Dr Paoletti's experiments, see pp. 156-157]

# Effects on offspring of maternal malnutrition in the rat

L. SVENNERHOLM, C. ALLING, Å. BRUCE, I. KARLSSON and O. SAPIA*

*Psychiatric Research Centre, Department of Neurochemistry, University of Göteborg*

A diminished brain weight, a diminished content of DNA and diminished concentrations of cholesterol and cerebrosides in the brain have been found in human infants who have died from marasmus (Wigglesworth 1969). The severe malnutrition at this age has invariably been due to protein-calorie malnutrition. There are no reports of a deficiency of essential fatty acids in such infants. In a number of infants suffering from protein malnutrition we found normal values for the linoleic acid content of plasma lecithin. But during treatment of the infants with a diet rich in protein the plasma concentration of lecithin linoleic acid dropped and that of eicosatrienoic acid (20:3 (*n*–9)) rose (Svennerholm, unpublished observations).

In Swedish newborns the sum of the concentrations of fatty acids of the linoleic and linolenic acid series (essential fatty acids) in blood phosphoglycerides was the same as in adults (Olegård and Svennerholm 1970). However, the concentration of linoleic acid in adipose tissue was very low at birth, and breast-fed 3-month-old infants had a significantly lower level of fatty acids of the linoleic and linolenic acid series in blood phosphoglycerides than one-year-old infants or adults (Olegård and Svennerholm 1971). In 3-month-old infants fed cow's milk the concentration of linoleic acid (18:2) was extremely low and that of 20:3 (*n*–9) very high in serum lecithin (Olegård and Svennerholm, unpublished observations).

The plasma studies indicated that in humans a suboptimal level or deficiency of essential fatty acids might occur during the early postnatal period. In the design of our animal experiments we have tried to simulate the dietary situation which may be encountered in families living under poor socio-economic conditions. Thus the animals have received a dietary supply of essential fatty

---

* *Present address:* Departamento de Quimica Biologica, Facultad de Farmacia y Bioquimico, Universidad de Buenos Aires, Argentina.

acids which was suboptimal but large enough to allow a rather normal fertility and survival of the offspring during lactation.

Only a few studies have been made in which the effect of prenatal and early postnatal EFA deficiency has been determined. Steinberg, Clarke and Ramwell (1968) fed weanling female rats a completely fat-free diet until they were mated and studied the weight of the brain and its lipid composition in the neonates. Berg-Hansen and Clausen (1969) and Paoletti and associates (Galli, White and Paoletti 1970, 1971; White, Galli and Paoletti 1971) also fed a fat-free diet, from about one week before delivery. When EFA restriction of the maternal diet is started during pregnancy the EFA supply to the offspring during gestation and lactation will depend largely on the previous maternal diet and it is questionable whether or when a deficiency will occur in the progeny. Other factors that can be criticized in previous studies are that the dietary change has not been limited to a reduction of EFA, but in general has been a drastic reduction of dietary fat; that the ratio of linoleic acid to linolenic acid has been different in the control and experimental diets; and that the sex of the animal studied has not always been given. In our nutritional studies we have tried to avoid these pitfalls by using constant calorie percentages of fats in all diets, by starting the dietary change in an earlier generation, and by comparing only animals of the same sex after the age of 30 days.

## MATERIALS AND METHODS

Rats of the Sprague-Dawley strain were allowed to eat the experimental diets *ad libitum*. The rats were mated at the age of 90 days. All the litters were reduced to six on the day of birth. The litters were weighed every 2nd day after the 5th day and every 5th day after the 21st day. Only animals with a weight within $\pm$ 2 S.D. of the mean weight were used for biochemical analyses (see Figs. 2 and 3). Four litters were used from each of the dietary groups for the biochemical studies.

All the assay methods have been used in our laboratory for a long time (Svennerholm 1964, 1968). A detailed description of the procedures adopted in this study is given in another report (Alling *et al.*).

## DIET AND GROWTH

It was established in our previous studies (Alling and Svennerholm 1970) that the pre-experimental diet of the dam was of primary importance for the accretion of EFA in the foetus and in the neonatal rat. When dietary EFA was reduced from 3.0 cal % to 1.0 cal % in the weanling rat, the concentration of polyenoic acids of the carcass did not become constant before adult age in the second generation.

The dietary concentration of 0.75 cal % linoleic + linolenic acid in the low-EFA group was chosen on the basis of several preliminary experiments. A reduction from 3.0 cal % to 1.0 cal % produced no clinical symptoms and only minor biochemical signs of EFA deficiency. A further reduction of linoleic + linolenic acid to 0.75 cal % reduced the fatty acids of the linolenic acid series and increased the 20:3 (*n*–9) in the tissue lipids of the dams. The fertility (Table 1) was only slightly reduced but the mortality of the newborns increased. Approximately 50 % of the offspring died between birth and the end of the lactation period (Table 2). At the time of the study, no temperature- and humidity-controlled room was available.

TABLE 1

Number of rats in the litters at delivery

| *Dietary group* | *Number of rats* | |
|---|---|---|
| | *Mean* | *S.D.* |
| Low EFA (0.74 cal %) | | |
| Low protein (8.0 cal %) (n=8) | 8.0 | 1.31 |
| High protein (16.0 cal %) (n=5) | 9.0 | 1.00 |
| High EFA (3.0 cal %) | | |
| Low protein (8.0 cal %) (n=6) | 8.5 | 1.87 |
| High protein (16.0 cal %) (n=7) | 10.3 | 1.60 |

High EFA:low protein < high protein ($P < 0.05$).

TABLE 2

Early postnatal mortality among offspring of rat dams on low and high dietary levels of essential fatty acids

| | *Maternal EFA Cal % of linoleate + linolenate 4:1* | |
|---|---|---|
| | *4.78* | *0.74* |
| Number of females for breeding | 17 | 11 |
| Number of litters born | 17 | 11 |
| Percentage mortality from birth to 21st day | 0 | 45 |

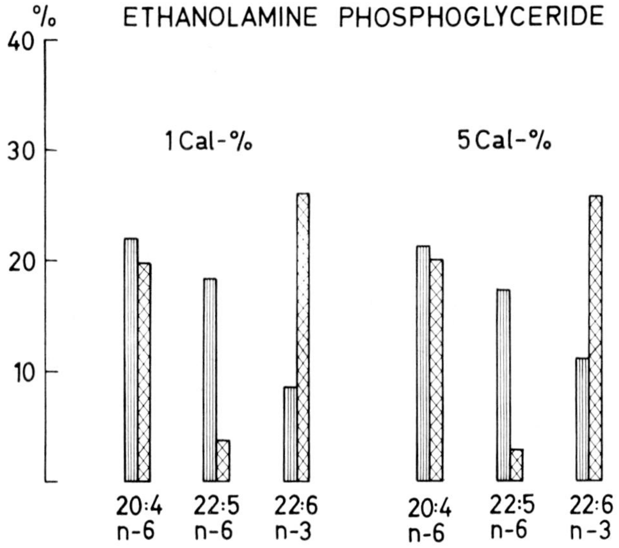


FIG. 1. Concentration of the major fatty acids in the linoleic and linolenic acid series of brain ethanolamine phosphoglycerides in 21-day-old rats given 1 and 5 cal % of EFA, respectively. Values are given as weight percentage of methyl esters of total fatty acids.

⊠ = ratio of linoleic acid to linolenic acid, 85:15.

▥ = ratio of linoleic acid to linolenic acid, 98:2.

The concentration of linoleic + linolenic acid in the high-EFA diet has been varied between 3 and 5 cal %. According to Pudelkiewicz, Seufert and Holman (1968) this amount is too high, but it was obvious from our pilot studies that the requirement of EFA of the rat was higher during gestation and lactation than was found by these authors for adult rats. No symptoms of toxicity were recorded even when as much as 10 cal % EFA was given for a year (Alling and Svennerholm 1970).

The ratio of linoleic acid to linolenic acid in the diet greatly influences the fatty acid pattern of the tissue lipids (Fig. 1; Mohrhauer and Holman 1963*b*; Walker 1967). Our preliminary studies revealed that in the brain lipids the relative percentages of 22:5 (*n*–6) and 22:6 (*n*–3) were strongly influenced by a change in the dietary linoleate/linolenate ratio, while even fairly wide variation of the concentration of EFA had little or no effect on the fatty acid composition. The diets were therefore composed in such a way as to have exactly the same ratio, although the concentration of EFA was varied.

A high and a low dietary level of EFA have been used together with a high and a low level of protein. Thus, we have studied four dietary (Table 3) groups of rats from birth up to the age of 90 days. At first we used casein supplemented

TABLE 3

Calorie percentage of the diets containing high or low protein

| | *High EFA* | | *Low EFA* | |
|---|---|---|---|---|
| | *High protein* | *Low protein* | *High protein* | *Low protein* |
| Protein (fish protein-EFP 90) | 16.0 | 8.0 | 16.0 | 8.0 |
| Carbohydrate | 62.9 | 71.0 | 62.9 | 71.0 |
| Corn starch | 58.0 | 66.1 | 58.0 | 66.1 |
| Sucrose | 4.9 | 4.9 | 4.9 | 4.9 |
| Fat | 21.0 | 21.0 | 21.0 | 21.0 |
| Linoleic acid 18:2(*n*–6) | 2.4 | 2.4 | 0.60 | 0.60 |
| Linolenic acid 18:3(*n*–3) | 0.6 | 0.6 | 0.15 | 0.15 |
| Sum of 18:2(*n*-6) and 18:3(*n*–3) | 3.0 | 3.0 | 0.75 | 0.75 |

with methionine as protein source, but more reproducible results were obtained with a fish protein (EFP-90 Astra Nutrition, Mölndal, Sweden), which was used in all subsequent studies. Also the basic fat, coconut fat, was replaced by hydrogenated lard. The growth curves (Figs. 2 and 3) were studied in six to eight litters in each dietary group. In the high-protein groups body weight was lower in the low-EFA than in the high-EFA group up to the age of about 90 days. In some litters an EFA-free diet was started on the 18th day. In these litters the body weight did not differ from that on the low-EFA diet. In the low-protein groups the differences in body weight between high and low-EFA

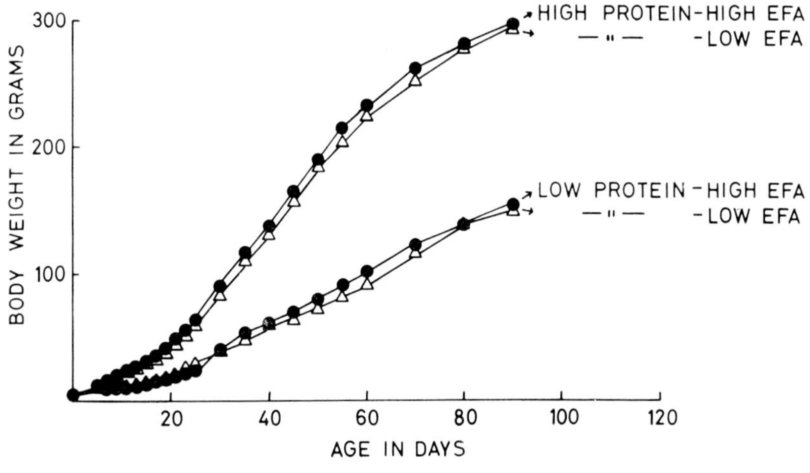


FIG. 2. Growth curve for male rats on four different diets up to the age of 90 days.

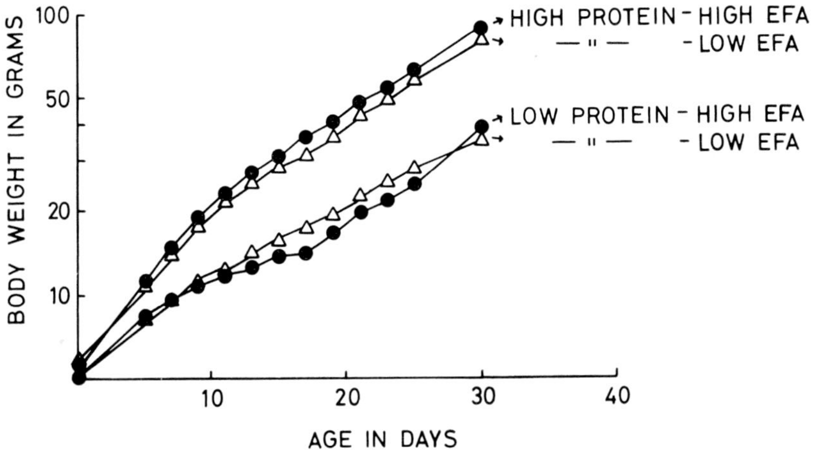


FIG. 3. The same growth curve as in Fig. 1, showing the first 30 days only.

groups also disappeared, but during the first 30 days the weight was slightly higher in the low-EFA group. The variations in weight between individuals were much larger for the low-protein groups.

Although the low-EFA rats in the high-protein litters had lower body weights than the high-EFA rats, there was no difference in brain weight between the two groups from birth up to 30 days. These results are in contrast to those reported by Paoletti and associates (White, Galli and Paoletti 1971), who found not only a significant diminution of body weights in the EFA-deficient rats but also a significant diminution of the brain weights. We consider their results uncertain because of the small number of rats examined, the abnormal curve for the body weights of the controls, and the widely fluctuating figures found for the brain weights with increasing age.

## ESSENTIAL FATTY ACID DEFICIENCY AND BRAIN LIPIDS

The effect of a low dietary intake of EFA by the mothers on the brain lipid composition has been studied in the cerebrum in four litters of six 21-day-old rats of both sexes and compared with a control group of the same size. The two diets were identical except in fatty acid composition (Table 4).

The protein, phospholipid, cholesterol and total fatty acid content of the brain was the same in the low and high-EFA groups (Table 5). Only cerebrosides were significantly lower in the low-EFA group ($P < 0.05$). A deficiency of myelin lipids or a delay in their formation has been the most characteristic

TABLE 4

Calorie percentage of the diets containing high casein levels

| | *High EFA* | *Low EFA* |
|---|---|---|
| Protein (casein) | 18.3 | 18.3 |
| Carbohydrate (wheat starch) | 60.2 | 60.2 |
| Fat | 21.5 | 21.5 |
| Linoleic acid, 18:2(*n*–6) | 3.80 | 0.58 |
| Linolenic acid, 18:3(*n*–3) | 0.98 | 0.16 |
| Sum of 18:2(*n*–6) + 18:3(*n*–3) | 4.78 | 0.74 |

TABLE 5

Constituents of cerebrum, liver, muscle and serum, in offspring of rats fed high and low-EFA diets

| | *High EFA* | | *Low EFA* | |
|---|---|---|---|---|
| | *Mean* | *S.D.* | *Mean* | *S.D.* |
| Body weight, g | 49.1 | 1.96 | 43.1 | 4.31* |
| Cerebrum | | | | |
| Weight, g | 1.00 | 0.061 | 1.00 | 0.054 |
| Protein, mg/g | 104 | 4.36 | 102 | 3.82 |
| Lipid-P, μmol/g | 55.7 | 1.43 | 54.5 | 2.59 |
| Total fatty acids, μmol/g | 105 | 6.43 | 98 | 5.06 |
| Cholesterol, μmol/g | 30.6 | 2.77 | 30.0 | 2.45 |
| Lipid-*N*-acetylneuraminic acid μmol/g | 3.2 | 0.13 | 3.1 | 0.32 |
| Cerebrosides, μmol/g | 2.8 | 0.28 | 2.3 | 0.34* |
| Liver | | | | |
| Weight, g | 2.03 | 0.09 | 1.92 | 0.15 |
| Protein, mg/g | 158 | 4.25 | 145 | 9.63* |
| Lipid-P, μmol/g | 39.4 | 2.54 | 36.7 | 1.91 |
| Triglycerides, μmol/g | 15.0 | 2.70 | 20.8 | 2.05** |
| Muscle | | | | |
| Lipid-P, μmol/g | 17.9 | 0.46 | 17.0 | 0.35** |
| Serum | | | | |
| Lipid-P, μmol/ml | 4.44 | 0.27 | 4.10 | 0.36 |
| Triglycerides, μmol/ml | 1.07 | 0.48 | 0.78 | 0.18 |

* $P < 0.05$; ** $P < 0.01$.

finding in brain in association with protein-calorie malnutrition (Dobbing 1964; Dobbing and Widdowson 1965; Geison and Waisman 1970). This study has shown that EFA deficiency will also lead to this result. The amount of gangliosides, measured as lipid-*N*-acetylneuraminic acid, has been used as an index of the outgrowth of the neurons. The figures for lipid-*N*-acetylneuraminic acid are identical in the two groups. Normal concentrations of brain gangliosides have also been found in protein-calorie malnutrition (Geison and Waisman 1970).

## FATTY ACID COMPOSITION OF BRAIN AND OTHER ORGANS

Comparison of the fatty acid patterns (Table 6) of the maternal diets with those of triglycerides in the adipose tissue and of the liver of the offspring reveals some characteristic findings. The concentration of linoleate and linolenate in the diet is significantly higher than in the triglycerides of the offspring. The short-chain fatty acids 12:0 and 14:0 are severely reduced in the offspring.

A striking finding was the marked similarity in fatty acid composition of the brain lipids (Figs. 4 and 5) from the two dietary groups. With the exception of a small but significant increase of 20:3 (*n*–9) in total lipids, ethanolamine phosphoglyceride and choline phosphoglyceride, and the increase of 22:5 (*n*–6) in total lipids and ethanolamine phosphoglyceride in the low-EFA group, there were no significant differences between the individual fatty acids of the brain lipids. An increased concentration of 20:3 (*n*–9) as a result of EFA deficiency was first reported by Mohrhauer and Holman (1963*a*), but there are only a few studies on the effect of maternal diet on the EFA level in the brain

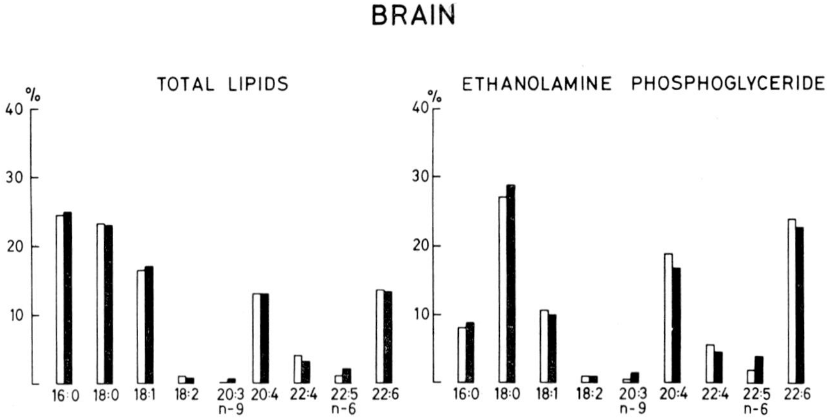


FIG. 4. Fatty acid composition of brain total lipids and brain ethanolamine phosphoglycerides. Open bars, high-EFA group. Solid bars, low-EFA group. Values are given as weight percentage of methyl esters.

TABLE 6

Fatty acid composition of triglycerides in maternal diet and in tissues of the offspring

| *Fatty acid* | *Diet* | | *Adipose tissue* | | *Serum* | | *Liver* | |
|---|---|---|---|---|---|---|---|---|
| | *High EFA* | *Low EFA* | *High EFA* | *Low EFA* | *High EFA* | *Low EFA* | *High EFA* | *Low EFA* |
| 12:0 | 27.1 | 40.3 | 13.6 | 15.3 | 10.4 | 13.0 | 1.5 | 2.5 |
| 14:0 | 16.7 | 24.8 | 12.8 | 15.9 | 9.7 | 13.5 | 8.0 | 10.2 |
| 16:0 | 11.5 | 14.0 | 26.0 | 31.4 | 23.7 | 30.0 | 28.6 | 36.4 |
| 16:1 (*n*–7) | trace | trace | 3.1 | 5.3 | 3.3 | 5.6 | 3.9 | 7.5 |
| 18:0 | 4.5 | 4.3 | 3.8 | 3.5 | 4.3 | 4.2 | 3.5 | 4.2 |
| 18:1 (*n*–9) | 14.3 | 9.7 | 25.0 | 26.8 | 28.8 | 31.1 | 35.5 | 37.9 |
| 18:2 (*n*–6) | 19.0 | 2.9 | 13.1 | 1.4 | 16.0 | 1.8 | 16.9 | 1.2 |
| 18:3 (*n*–3) | 4.9 | 0.8 | 2.7 | 0.6 | 3.6 | 0.8 | 2.3 | 0.3 |

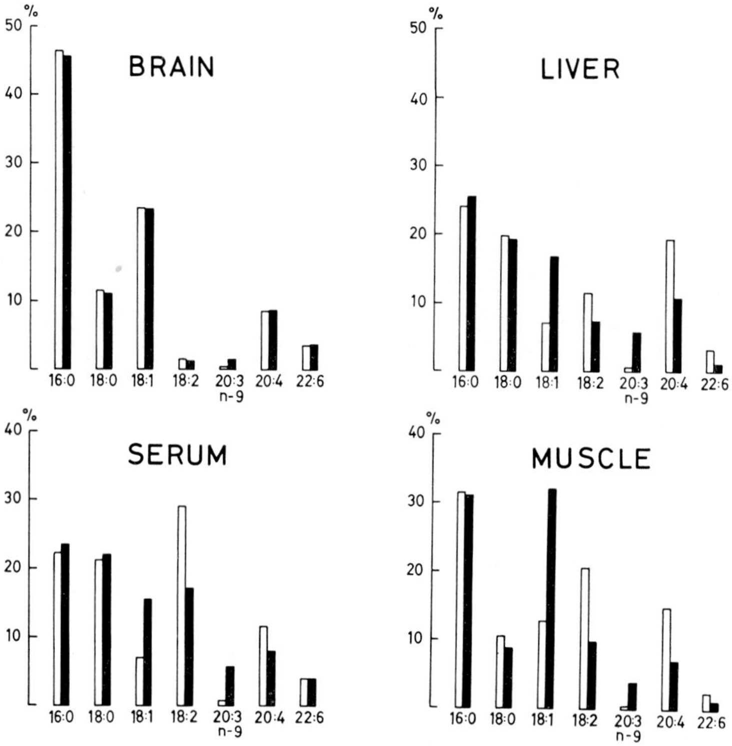


FIG. 5. Fatty acid composition of lecithins in brain, liver, muscle and serum. Open bars, high-EFA group. Solid bars, low-EFA group. Values are given as weight percentage of methyl esters.

lipids of the offspring. In the study by Steinberg, Clarke and Ramwell (1968) weanling female rats were given a fat-free diet and were mated 2 months later. Large alterations were reported in the fatty acid composition of the brain lipids of the newborn offspring, but the incompatible figures given for ethanolamine phosphoglycerides and total lipids reduce the value of the findings. White, Galli and Paoletti (1971) started to give dams an EFA-deficient diet 5 days before delivery. The diet contained only 0.12% of lipids in which linoleate and linolenate constituted 5.9 and 1.7%, respectively. In the control diet the corresponding figures for linoleate and linolenate were 44 and 1.2%. They also found minor changes in the fatty acid composition of brain ethanolamine phosphoglycerides. There was a slight diminution of fatty acids of the linoleic acid series from the 10th day and an increase of 20:3 (*n*–9) from the 30th day. Fatty acids of the linolenic acid series were unchanged up to the age of 90 days.

The fatty acid composition of the tissue phosphoglycerides showed large differences in our study. In lecithins of liver, muscle and serum concentrations of 18:2 (*n*–6), 20:4 (*n*–6) and 22:6 (*n*–3) were significantly lower ($P < 0.01$) in the low-EFA group, with the exception of 22:6 (*n*–3) in serum, which was the same in the two groups. There was a rise of 20:3 (*n*–9) and 18:1 ($P < 0.001$) in liver, muscle and serum in the low-EFA group. Only minor changes were found among the saturated fatty acids.

## SUMMARY

The effect of a low essential fatty acid (EFA) diet during gestation and lactation on body growth, brain weight and lipid and fatty acid composition of brain and other organs in the offspring was studied. Groups of Sprague-Dawley rats were raised on diets with high and low concentrations of proteins. The concentration of fat was the same in all the groups, but the concentration of linoleate + linolenate was 3 or 5 cal % (high-EFA group) or 0.75 cal % (low-EFA group). In the low-EFA groups the litter size was not significantly smaller than in the high-EFA groups, but the mortality of the offspring from birth to the 21st day of age was 45 %, when the temperature and humidity of the animal room were not controlled. Body weight was slightly lower in the low-EFA group on a high-protein diet, but the EFA concentration did not influence the body weight of the animals on a low-protein diet. Brain weight did not vary with dietary EFA concentration.

The lipid and fatty acid compositions of the brain were determined for high and low-EFA with high dietary protein. Though the low level of EFA had been given for three generations, there was a remarkable similarity between the brain lipids in the two groups. In the low-EFA group there was a diminution of cerebrosides, but other lipid classes did not show any significant difference. The brain lipids of the low-EFA group showed a significant increase of 20:3 (*n*–9), while none of the other polyenoic acids showed any significant change except for 22:5 (*n*–6), which was increased. In the lecithins of liver, muscle and serum, the fatty acids of the linoleic and linolenic acid series were extensively reduced in the low-EFA group with a concomitant increase of 18:1 and 20:3 (*n*–9).

## ACKNOWLEDGEMENTS

We are very much indebted to Dr H. Wendéus, Astra Nutrition, Mölndal, Sweden, for the gift of fish protein EFP-90, to Dr R. Ohlsson, Karlsham

Oljefabriker, Sweden, for the hydrogenated lard and to Dr L. Wedberg, AB Ferrosan, Malmö, for the vitamins. The skilful technical assistance of Mrs Karin Andersson and Mrs Kristina Rinäs is gratefully acknowledged.

This work was supported by grants from the Swedish Medical Research Council (Project nos. B70-13X-627-06B, B71-13X-627-07C).

## References

ALLING, C., BRUCE, Å., KARLSSON, I., SAPIA, O. and SVENNERHOLM, L. (1972) *J. Nutr.* in press
ALLING, C. and SVENNERHOLM, L. (1970) In *Proceedings of the 6th International Congress of Neuropathology*, pp. 91-92. Masson, Paris
BERG-HANSEN, J. and CLAUSEN, J. (1969) *Z. Ernährungswiss.* **9**, 278-289
DOBBING, J. (1964) *Proc. R. Soc. B* **159**, 503-509
DOBBING, J. and WIDDOWSON, E. M. (1965) *Brain* **88**, 357-366
GALLI, C., WHITE, H. B., JR and PAOLETTI, R. (1970) *J. Neurochem.* **17**, 347-355
GALLI, C., WHITE, H. B., JR and PAOLETTI, R. (1971) In *Chemistry and Brain Development*, pp. 425-435, ed. R. Paoletti and A. N. Davison. Plenum Press, New York and London
GEISON, R. L. and WAISMAN, H. A. (1970) *J. Nutr.* **100**, 315-324
MOHRHAUER, H. and HOLMAN, R. T. (1963*a*) *J. Neurochem.* **10**, 523-530
MOHRHAUER, H. and HOLMAN, R. T. (1963*b*) *J. Lipid Res.* **4**, 151-159
OLEGÅRD, R. and SVENNERHOLM, L. (1970) *Acta Paediatr. Scand.* **59**, 637-647
OLEGÅRD, R. and SVENNERHOLM, L. (1971) *Acta Paediatr. Scand.* **60**, 505-511
PUDELKIEWICZ, C., SEUFERT, J. and HOLMAN, R. T. (1968) *J. Nutr.* **94**, 138-146
STEINBERG, A. B., CLARKE, G. B. and RAMWELL, P. W. (1968) *Dev. Psychobiol.* **1**, 225-229
SVENNERHOLM, L. (1964) *J. Neurochem.* **11**, 839-853
SVENNERHOLM, L. (1968) *J. Lipid Res.* **9**, 570-579
WALKER, B. L. (1967) *Lipids* **2**, 497-500
WHITE, H. B., JR, GALLI, C. and PAOLETTI, R. (1971) *J. Neurochem.* **18**, 869-882
WIGGLESWORTH, J. S. (1969) *Dev. Med. Child. Neurol.* **11**, 792-803

## Discussion

*Menkes:* What is known about the factors controlling the synthesis of eicosatrienoic acid?

*Svennerholm:* The rats which received a low-EFA diet had, at the age of 21 days, 12% of 20:3 (*n*–9) in liver lecithin, but less than 0.5% in the liver triglycerides. The two lipids have the same precursor, diacylglycerol. The control mechanism does not seem to be only the tissue concentration of 18:2 and 18:3. With reference to what Professor Chapman said earlier, the lipid membrane requires a certain fatty acid composition of the polar lipids which form the membrane. Lipids will be biosynthesized with the available fatty acids but will not be incorporated in the membrane. A deficiency of 18:2 will lead to a diminished formation of 20:4 (*n*–6), which is a necessary component of all membrane lipids. 20:3 (*n*–9) will then be formed because it shows the largest similarities to 20:4 and has double bonds in three positions in common with 20:4.

*Menkes:* Holman showed that a number of saturated and unsaturated fatty acids inhibit chain elongation and desaturation of fatty acids such as linoleic acid (Mohrhauer *et al.* 1967). Could the trigger for synthesis of 20:3 (*n*–9) be a loss of some of the other polyunsaturated fatty acids?

*Svennerholm:* Holman has suggested that a low tissue concentration of 18:2 and 18:3 will initiate the formation of 20:3 (*n*–9). He might be right, but I think that a low concentration of 20:4 (*n*–6) or 20:5 (*n*–3) is the primary trigger for the synthesis of 20:3.

*Houtsmuller:* Brenner and Holman have both studied this problem. There is a competition between several unsaturated fatty acids for the enzymes of chain elongation and unsaturation. Linolenic acid is preferred, then linoleic and then oleic acid. If linoleic acid is present, oleic acid will be less elongated or desaturated (see Dhopeshwarkar and Mead 1961; Holman 1964; Brenner, de Tomas and Peluffo 1965).

*Svennerholm:* Arachidonic acid is most potent of all fatty acids in depressing the formation of 20:3 (*n*–9).

*Houtsmuller:* And high levels of linoleic acid depress the synthesis of arachidonic acid.

*Crawford:* We have fed guinea-pigs on low and high protein diets. We were interested in particular in the effect of specific amino acids like histidine and arginine which are present in certain foods in very high concentrations. We added extra histidine to the stock diet and found that this accelerated growth, and led to larger litters. When we added histidine to the low-protein diet we depressed their growth markedly, over and above the retardation of the low-protein diet itself (Gale and Crawford 1969). We thought we had perhaps demonstrated an extra requirement for histidine in the guinea-pig, until 2 years later we found that the guinea-pigs that had grown fast also died fast, so there were two ends of the scale. We still have the control guinea-pigs alive who were fed the normal diet.

In your experiments, Dr Svennerholm, you have compared the effects of the same amount of essential fatty acids in both high and low-protein diets. From our results, we wondered whether, if you accelerate protein synthesis without changing the essential fatty acids, you may not be providing enough polyunsaturated fatty acids for simultaneous construction of phospholipids, so that phospholipid and protein can be stuck together to construct membranes.

Might this also explain your results on growth, EFA and protein? In a sense, could protein synthesis leave phospholipid synthesis behind?

*Svennerholm:* This is our own explanation. We see a smaller increase of trienoic acids in liver and serum in association with a low than with a high-protein diet in animals given a low supply of linoleic acid.

*von Muralt:* Is nutritional damage to the protein matrix of the brain into which the lipids are incorporated more serious than a lack of essential fatty acids?

*Svennerholm:* I would not say so. We have found that a low level of essential fatty acids in the maternal diet will result in a mortality of almost 50% of the offspring. This high mortality is mainly caused by an increased permeability of the skin to water, owing to the EFA deficiency. In our experiments the cerebral membranes undergo only minor changes, which might depend on an adaptation to the low EFA level. But Professor Paoletti, who drastically reduced the fatty acid content of the diet, found rather large changes in the lipid and fatty acid composition of brain.

*Crawford:* Dr A. J. Sinclair in my laboratory has been doing experiments on EFA deficiency in rats. I was very interested to see that you took 0.75% of calories as the low level for your diet, because we went even lower than that (0.33% of calories) and our experience agrees with what you found, namely that at about 0.7% of calories the offspring survive but below, there is a marked increase in mortality of the newborn pups. By coincidence, we have used the same ratio of linoleic to linolenic acids as you have. At this low level of 0.33%, fed to the pregnant rats, we can expect roughly an 80% mortality of the offspring by 2 weeks. We do seem to find more marked changes in both liver and brain lipids in the animals that die compared with those that survive. I wonder what your experience was at this lower level?

*Svennerholm:* We have been able to reduce our figures for the mortality of the offspring on 0.75% EFA by doing all the studies in temperature- and humidity-controlled rooms. We have also started to feed our female rats, which have been on the 0.75% EFA diet, with a diet containing no EFA at mating, and our survival figures have drastically fallen again. We have not and will not study the animals that died during the experiments because we can never know the cause of death. For more than 15 years we have determined the lipids in organs obtained at autopsy of infants and children. We have found it impossible to draw any conclusions from these determinations unless we can relate the results to the clinical record and the patho-anatomical changes. The results of the brain analyses in an infant of a given weight will be different if the infant is premature or dysmature (small-for-date). I am also very sceptical about the studies of some malnutrition research workers who have compared results of analyses of brains from infants who have died from marasmus with results obtained in a different country from infants who have died in accidents, and have claimed that the differences depend on the deficient diet. In our animal experiments we wish to work with 'clean' groups, when possible.

*Winick:* At what age do the young of EFA-deficient mothers die?

*Svennerholm:* They die at any age, but most often within the first few days.

*Crawford:* Our pups also appear quite normal but they still die. By examining the pups which we kill but which we expect to die, we have shown changes in liver lipids. So they look normal from the outside but are in fact smaller and are abnormal.

*Bernsohn:* Do the mothers on deficient diets eat their young?

*Svennerholm:* The mothers on the low-protein diet eat their young, but very seldom if they are on the low-EFA diet, unless the young have died.

*Mead:* One important general point seems to be that in order to establish essential fatty acid deficiency, you must have cell division, or the symptoms are not manifest. So one would assume that in the adult brain, for example, in which cells are not dividing rapidly, you wouldn't get signs of essential fatty acid deficiency.

*von Muralt:* Would this explain the difficulties of demonstrating EFA deficiency in humans? The vulnerability is restricted to the period of rapid cell growth, which in humans happens before 18 months of age.

*Lloyd:* Investigators who are convinced that there is an essential fatty acid deficiency state seem to be describing it at all ages; however, some cell division presumably goes on in the elderly.

*Winick:* What do you base the statement on, that one needs cell division?

*Mead:* There is a lot of information. The younger one puts an animal on a diet deficient in essential fatty acids, the earlier and the more drastic are the symptoms. If one puts an adult rat on an EFA-deficient diet he doesn't suffer deficiency symptoms at all unless the calories are reduced to the point where his weight is reduced, and he is then put on the deficient diet. Then he shows the symptoms as he regains his weight, but not until then. So if you decrease the calories at the same time as you decrease the essential fatty acids, the symptoms appear when you let the rat grow. In man we may find the same thing.

*Herschkowitz:* If that is true, then a lower number of microneurons should be observed in rats deprived of fatty acids postnatally, since these cells are known to divide postnatally.

*Mead:* I don't think that has been studied.

*Bovet:* Would cross-fostering and the artificial reduction of the number in the litter have an effect on the mortality of the newborn, Professor Svennerholm?

*Svennerholm:* We have not done such experiments.

*Winick:* What happened to offspring of rats who were protein-malnourished and deprived of EFA during pregnancy? Did the mortality stay the same?

*Svennerholm:* There was no difference in mortality between the offspring of protein-deficient and protein + EFA-deficient mothers.

*Dobbing:* One has the impression from ethologists that survival in the first few days of life is perhaps even more dependent on maternal behaviour and attention than on nutritional factors. Have you observed differences in maternal behaviour, such as in nesting and mothering?

*Svennerholm:* We have observed our rats carefully, but we have not been able to find any behavioural differences. Steinberg, Clarke and Ramwell (1968) reported that EFA-deficient young die within the first 24 hours of birth because of lack of nesting and mothering.

*Dobbing:* But some of your animals did die in the early postnatal period and it's conceivable that the aetiology of their death is different.

*von Muralt:* There seems to be a discrepancy between the experiments and results of Dr Paoletti and those of Dr Svennerholm. Why are they different?

*Davison:* I wonder whether it's possible that Professor Paoletti is studying the animals that would die in the type of experiment described by Professor Svennerholm. Professor Paoletti, how many of the rats that are born alive in your experiments actually survive? Because if a high proportion survive, then these are potential candidates for death in Dr Svennerholm's situation. If one added in the data from the animals dying in Dr Svennerholm's work, it might explain the discrepancy in the results.

*Paoletti:* In our experiments the survival rate is much higher than in the experiments described by Dr Svennerholm. The rates of death in the control and deficient groups are not very different.

*Davison:* This would fit in with this explanation.

*Svennerholm:* I do not think that the results are incompatible. The experiments were designed in completely different ways and Professor Paoletti found differences at an age which was not studied by us. We wished to study the effect of a low intake of EFA on the development of the brain in animals which have been adapted to the low level for two generations. Dr Paoletti made a drastic reduction in the supply of fat to the mothers during pregnancy, which means that the offspring were exposed to a continuous reduction of the supply of EFA until weaning, after which the young were fed a practically fat-free diet. We made our biochemical determinations when the animals were 21 days old, while Professor Paoletti studied animals aged 30, 60 and 90 days. The lipid changes that he described did not occur until after the age of 30 days. We have found linoleic acid to be a vital requirement during intrauterine and early postnatal life in the rat. If the linoleic acid supply to the animals is too low, they will die from water and electrolyte imbalance. The adult rat sccms to bc less sensitive to essential fatty acid deficiency and therefore several people have been able to induce rather large fatty acid changes in brain lipids of the type described by Professor Paoletti. The other changes described by Professor Paoletti, such as the reduced body weight and the diminished brain weight, have not been proved to have been caused by the EFA deficiency. The small number of animals, the wide variation of the results obtained in control and fat-deficient rats, and the drastic reduction in the fat supply are all factors which have to be checked before any conclusions can be drawn on the effect of EFA deficiency on body and brain weight.

*Bernsohn:* How do the results presented fit in with the data that Holman reported on deficiency of individual fatty acids (Mohrhauer and Holman 1963)? His rats were put on a deficient diet at weaning and carried through to about 90 days. He showed marked decreases in the corresponding series of fatty acids.

*Svennerholm:* The experimental designs of Mohrhauer and Holman (1963) are more similar to those described by Professor Paoletti. They gave their rats a fat-deficient diet and supplemented the diet with pure fatty acids. They found that the level of 20:3 (*n*–9) could be reduced by the addition of linoleic, linolenic and arachidonic acid, the latter being most potent. Linolenate was shown to inhibit the conversion of linoleate to arachidonate. The intimate relationship between 22:5 (*n*–6) and 22:6 (*n*–3) demonstrated in our study could not be shown by Mohrhauer and Holman: this may be due to the relatively higher concentration of linolenate used in their studies.

*Paoletti:* We were unable to find any consistent study made during the period of lactation and at the end of pregnancy on essential fatty acid deficiency when we started our own studies 3 years ago. This period of development had apparently been overlooked by previous investigators.

## References


BRENNER, R. R., DE TOMAS, M. E. and PELUFFO, R. O. (1965) *Biochim. Biophys. Acta* **106**, 640-642

DHOPESHWARKAR, G. A. and MEAD, J. F. (1961) *J. Am. Oil Chem. Soc.* **38**, 297

GALE, M. M. and CRAWFORD, M. A. (1969) *Trans. R. Soc. Trop. Med. Hyg.* **63**, 826

HOLMAN, R. T. (1964) *Fed. Proc. Fed. Am. Soc. Exp. Biol.* **23**, 1062

MOHRHAUER, H., CHRISTIANSEN, K., GAN, M. V., DEUBIG, M. and HOLMAN, R. T. (1967) *J. Biol. Chem.* **242**, 4507

MOHRHAUER, H. and HOLMAN, R. T. (1963) *J. Neurochem.* **10**, 523-530

STEINBERG, A. B., CLARKE, G. B. and RAMWELL, P. W. (1968) *Dev. Psychobiol.* **1**, 225-229

# Polyenoic fatty acid metabolism of phosphoglycerides in developing brain

JOSEPH BERNSOHN and STEVEN R. COHEN

*Neuropsychiatric Research Laboratory, Veterans Administration Hospital, Hines, Illinois and*
*Department of Biochemistry and Biophysics, Loyola University, Stritch School of Medicine, Maywood, Illinois*

The lipid composition of brain is unique in a number of quantitative features, one of which is the high concentration of polyenoic fatty acids (PFA) in the phospholipid fraction. This is true of the ethanolamine (EPG) and serine (SPG) phosphoglycerides and to some extent of the inositol phosphatides. Arachidonic (20:4) and docosahexaenoic acid (22:6) constitute over 30% of the total fatty acids of these fractions in human brain (O'Brien and Sampson 1965). Since EPG and SPG constitute about 45% of the chick brain phosphatide fraction at 20 days of embryonic development (Miyamoto, Stephanides and Bernsohn 1966), it is apparent that the PFA represent a considerable fraction of the total brain phospholipid fatty acids. Of the two major PFA mentioned, 20:4 belongs to the *n*–6 series and 22:6 to the *n*–3 series fatty acids. It has been shown *in vitro* and *in vivo* in the rat liver (Klenk 1961) and in the embryonic chick (Miyamoto, Stephanides and Bernsohn 1967*a*) that no interconversion occurs between the two series and that for the deposition of these two polyenoic acids, the fatty acids themselves or a suitable precursor must be provided. The two major dietary precursors are linoleic acid for PFA of the *n*–6 series and linolenic acid for those of the *n*–3 series. In the absence of the precursors, the corresponding PFA of that series are not synthesized, to any extent (Mohrhauer and Holman 1963).

From these considerations and on the assumption that the high concentration of 22:6 in brain phospholipids has a function, it was postulated that either a diet deficient in *n*-3 fatty acids, or a defect in the metabolic pathway leading to biosynthesis of 22:6 from suitable precursors during the period of active myelination, might be an aetiological factor in demyelination processes in man (Bernsohn and Stephanides 1967). It was postulated that a suboptimal availability of *n*–3 fatty acids during the period of rapid deposition of myelin could lead to the formation of myelin which might be unable to maintain its structural stability and would ultimately break down. The *n*–3 series of fatty acids was considered because of the limited possibility of incurring an *n*–6 deficiency in the diet, and from epidemiological data. The time interval between myelin synthesis and its ultimate breakdown could be attributed to the slow turnover of myelin. Epidemiological studies have shown that the basis for demyelinating disease in man is established early in the lifetime of the individual (Alter, Liebowitz and Speer 1966), though its overt manifestations do not usually occur until late in the second decade or early in the third decade of life (McAlpine, Lumsden and Acheson 1963).

It is generally accepted that myelin is biosynthesized as an extrusion of the plasma membrane of the oligodendroglial cell (Peters, Palay and Webster 1970). The elaboration of myelin could involve the metabolic machinery of the oligodendrocytes and a *milieu* deficient in *n*–3 fatty acids during the period of active myelination could result in the production by the cell of myelin defective in some aspect and incapable of the necessary stability for the lifetime of the individual. This would imply that the oligodendrocyte rather than myelin itself would be the primary target during periodic deficits in *n*–3 fatty acids. During periods of deficiency the biosynthetic role of the oligodendrocyte might be impaired and thus result in an end-product, namely myelin, which differed from that produced when all necessary precursors are available.

A study was therefore undertaken of the biosynthesis of PFA in developing chick brain from suitable precursors. The role of glial cells was also studied, but the separation procedures for the isolation of glial-enriched fractions proved difficult to apply to embryonic chick brain and the developing rat brain was used in this phase of the work.

## METHODS

### *Isolation and incubation procedures*

Brains were removed from chick embryos, washed in 0.25 M-sucrose and slices weighing about 200 mg were prepared using a Stadie-Riggs slicer. The slices were incubated in a Dubnoff incubator at 37°C with air as the gas phase in a medium containing 10 μmol ATP, 3 μmol NADH, 2 μmol NADPH, 100 μmol phosphate buffer, pH 7.3, 11 μmol glucose, and 2.5 μCi [1,3-$^{14}$C] malonyl-CoA (9.4 mCi/mmol) or 4 μCi [1-$^{14}$C]acetyl-CoA (58.1 mCi/mmol), to a total volume of 2.0 ml. At the end of one hour the slices were washed 3 times with 0.9% NaCl solution and then lyophilized. The dried tissue was extracted with 20 volumes of $CHCl_3$:$CH_3OH$ (2:1) and chromatographed on a silicic acid column. The neutral lipids were eluted with $CHCl_3$ and the phospholipids with $CH_3OH:CHCl_3$ (80:20). The phospholipids were intra-esterified with $BF_3:CH_3OH$ as previously described (Bernsohn, Stephanides and Norgello 1971) and then subjected to gas-liquid chromatography.

Microsomes were obtained from embryonic chick brain by homogenization with 5 volumes of 0.32 M-sucrose in Tris-HCl buffer, pH 7.0. The homogenate was centrifuged at 1350 **g** for 15 minutes, the residue washed and centrifuged again and the supernatants combined and centrifuged at 12 500 **g** for 20 minutes to yield the crude mitochondrial fraction. The supernatant was centrifuged at 15 000 **g** for 15 minutes, the pellet discarded, and the resultant supernatant was centrifuged at 90 000 **g** for 70 minutes to yield the crude microsomal fraction. This fraction was washed in 0.32 M-sucrose in Tris-HCl and centrifuged at 109 000 **g** for 60 minutes to yield the microsomes. These particulates were incubated in air as the gas phase in a medium containing 3.2 μmol NADH, 2.75 μmol NADPH, 16 μmol ATP, 16 μmol $MgCl_2$, 200 μmol phosphate buffer, pH 7.4, [1-$^{14}$C]linoleyl-CoA containing 0.1-1.0 μCi, in a total volume of 1.2 ml. After incubation for one hour at 37°C in a Dubnoff shaking water bath, the microsomes were lyophilized, extracted, esterified and chromatographed as described above.

Neuronal soma and neuroglial fractions were isolated essentially by the method of Norton and Poduslo (1970). Rat brain minus cerebellum was sliced in a McIlwain tissue chopper and the brain slices were incubated in Krebs-Ringer phosphate buffer, pH 7.4, to which 11 mM-glucose and 10 μCi of [1-$^{14}$C]sodium acetate (specific activity 59 mCi/mmol) had been added. After one hour of incubation the slices were washed twice in a medium of 5% glucose, 5% fructose, 1% bovine serum albumin and 10mM-phosphate buffer, pH 6.0. After an hour of incubation under 100% $O_2$ in the above medium to which 1% trypsin was added, the slices were suspended in 0.9 M-sucrose and filtered through sieves of pore size 150 and 74 μm. The resultant suspension was layered over a 2.0 M, 1.55 M, and 1.35 M sucrose gradient and centrifuged at 3300 **g** for 10 minutes. All sucrose solutions were made in the hexose-albumin-phosphate media and adjusted to pH 6.0. The material at the 2.0 M-1.55 M sucrose interface was collected, diluted with medium and centrifuged at 630 **g** for 10 minutes to yield the neuronal fraction in the pellet. The material at the 0.9 M-1.35 M sucrose interface was collected, diluted with medium, layered over a gradient of 0.9 M and 1.4 M sucrose and centrifuged at 3300 **g** for 20 minutes. The material at the 0.9 M-1.4 M sucrose interface was collected, diluted with medium and centrifuged at 630 **g** for 10 minutes. The neuroglial-enriched fraction was recovered in the pellet and was astroglia principally. The nature of the two preparations is shown in Fig. 1.

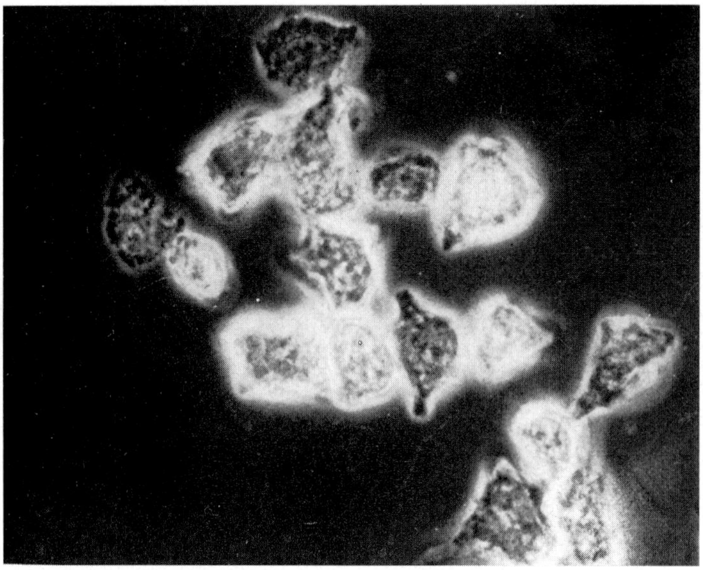

FIG. *1a*. Neuronal-enriched fraction, prepared as described. Phase-contrast microscopy × 750.

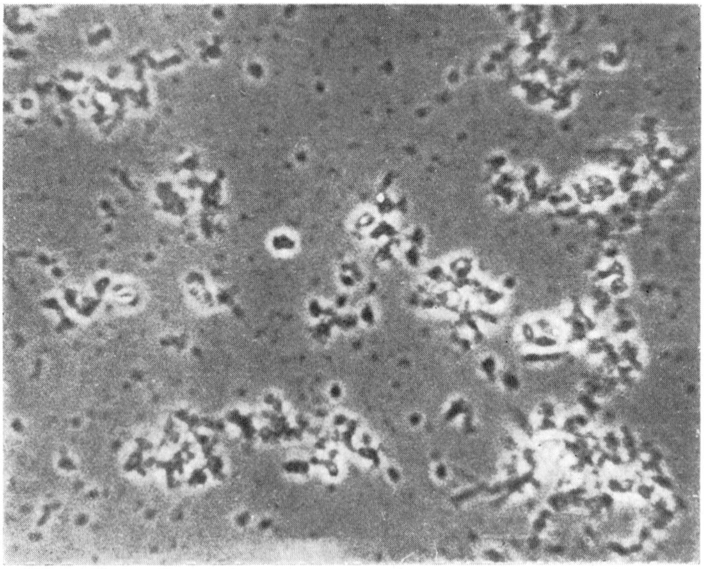

FIG. *1b*. Astroglial-enriched fraction, prepared as described. Phase-contrast microscopy × 500.

*Gas-liquid chromatography*

For analytical purposes a Model 2100 Varian flame ionization gas chromatograph with Model # 475 Integrator was used. Separations were achieved with a 15% EGSS-X (organosilicone-ethylene succinate copolymer; Applied Science Labs., State College, Pa.) column packed with Gas-Chrom P (Applied Science Labs., State College, Pa.) as the stationary phase at 190°C and helium as the carrier gas. Peaks were identified by retention times and comparison with authentic fatty acids. Radio gas chromatography was performed on a Packard gas chromatograph equipped with an ionization detector using a 5% DEGS (diethylene glycol succinate) column on an Anachron SD support obtained from Analabs, North Haven, Conn. The individual fatty acids were collected on separate cellulose cartridges containing terphenyl coated with 5% 550 Dow-Corning on a rotating Packard fraction collector. To visualize the peaks an inactive standard lipid extract from chick brain was methylated and added as carrier to the sample before fractionation.

*Scintillation counting*

The cartridges were extracted in the scintillation fluid which consisted of 98% PPO (diphenyl oxazole)–2% POPOP (1,4-bis[2-(5-phenyloxazoyl)]benzene) dissolved in toluene (5 g/100 ml). A Packard Tri-Carb ambient-temperature scintillation counter was used for radioactivity counting. Counting efficiency for $^{14}C$ was greater than 80%.

Linoleyl-CoA was synthesized according to Kornberg and Pricer (1953) and the purity of the compound was checked by thin-layer chromatography on Silica Gel HRB (E. Merck AG, Darmstadt, Germany) with $CH_3Cl$:$CH_3OH$:$H_2O$ (65:25:4) in a controlled humidity chamber (Colli, Hinkle and Pullman 1969).

RESULTS

*In vivo*

The concentrations of PFA in chick embryonic brain are relatively constant during the developmental period, but because of brain growth, a net increase in PFA occurs. It was necessary to determine whether this deposition of PFA in brain was due to biosynthesis or represented transport of preformed fatty acids either from the yolk or from non-neural sources. A series of labelled precursors was injected into the yolk sac of 10-day-old chick embryos and the phosphoglyceride fatty acids separated into saturated, monoenoic and dienoic, and polyenoic fractions after 48 hours. Most of the radioactive acetate and the saturated fatty acids were recovered from the saturated fatty acid fraction; about 10% of the original material showed some evidence of desaturation, but only 3.6-4.0% was recovered in the PFA fraction (Table 1). With linoleate,

TABLE 1

Incorporation of 1-$^{14}$C-labelled compounds into phosphoglyceride fatty acids of chick embryonic brain

| *Compound injected* | *% of radioactivity in fatty acids* | | |
|---|---|---|---|
| | *Saturated* | *Monoenoic and dienoic* | *PFA* |
| Acetate | 88.9 | 7.6 | 4.0 |
| Myristate | 85.8 | 10.3 | 3.7 |
| Palmitate | 86.3 | 10.8 | 3.6 |
| Stearate | 84.2 | 11.6 | 4.2 |
| Linoleate | 35.8 | 39.7 | 24.8 |
| Linolenate | 46.4 | 9.2 | 44.5 |

Labelled precursor containing 4.4 μCi was injected into the yolk sac of 10-day-old embryos and the brains analysed 48 hours after injection.

24.8% was found in the PFA, with almost all of the activity appearing in the *n*–6 series, while 44.5% of the linolenate label was in the PFA fraction. However, about 10% of the linolenate label was recovered in arachidonic acid, the rest in the *n*-3 series. The presence of radioactivity in arachidonic acid may have been due to elongation with radioactive acetate formed by oxidation of linolenic acid.

### *In vitro*

While the data obtained *in vivo* indicated that the chick embryo could synthesize PFA at 10 days of age, the possibility that the fatty acids were synthesized elsewhere and transported to the brain could not be excluded. To study this problem, slices of 14-day-old chick embryonic brain were incubated with either labelled acetate, [1-$^{14}$C]acetyl-CoA or [1,3-$^{14}$C]malonyl-CoA. The results are shown in Table 2.

TABLE 2

Incorporation of $^{14}C$-labelled precursors in phospholipid fatty acids of chick embryonic brain slices (14 days)

| *Substrate* | *Incorporation into* | | |
|---|---|---|---|
| | *C14-C18* | *PFA* | *C14-18/PFA* |
| [1-$^{14}$C]Na-acetate | 3780* | 78 | 48.2 |
| [1-$^{14}$C]acetyl-CoA | 66 | 15 | 4.4 |
| [1,3-$^{14}$C]malonyl-CoA | 1321 | 67 | 19.7 |

* pmoles substrate incorporated/min/mg lipid P. Medium contains 11 mmol of glucose.

[1-$^{14}$C]acetate was incorporated more rapidly than either [1-$^{14}$C]acetyl-CoA or [1,3-$^{14}$C]malonyl-CoA, presumably because it was transported into the slice more rapidly than the CoA derivatives. Malonyl-CoA was utilized more rapidly than acetyl-CoA. With all three substrates the major activity was recovered in the $C_{14}$-$C_{18}$ fraction. However, with acetyl-CoA the ratio of short-chain acids to PFA was 4.4, whereas with malonyl-CoA this ratio was 19.7. Thus malonyl-CoA appeared to be the substrate of choice for synthesis of shorter-chain fatty acid in brain slices while acetyl-CoA was incorporated into PFA to a greater extent. This appears to corroborate existing information on the roles of malonyl-CoA and acetyl-CoA in the production of PFA in brain (Aeberhard and Menkes 1968). Since the slices contained malonyl-CoA decarboxylase and acetyl-CoA carboxylase activities which can interconvert the two CoA esters, a more detailed analysis of the data is not possible.

When the incorporation of radioactive [1-$^{14}$C]acetyl-CoA and [1,3-$^{14}$C]-malonyl-CoA into the $C_{14}$-$C_{18}$ fatty acids is examined (Table 3), with the

TABLE 3

Incorporation of [1-$^{14}$C]acetyl-CoA and [1,3-$^{14}$C]malonyl-CoA into phospholipid fatty acids of chick embryonic brain (14 days)

| *Fatty acid* | *Radioactivity % of total fraction* | | *Relative specific activity** | |
|---|---|---|---|---|
| | *Acetyl-CoA* | *Malonyl-CoA* | *Acetyl-CoA* | *Malonyl-CoA* |
| 14:0 | 11.6 | 0.3 | 5.8 | 0.1 |
| 16:0 | 42.7 | 23.6 | 1.0 | 0.5 |
| 16:1 | 26.0 | 18.6 | 4.6 | 3.4 |
| 18:0 | 11.9 | 50.2 | 0.6 | 4.6 |
| 18:1 | 2.7 | 5.6 | 0.1 | 0.2 |
| 18:2 | 1.2 | 1.0 | 0.3 | 0.3 |

* Relative specific activity $= \dfrac{\%\text{ radioactivity in fatty acid}}{\%\text{ of total fatty acids.}}$

former precursor the major activity, 42.7%, is found in 16:0, and 11.9% occurs in 18:0. With [1,3-$^{14}$C]malonyl-CoA, 50.2% of the activity is recovered from 18:0 and 23.6% from 16:0, with only little activity in 18:1 and 18:2. The increased radioactivity in 18:0 found with malonyl-CoA could reflect the utilization of that CoA ester by microsomes for fatty acid synthesis. The microsomes are a particulate fraction which is the site of localization of gangliosides (Wherret and McIlwain 1962), whose fatty acid moiety consists principally of 18:0. In the PFA fraction, acetyl-CoA activity is incorporated largely into 20:4 and 22:4, where 74.6% of the radioactivity is found (Table 4).

TABLE 4

Incorporation of [1-$^{14}$C]acetyl-CoA and [1,3-$^{14}$C]malonyl-CoA into phospholipid fatty acids of chick embryonic brain (14 days)

| *Fatty acid* | *Radioactivity % of total fraction* | | *Relative specific activity** | |
|---|---|---|---|---|
| | *Acetyl-CoA* | *Malonyl-CoA* | *Acetyl-CoA* | *Malonyl-CoA* |
| 20:3 (*n*–9) + (*n*–6) | 6.4 | 2.8 | 1.4 | 0.3 |
| 20:4 | 11.7 | 6.4 | 0.4 | 0.2 |
| 20:4 (*n*–3)** | 44.9 | 3.6 | — | — |
| 20:5 | 4.8 | 8.4 | — | — |
| 22:4 | 18.0 | 30.8 | 2.2 | 3.0 |
| 22:5 (*n*–6) | 2.4 | 18.4 | 0.1 | 0.8 |
| 22:5 (*n*–3) | 8.0 | 20.8 | 2.6 | 6.9 |
| 22:6 | 3.3 | 6.4 | 0.2 | 0.2 |

* Relative specific activity $= \dfrac{\text{\% radioactivity in fatty acid}}{\text{\% of total fatty acids.}}$

** Tentative identification.

Of interest is a fatty acid which is tentatively identified as 20:4 (*n*–3), where 44.9% of the label of the PFA fraction occurs after one hour of incubation. A portion of the chromatograph is shown in Fig. 2, where this fatty acid is identified. This peak was collected, hydrogenated and rechromatographed and shown to be a $C_{20}$ acid. A 20:4(*n*–3) fatty acid has been described by Ackman (1969) in fish oil. In view of its position on the chromatographic tracing it is difficult to assign any other structure to this peak. Malonyl-CoA appears to give a different labelling pattern; the $C_{22}$ acids appear to be the predominant radioactive fatty acids, 62% of the $^{14}$C being found there. Although the patterns differ, it is apparent that 14-day-old chick embryonic brain can elaborate PFA (Table 4).

It has been demonstrated (Aeberhard and Menkes 1968) that microsomes from rat brain utilize malonyl-CoA for PFA elongation. To determine whether any changes in PFA metabolism occurred in the brain during development,

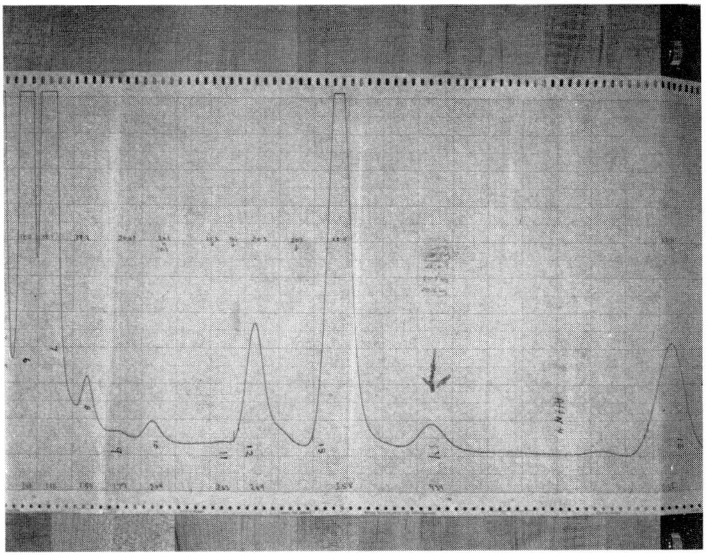

FIG. 2. A portion of the gas chromatographic tracing showing the fatty acid peak described in the text and tentatively identified as 20:4(*n*–3).

TABLE 5

Distribution of phosphoglyceride fatty acids in mitochondria and microsomes of chick embryonic brain (12 days)

| *Fatty acid* | *Mitochondria* | *Microsomes* |
|---|---|---|
| 14:0 | 3.0 | 1.6 |
| 16:0 | 22.1 | 21.9 |
| 16:1 | 2.8 | 3.7 |
| 18:0 | 19.3 | 15.3 |
| 18:1 | 15.9 | 15.0 |
| 18:2 | 3.5 | 2.7 |
| 20:1 + 18:3 | 1.3 | 1.1 |
| 20:2 | 0.2 | tr |
| 20:3 (*n*–9) + (*n*–6) | 0.3 | 2.7 |
| 20:4 (*n*–6) | 12.1 | 14.4 |
| 20:4 (*n*–3)* | 1.1 | 0.8 |
| 20:5 | tr | tr |
| 22:4 | 1.6 | 3.1 |
| 22:5 (*n*–6) | 2.1 | 4.5 |
| 22:5 (*n*–3) | 1.1 | 0.1 |
| 22:6 | 13.8 | 12.0 |

* Tentative identification.

brain microsomes from 12-day and 20-day chick embryos were prepared.

The distribution of phosphoglyceride fatty acids among mitochondria and microsomes of the embryonic chick brain is shown in Table 5. The high concentrations of 20:4 and 22:6 noted for these particulates in other species are evident here. The biosynthetic mechanism was studied using [1-$^{14}$C]linoleyl-CoA as a precursor with malonyl-CoA added as a 'primer'.

With 0.1 to 1.0 $\mu$Ci of [1-$^{14}$C]linoleyl-CoA in the incubation medium about 63.0% and 43.9% of the counts were incorporated into the phosphoglyceride fraction in the 12-day-old and 20-day-old embryonic brain respectively. About 85-90% of the radioactivity was incorporated as linoleic acid. The distribution of the remainder of the $^{14}$C is shown in Table 6. Of interest is the fact that

TABLE 6

Incorporation of [1-$^{14}$C]linoleyl-CoA into phospholipid fatty acids of chick embryonic brain

| *Fatty acid* | *% of total radioactivity** | |
|---|---|---|
| | *12 days* | *20 days* |
| 14:0 | 0.4 | 0.5 |
| 16:0 | 21.9 | 25.7 |
| 16:1 | 1.2 | 1.0 |
| 18:0 | 0.6 | 0.6 |
| 18.1 | 3.0 | 9.7 |
| 18:3 | 10.1 | 11.4 |
| 20:1 + 18:3 | 4.3 | 2.8 |
| 20:3 (*n*–9) + (*n*–6) | 9.2 | 7.2 |
| 20:4 | 5.6 | 7.1 |
| 20:4 (*n*–3)** | 23.4 | 7.3 |
| 20:5 | 2.3 | 3.3 |
| 22:4 | 3.0 | 4.4 |
| 22:5 (*n*–6) | 5.6 | 10.8 |
| 22:5 (*n*–3) | 4.3 | 5.4 |
| 22:6 | 4.6 | 5.4 |

* Exclusive of 18:2. ** Tentative identification.

21.9% and 25.7% of the label is found in palmitic acid in the younger and older embryonic brain respectively. Another major site of incorporation is 18:3 (*n*–6), which has been shown to be intermediate in the biosynthesis of 20:4 (Klenk 1965). The fatty acid mentioned in the work on brain slices and tentatively identified as 20:4 (*n*–3) is actively labelled in the 12-day-old embryonic brain, where 23.4% of the activity is localized, while 7.3% is recovered in this fatty acid in the 20-day-old chick embryonic brain (Table 6). The pattern of labelling is otherwise not significantly different for the two age groups.

*Neuronal and glial preparations*

Table 7 shows the uptake of [1-$^{14}$C]acetate into neuronal and glial preparations obtained from rat brain at 10 and 20 days postnatally. The earlier period shows a more rapid uptake of activity in both preparations with the glial preparation somewhat more active. The activity in both fractions falls at 21 days with the glial fraction diminishing to less than 10% of its 10-day value. The activity of the neuronal fraction at this period is about one-third of the 10-day value, and is 2½ times greater than that of the glia. The ratio of neuronal to glial activity changes from 0.68 at 10 days to 2.47 at 21 days.

TABLE 7

Incorporation of [1-$^{14}$C]acetate into phosphoglyceride fatty acids of neuronal and glial preparations of developing rat brain

| *Age days* | *Neuronal* | *Glial* | *Ratio N/G* |
|---|---|---|---|
| 10 | 4875* ± 1475 (3) | 7125 ± 1125 (2) | 0.68 |
| 21 | 1514 ± 264 (4) | 612 ± 47 (4) | 2.47 |

* C.p.m./μmol lipid P.
Numbers in parentheses are numbers of experiments.

The distribution of the radioactivity in the fatty acid fraction shows no differences in labelling patterns between the two cell types (Table 8). In both glial and neuronal fractions the major activity in the PFA fraction is found in 22:4. The other principal areas of radioactivity are in 16:0 and 18:0, with the remaining activity distributed among the various fatty acids at a low level.

## DISCUSSION

It has been demonstrated *in vivo* and *in vitro* that embryonic chick brain can synthesize fatty acids before the period of active myelination. Of interest is the finding that with [1-$^{14}$C]acetyl-CoA as a marker, a fatty acid can be isolated that has been tentatively identified as 20:4 (*n*–3) which contains more of the radioactivity than any other fatty acid after one hour of incubation. This fatty acid may be an intermediate in 22:6 synthesis. It has been reported to be present in cod-liver oil (Ackman 1969) and in chick muscle (Miller *et al.* 1967). Stoffel (1965) has also reported its synthesis from 18:4 (*n*–3). When labelled linoleyl-CoA was used, a large part of the radioactivity could also be recovered in the peak described. Since carboxyl radioactivity was not measured, it was not

TABLE 8

Incorporation of [1-$^{14}$C]acetate into phosphoglyceride fatty acids of neuronal and glial preparations of developing rat brain, as percentage of total radioactivity

| Fatty acid | *10-day brain* | | *21-day brain* | |
|---|---|---|---|---|
| | *Neuronal* | *Glial* | *Neuronal* | *Glial* |
| 14:0 | 6.0 | 13.3 | 4.7 | 1.5 |
| 16:0 + 16:1 | 49.5 | 32.0 | 15.6 | 23.3 |
| 18:0 | 11.3 | 6.9 | 30.7 | 10.3 |
| 18:1 | 3.5 | 3.2 | 4.7 | 8.9 |
| 18:2 | 1.9 | 1.3 | 3.6 | 1.5 |
| 18:3 + 20:1 | 2.6 | 1.6 | 4.9 | — |
| 20:3 (*n*–9) + (*n*–6) | 1.8 | 0.6 | 2.2 | — |
| 20:4 | 2.1 | 3.1 | 5.7 | 3.8 |
| 20:4 (*n*–3) | — | 2.1 | 1.2 | 4.5 |
| 22:4 | 19.0 | 24.0 | 23.4 | 20.0 |
| 22:5 (*n*–6) | 0.8 | — | 4.0 | 3.9 |
| 22:5 (*n*–3) | 1.1 | 3.6 | 2.2 | 1.0 |
| 22:6 | 1.2 | 1.5 | 3.1 | 2.1 |

possible to determine how 18:2 is converted to this compound. However, the identification of the fatty acid is not definite, and so any explanation must be speculative. That differences were obtained in the glial and neuronal fractions of rat brain could be accounted for by differences in experimental conditions. The recovery of 18:2 radioactivity in 16:0 was also unexpected. However, in a series of papers, Dhopeshwarkar and Mead (1970, 1971*a*, *b*) report similar results in brain after giving labelled 18:1, 18:2 and 18:3 to rats. They found a high relative carboxyl activity in 16:0 and concluded that this might be due to exchange of radioactive carboxyl. If so, perhaps a similar mechanism accounts for the presence of radioactivity in the unknown fatty acid we have described derived from 18:2. That both the brain slice and the microsomal preparations gave similar results despite the use of different precursors is of some interest.

Much of the work on brain cell types has indicated that the neuronal fraction has the most active metabolism. Satake and Abe (1965) showed that neuronal proteins were labelled more rapidly than the proteins of glial cells and Blomstrand and Hamberger (1969) found neurons to be three times as active as glial cells in incorporating amino acids into proteins. Freysz, Bieth and Mandel (1969) found that neuronal phospholipids turned over more rapidly than glial phospholipids as measured by incorporation of $^{32}$P. Jarlstedt and Hamberger (1971), however, showed no differences in RNA labelling between the two cell types after 1 hour, using [$^{3}$H]uridine. None of the studies cited deals with developing brain. Our studies indicate that [1-$^{14}$C]acetate is incorporated more rapidly into phosphoglyceride fatty acids of glial cells than into neurons at 10 days of postnatal brain development in the rat. At 21 days of life, when the period of active myelination has passed, neurons incorporate acetate more actively than glia, though both cell types are less active at this age than at the earlier period. This indicates that fatty acid biosynthesis in glial cells may be related to the demands of the organism for fatty acids, engendered by myelin deposition. It can be seen from the data on fatty acid distribution that the *n*–3 series fatty acids are poorly labelled compared to *n*–6 fatty acids. That acetate is a poor precursor for elongation to 22:6 has been reported earlier (Miyamoto, Stephanides and Bernsohn 1967*b*). This could result from the lack of available 18:3 necessary for 22:6 production. If malonyl-CoA is the preferred substrate for this elongation mechanism, the conversion of acetate to malonyl-CoA could be limiting, since in the absence of citrate, acetyl-CoA carboxylase seems to be a rate-limiting step in fatty acid synthesis (Martin and Vagelos 1962).

Thus the biosynthesis of polyenoic fatty acids in developing brain appears to show distinctive features during the period of active formation of myelin. The incorporation of labelled precursors at an early period of brain development into a fatty acid that has not been reported to play a significant part in PFA biosynthesis in other organs or in adult brain, is to be noted. In addition, the active incorporation of labelled acetate into phosphoglyceride fatty acids by glial cells from the rat at a period just before myelination, and the diminution in this activity after the active period of myelin deposition, might have significant implications in this system.

## SUMMARY

The role of polyenoic fatty acid synthesis in developing brain was studied in order to investigate the relationship between fatty acids and myelin deposition. In the chick embryonic brain polyenoic acids were synthesized *in vivo* and *in vitro* at an early stage of development. Under the experimental conditions described, active incorporation occurs from [1-$^{14}$C]acetyl-CoA into a fatty acid fraction which has been tentatively identified as 20:4 (*n*–3). With [1-$^{14}$C]linoleyl-CoA, palmitic acid was found to be the most active fatty acid apart from linolenic acid. Neuronal and glial preparations obtained from developing rat brain showed that at 10 days of age the glial fraction was more active than the neuronal fraction in the incorporation of [1-$^{14}$C]acetate into fatty acids. At 20 days of age both neuronal and glial preparations showed diminished activity, with the glial fractions incorporating about 10% of the activity incorporated at 10 days. No differences in fatty acid labelling were observed between the two fractions.

## References

ACKMAN, R. G. (1969) In *Methods in Enzymology*, vol. 14, p. 344, ed. J. M. Lowenstein. Academic Press, New York
AEBERHARD, E. and MENKES, J. H. (1968) *J. Biol. Chem.* **243**, 3834
ALTER, M., LIEBOWITZ, V. and SPEER, J. (1966) *Arch. Neurol.* **15**, 234
BERNSOHN, J. and STEPHANIDES, L. M. (1967) *Nature* (*Lond.*) **215**, 821
BERNSOHN, J., STEPHANIDES, L. M. and NORGELLO, H. (1971) *Brain Res.* **28**, 327
BLOMSTRAND, M. C. and HAMBERGER, A. (1969) *J. Neurochem.* **16**, 1401
COLLI, W., HINKLE, P. C. and PULLMAN, M. E. (1969) *J. Biol Chem.* **244**, 6432
DHOPESHWARKAR, G. A. and MEAD, J. F. (1970) *Biochim. Biophys. Acta* **210**, 250
DHOPESHWARKAR, G. A. and MEAD, J. F. (1971*a*) *Biochim. Biophys. Acta* **231**, 8
DHOPESHWARKAR, G. A. and MEAD, J. F. (1971*b*) *Biochim. Biophys. Acta* **239**, 162
FREYSZ, L., BIETH, R. and MANDEL, P. (1969) *J.Neurochem.* **16**, 1417
JARLSTEDT, J. and HAMBERGER, A. (1971) *J. Neurochem.* **18**, 921
KLENK, E. (1961) In *Drugs Affecting Lipid Metabolism*, p. 21, ed. S. Garattini and R. Paoletti. Elsevier, Amsterdam
KLENK, E. (1965) *J. Am. Oil Chem. Soc.* **42**, 580
KORNBERG, A. and PRICER, W. E. (1953) *J. Biol. Chem.* **204**, 345
MARTIN, D. B. and VAGELOS, P. R. (1962) *J. Biol. Chem.* **237**, 1787
MCALPINE, D., LUMSDEN, C. E. and ACHESON, E. D. (1963) In *Multiple Sclerosis, a Reappraisal*, p. 18. Williams and Wilkins, Baltimore
MILLER, D., GRUGER, E. H., Jr, LEONG, K. C. and KNOBL, G. M., JR (1967) *Poultry Sci.* **46**, 438
MIYAMOTO, K., STEPHANIDES, L. M. and BERNSOHN, J. (1966) *J. Lipid Res.* **7**, 664
MIYAMOTO, K., STEPHANIDES, L. M. and BERNSOHN, J. (1967*a*) *J. Neurochem.* **14**, 227
MIYAMOTO, K., STEPHANIDES, L. M. and BERNSOHN, J. (1967*b*) *J. Lipid Res.* **8**, 191
MOHRHAUER, H. and HOLMAN, R. (1963) *J. Neurochem.* **10**, 523
NORTON, W. T. and PODUSLO, S. E. (1970) *Science* **167**, 1144
O'BRIEN, J. S. and SAMPSON, E. L. (1965) *J. Lipid Res.* **6**, 545
PETERS, A., PALAY, S. L. and WEBSTER, F. H. DE (1970) *The Fine Structure of the Nervous System*, pp. 125-126. Harper and Row, New York
SATAKE, M. and ABE, S. (1965) *J. Biochem.* (*Japan*) **59**, 72
STOFFEL, W. VON (1965) *Colloq. Ges. Physiol. Chem.* no. 16, 64
WHERRET, J. R. and MCILWAIN, H. (1962) *Biochem. J.* **84**, 232

## Discussion

*Menkes:* Dr. Bernsohn, in Table 4 you showed that on incubation of chick embryonic brain slices with malonyl-CoA, there was a very high relative specific activity (6.9) for 22:5 (*n*–3). Can you explain that?

*Bernsohn:* I think this high specific activity may be due to high turnover, but also the low concentration of 22:5 (*n*–3) in the brain tends to elevate the value for relative specific activity.

*Ansell*: The transfer of lipid components from one membrane to another was discussed earlier by Professor Davison (pp. 73-83). In your experiments with isolated astroglial cells and neurons, have you considered labelling the astroglial cells, incubating them with neurons and seeing whether lipids are transferred from one cell type to the other? In addition, have you seen which lipids were labelled by the incorporation of fatty acids?

*Bernsohn:* So far we have separated the cell types after labelling and incubation, because when we fractionated first we ran into problems of the morphology and fragility of the cells. In Norton's technique (Norton and Poduslo 1970) the cells are incubated in trypsin and this makes them vulnerable to further manipulations. Probably we could reincubate the cells, mixing labelled neurons with a fresh glial preparation or *vice versa*, to see if exchange of radioactive material occurs. We have some data on the incorporation of long-chain fatty acids into the various phospholipid classes.

*Ansell:* I realize that the re-isolation of neurons and glia from the mixture would be difficult. You might have to use a radioautographic procedure or something of this sort.

*Bernsohn:* One of the steps in the isolation depends on the ability of the two types of cells to separate on different sucrose density gradients, and they may retain that property. It has been reported by Hemminki, Huttunen and Jarnefelt (1970) that of the various separation techniques, Norton's method yielded cells which showed the best protein synthesis and had the best oxygen uptake.

*Davison:* A fundamental issue raised by Dr Bernsohn is the hypothesis that an abnormal fatty acid may be incorporated into the brain and stay there for the life of the animal, or that there may be a lack of essential fatty acid in the brain, which would again remain for the life of the animal, and make the brain susceptible to disease processes. The basis for this idea is that the entry of fatty acids into the adult brain has long been known to be very slow, and Dr Mead's experiments support this, even though he has shown that fatty acids in trace amounts can get in from the blood. Secondly, metabolism of fatty acids within the brain by β-oxidation is very restricted. So that if a long-chain fatty acid molecule gets in, it will be likely to stay.

Two things are contrary to this idea. The first we have heard from Professor Paoletti, that in his rats the effect of unsaturated fatty acid deficiency was reversible. If that is true, it is contrary to current views, and it is important to confirm whether or not the deficiency is reversible. The second point is our finding that phospholipid molecules and fatty acids can exchange readily with all membranes in the brain. If this is true, any deficiency, such as you suggest might occur in multiple sclerosis, would be distributed throughout the whole of the myelin sheath. As a result it would be very difficult to explain the pathology of multiple sclerosis, where the lesions are randomly spaced in time and in region of the central nervous system.

*Bernsohn:* There are a number of ways of looking at this, and when we first proposed this hypothesis we assumed that the defect in multiple sclerosis lay in the lipid composition of myelin. We have to retreat on this particular point, and what I'd like to propose is that the defect is not necessarily in the fatty acid composition of myelin itself. It seems reasonable to think that if a certain biochemical *milieu* of *x* factors has to be present for oligodendrocytes to elaborate normal myelin, and the absence of any one factor during this period could upset the metabolic machinery of the oligodendrocyte, then the end product, myelin, of the inadequate metabolic machinery could be defective anywhere, not necessarily in the lipid composition or the fatty acid composition. Perhaps even the protein may be abnormal, and a defective protein molecule is laid down. The conventional histological stain, usually the Weigert stain, for demonstrating myelin in fact probably shows the disappearance of proteolipid in demyelination. Of course, we know the lipids change too, but the point is that the basic machinery required to elaborate normal myelin may be defective in the oligodendrocyte to start with. We don't know what the ultimate basic defect in the myelin is, but it doesn't have to be restricted to fatty acid composition.

*Davison:* That hypothesis doesn't explain the random nature of the lesion.

*Bernsohn:* It didn't, until Dr Dobbing remarked that myelination occurs in tracts. If we're talking about episodic deficits, if there was such a deficit at a time when a tract was being myelinated, one tract could be defective and the one next to it might be normal.

*Dobbing:* Myelination happens in tracts, certainly, but not in plaques. The tract is a long thing, going right down the spinal cord, and demyelinating disease occurs in plaques, which are presumably spherical lesions.

*Menkes:* Any theory of multiple sclerosis has to take into account that there are two factors in operation. There is undoubtedly an environmental factor which is almost certainly a virus, plus something else which could very well be prenatal dietary changes making certain areas of the brain more susceptible to the virus. The location of plaques in the vicinity of blood vessels may reflect the site of the auto-immune reaction. This does not explain why not everyone who contracts a virus such as measles (a measles-like virus has been proposed as the inciting cause), develops multiple sclerosis. There has to be another factor. Your theory's as good as any!

*Bernsohn:* Clausen and Møller (1967) found that when rats were raised on a diet deficient in essential fatty acids and then subjected to allergic encephalomyelitis antigen, they developed the disease at much smaller doses of the antigen than the normal rat.

*Chapman:* You are suggesting that some fatty acid is present in the myelin which then encourages some molecular processes to occur, causing the destruction of the myelin membrane system. What is known about the details of the breakdown process?

*Davison:* One of the latest views (Adams, Hallpike and Bayliss 1971) is that the basic protein cementing together the myelin lamellae is attacked by proteolytic enzymes, because it can be shown that the inter-period lines disappear early in the demyelinating process (Dickinson *et al.* 1970). It looks as if the basic protein, which has been shown to be deficient in areas of actively demyelinating tissue, is one of the things that disappears, not primarily the lipid.

*Chapman:* Are cholesterol esters produced?

*Davison:* Cholesterol esters are produced some time afterwards in the initial attack. I think Professor Bernsohn has a very ingenious and interesting idea, but I don't accept it as a possible factor in multiple sclerosis. It doesn't explain the possible reversibility of the condition, because if Professor Paoletti's work is correct, you should be able to reverse a deficiency by feeding polyunsaturated acids. Quite a lot of clinical work has been done on the basis of Dr Bernsohn's hypothesis, feeding fish liver oils and so on to patients with multiple sclerosis, and there has been no dramatic improvement in the course of the disease. Yet from Professor Paoletti's results one would have expected quite a rapid reversal, if the deficiency in the myelin is an essential fatty acid deficiency.

*Bernsohn:* I'm not necessarily prepared to accept the idea that a reversal of the defect in the essential fatty acid composition would alter the demyelination process.

*Chapman:* Does your idea explain the molecular processes that occur? Just to say that the absence of some essential fatty acid causes multiple sclerosis doesn't help me to see the next steps in the argument.

*Bernsohn:* I can't argue that point, because I happen to agree with you! One of the merits of the hypothesis is that it correlates a number of epidemiological facts which hitherto have been unrelated haphazard observations. For example, there is a north-south gradient in the incidence of multiple sclerosis. People in northern latitudes have a higher incidence of the disease than those in warmer places. But this is not true of the Japanese or the Chinese, or of the Eskimos (Bernsohn and Stephanides 1967). Health officials in Canada have been unable to find multiple sclerosis in the Eskimo population (Bernsohn and Barron 1970). Nor does this north-south gradient apply to coastal areas. Even in areas of high incidence of the disease, people living on the coast have a lower incidence than those living inland. In northern Ireland, for example, where the incidence of multiple sclerosis is high, the incidence of the disease in Belfast is about half that of the inland areas (Millar 1971). All these peoples have available to them either a marine diet, or, as in Japan, soya bean oil is a dietary staple and is rich in linolenic acid.

There's a tendency for people of the managerial classes in England to have a higher incidence of the disease than working-class people (Miller, Ridley and Schapira 1960), a reflection of the fact that the managerial class may use more animal fats which are low in polyunsaturates as a source of protein. The people in southern climates have available to them seed and fish oils.

There are other facts: the incidence of the disease tends to be higher within families than between families, and a genetic factor has been eliminated as a possible explanation. Such information indicates that there may be some environmental factor, and this could be nutritional and related to the dietary habits of the family group. Migration from a high-risk zone to a low-risk zone carries with it the risk of the country of origin, unless the person was under 15 years old at the time of migration (Alter, Liebowitz and Speer 1966). This would indicate that the disease is established early in the life of the individual, and this may be relevant to the vulnerability of the brain at an early period of development.

*Crawford:* This is similar to the contrast in the incidence of atherosclerosis between Africa and Europe. Professor J. N. P. Davies of Albany University told me that an American team had looked for evidence of multiple sclerosis in Africa, both clinically and in the records, with negative results. This is not a disease that should be missed.

*Bovet:* Professor Bernsohn used the term 'vulnerability': would it be better to talk about 'sensitivity', to take into account the fact that the same agent can have opposite effects? We are not all convinced that the brain is sensitive to nutritional deficiency, so it would be prudent to speak of possible positive effects of nutrition and not only of negative effects. In the future we hope to discover the complex equilibrium between body weight and mental capacity, in order to assist people to achieve rapid body growth, which may have some component affecting development of the brain.

*Crawford:* One point that should be borne in mind with regard to Professor Paoletti's results is that his animals were breast-fed and were therefore receiving a certain amount of long-chain polyunsaturated acids. So his experiments are not directly analogous to the situation in technically advanced countries where breast-feeding may not be done at all. It is difficult to argue from the experiments in rats, either negatively or positively, particularly with regard to reversibility, because in fact Dr Paoletti's situation is a low level of fatty acids until weaning and then the deficiency really starts.

*Davison:* But the reversibility was after 60 days (30 days of EFA deficiency and 30 days of normal diet).

*Crawford:* There is a different timing here, because myelination starts in the rat at about 15 days, and brain cell formation precedes myelination. It is unlikely that the reversibility in Paoletti's rats would restore brain cells if these were lost or not formed, even if the lipid patterns were corrected. A gain in brain weight at 60 days might be due to growth of white matter.

It may be that what is happening before myelination is critically important. We don't really know about reversibility of damaged brain cells in the rat because the experiment hasn't been done. An experiment that should be done is to put the rats on a fat-free milk.

*Chapman:* Couldn't one argue that the deficiency of essential fatty acid causes the production of some molecule, perhaps lysolecithin, which then affects myelin and that the myelin was essentially quite normal in the first place? If this is the case, to try to pin everything on some minor modification of fatty acid of the myelin may not be the right approach at all. We should try to get to the molecular details of what's happening.

*Paoletti:* It was recently observed in our laboratory that in some patients with multiple sclerosis, just before the outburst of the disease, there was a considerable increase of activity of a plasma enzyme, the cholesterol:lecithin acyltransferase. This would fit in with the finding that such patients have more plasma lysolecithin than normal. Is this a factor which affects membranes, especially myelin?

*Davison:* The cholesterol:lecithin acyltransferase activity in brain is very low, according to Eto and Suzuki (1972), so it would be unlikely that this could occur in brain tissue itself.

*Paoletti:* I agree with that, but I just wonder if the lysolecithin which is present in plasma may play some role in the onset of the disease. If so, it would be enough to have an increase of the enzyme in plasma.

*von Muralt:* Dr Bernsohn's conception of the oligodendroglial apparatus as a production line for myelin and the marked disturbance of production by a deficiency in one essential fatty acid recalls the *in vitro* experiments on lysosomal synthesis of, for instance, haemoglobin. Any disturbance in the balance of available amino acids has far-reaching effects on the synthesis.

*Crawford:* I am reminded of some work on yeast by Wallace, Huang and Linnane (1968). They found that if yeast is grown anaerobically in a purely carbohydrate medium, with no lipid, the mitochondria are poorly formed, globular and have very little in the way of internal cristae. If you then add lipid to the medium, internal membranous structures develop in the mitochondria. Many of the oxidative enzymes present in mitochondria are of course lying along the cristae and you can detect differences between these two types of mitochondria by the presence or absence of these enzymes. This is possibly pertinent to this discussion, in that it's not a question of the yeast surviving, because it survives whether it has lipid or not; but if you give it some lipid it does something slightly different from what it does if it hasn't got lipid.

*Mead:* In most of the cases of demyelination that we have been discussing, we are basically concerned with enzymes in the endoplasmic reticulum, and it is probably true to say that almost all these enzymes are lipoproteins, and if the lipoprotein is abnormal, the spatial relationship of the enzyme and substrate will not be correct. This could explain some of our difficulties: the defects are not a result of lipid metabolism *per se*, but of spatial relationships in the endoplasmic reticulum.

# References

ADAMS, C. W. M., HALLPIKE, J. F. and BAYLISS, O. B. (1971) *J. Neurochem.* **18**, 1479-1483

ALTER, M., LIEBOWITZ, V. and SPEER, J. (1966) *Arch. Neurol. (Chic.)* **15**, 449-462

BERNSOHN, J. and BARRON, K. D. (1970) In *Handbook of Clinical Neurology*, vol. 9, ed. P. J. Vinken and G. W. Bruyn. North-Holland, Amsterdam

BERNSOHN, J. and STEPHANIDES, L. M. (1967) *Nature (Lond.)* **215**, 821-823

CLAUSEN, J. and MØLLER, J. (1967) *Acta Neurol. Scand.* **43**, 375-388

DICKINSON, J. P., JONES, K. M., APARICIO, S. R. and LUMSDEN, C. E. (1970) *Nature (Lond.)* **227**, 1133-1135

ETO, Y. and SUZUKI, K. (1972) *J. Neurochem.* **19**, 117

HEMMINKI, K., HUTTUNEN, M. O. and JARNEFELT, J. (1970) *Brain Res.* **23**, 23-34

MILLAR, J. H. D. (1971) *Multiple Sclerosis*. Thomas, Springfield, Ill.

MILLER, H., RIDLEY, A. and SCHAPIRA, K. (1960) *Br. Med. J.* **2**, 343-345

NORTON, W. T. and PODUSLO, S. E. (1970) *Science* **167**, 1144-1146

WALLACE, P. G., HUANG, M. and LINNANE, A. D. (1968) *J. Cell Biol.* **37**, 207

# Lipid metabolism of brain tissue in culture

JOHN H. MENKES

*Division of Pediatric Neurology, University of California at Los Angeles and Veterans Administration Hospital, Brentwood*

In order to study the synthesis and turnover of myelin lipids with long half-lives a system had to be devised which would allow metabolic studies over prolonged periods. Homogenates and subcellular fractions of brain are suitable only for an investigation of cerebral lipids with short half-lives, whose principal localization is outside the myelin sheath and which are probably only secondarily involved in the demyelinating disorders (O'Brien 1965).

The development of methods for cultivating brain tissue *in vitro* provided a new and potentially useful system for the study of lipid metabolism under normal and pathological conditions. Mammalian cells in tissue culture derive most of their lipids from the serum customarily added to the growth medium. Growth of a number of cell strains can also be supported by chemically defined media which do not contain serum. Under these conditions cell lipids are synthesized from precursors added to the medium. Our initial studies indicated that brain explants remain metabolically active for several days in a chemically defined, serum-free medium and that they incorporate radioactive lipid precursors such as mevalonate and fatty acids into a number of lipid fractions (Menkes 1971).

In this report I shall review the metabolic data obtained on brain explants from immature and mature rats and contrast them with those obtained on tissues removed by surgical biopsy from patients with demyelinating and lipid storage diseases.

## METHODS

### *Cell cultures*

For the animal experiments, frontal poles from brains of immature rats of the Sprague-Dawley strain, aged 2 to 22 days, and mature animals, aged 5 to 6 months, were used. After removal from the cranium, tissue was left overnight at 4°C in 50 ml Hanks Salt Solution (Grand Island Biological Company, Berkeley, Calif.) containing 0.5 ml antibiotic–antimycotic solution 524 (Grand Island Biological Company, Berkeley, Calif.). The next day dura and blood vessels were carefully removed under a dissecting microscope, and the remaining tissue further cut into fragments approximately 1 mm in diameter. These were placed into plastic Falcon flasks (30 ml) (Becton, Dickinson and Co., Oxnard, Calif.). Four flasks were used for frontal lobes of a 3-day-old animal. Medium 199, 0.5 ml (Hyland Laboratories, Costa Mesa, Calif.), enriched with 20% (v/v) calf serum, 10% (v/v) egg ultrafiltrate and 300 mg of glucose per ml was added to all cultures. In addition, 1 ml of antibiotic–antimycotic solution 524 was added to each 100 ml of medium. The flasks were placed for 8 to 12 hours in a 37°C incubator under an atmosphere of 95% air – 5% $CO_2$. This allowed the fragments to adhere to the plastic. Five ml more of incubation medium were added, and the tissue was grown for 8 to 10 days at 37°C in an atmosphere of 95% air – 5% $CO_2$, with the medium being changed after 4 days.

Microscopic examination at that time showed outgrowth of multipolar glial cells from the margin of the explants. The outgrowth was better in explants obtained from 3- and 6-day-old animals than those derived from older rats. At the conclusion of the initial incubation the growth medium was removed and replaced with the experimental medium, 5 ml NCTC 109 (Hyland Laboratories) enriched with 300 mg glucose per ml and 1 ml of the antibiotic–antimycotic solution containing the labelled substrate.

Brain tissue obtained from patients at surgical biopsy of the non-dominant frontal lobe was treated in an identical manner.

In experiments designed to measure fatty acid uptake one of the following precursors was used: [1-$^{14}$C]stearic acid, 0.2 μCi (48.4 mCi/mmol) (Amersham-Searle, Des Plaines, Ill.); [1-$^{14}$C]palmitic acid, 0.2 μCi (10.0 mCi/mmol); [1-$^{14}$C]linoleic acid, 0.2 μCi (52.9 mCi/mmol) (Amersham-Searle, Des Plaines, Ill.); [1-$^{14}$C]lignoceric acid, 0.2 μCi (courtesy of Dr James Mead); and [1-$^{14}$C] sodium acetate, 0.10 mCi (50 mCi/mmol) (Mallinckrodt Chemical Co.). The fatty acids were added in the form of their albumin complexes prepared according to the method of Fillerup, Migliore and Mead (1958). Molar ratios of added free fatty acid : albumin of the order of 0.003 resulted in optimal microscopic appearance of explants.

### *Lipid extraction and fractionation*

At the termination of the experiment tissue from the four flasks was combined, cells were scraped off with a policeman, the medium was removed by centrifugation, and cells were washed three times with 0.15 M-NaCl. The tissue was homogenized in 3 ml of chloroform-methanol (2:1, v/v) and aliquots removed for determination of radioactivity and protein content (Gornall, Bardawill and David 1949).

The homogenate was filtered through a medium-porosity sintered glass funnel, portions were taken for counting and the solution was evaporated to dryness under nitrogen and placed overnight in a desiccator prior to fractionation on an anhydrous silica column. The lipids were suspended in 0.2 ml of chloroform containing 0.1 g of silicic acid and were then applied to a 0.5 × 6 cm silicic acid column (Sigma Chemical Co., St. Louis, Mo.) and fractionated according to the method of Sun and Horrocks (1969). Neutral lipids were eluted with 60 ml of chloroform; glycolipids were eluted with 50 ml of chloroform-acetone (1:1, v/v) followed by 50 ml of acetone; and phospholipids were eluted with 100 ml of methanol. Portions of each fraction were taken for determination of radioactivity; the remainder was separated by thin-layer chromatography.

Lipids in each fraction were separated by thin-layer chromatography on 20 × 20 cm plates. For the separation of neutral lipids, Silica Gel G (Merck, AG, Darmstadt, Germany) powder was slurried in 0.01 M-$Na_2CO_3$ and the plates were developed in hexane-ether (70:30, v/v) according to the procedure of Sun and Horrocks (1969). Glycolipids were separated on Silica Gel G with a solution of chloroform-acetone-methanol-water (60:20:20:1 by volume). Phospholipids were separated on Silica Gel H with chloroform-methanol-acetic acid-water (25:15:4:2 by volume), according to the method of Skipski, Peterson and Barclay (1964). Areas containing lipids were located by a brief exposure to iodine vapours and were scraped from the silica gel and transferred to a counting vial to which 15 ml of scintillation mixture [0.5% (w/v) 2, 5-diphenyloxazole (PPO) and 0.03% (w/v) 1,4-bis [2-(5-phenyloxazolyl]-benzene (POPOP) in toluene] and 0.6 g Cab-O-Sil (Snyder and Stephens 1962) were added. Uptake of radioactivity was a function of the amount of tissue incubated. Since this varied considerably between experiments, all data were expressed in terms of mg of tissue protein.

### *Identification of fatty acids*

For identification of the labelled fatty acids the lipid extract was dried under a stream of nitrogen. Fatty acid methyl esters were prepared by heating the dried sample at 100°C for 90 minutes with 14% (w/v) boron trifluoride in methanol (Morrison and Smith 1964). The fatty acids were extracted into hexane, purified by thin-layer chromatography on Silica Gel G plates developed with hexane-ether (9:1, v/v), and separated according to degree of unsaturation on silver nitrate-impregnated plates developed in chloroform (Morris 1966). Gas-liquid chromatography of each fraction was performed on columns of 16% (w/v) diethyleneglycol succinate on Gas Chrom Z as stationary phase (Applied Science Laboratories, State College, Pa.). Gas chromatography was carried out in a Barber-Coleman model 10 gas chromatograph with argon detector. The column was operated at 175°–195°C at 19 lb argon pressure. Peaks were identified by comparison with standard mixtures of fatty acid esters. Radioactive fatty acid methyl esters were collected from the gas chromatograph by means of a glass U-tube (4 mm in diameter) directly connected to the heated outlet and cooled in a dry-ice mixture. The fatty acid esters were rinsed from the collection tubes into a scintillation vial with 15 ml of scintillation mixture. Approximately 90% of the radioactivity injected into the column was recovered.

## RESULTS

### *Incorporation of fatty acids into tissue lipids*

Even when experimental conditions were well standardized the total fatty acid uptake varied considerably between experiments. In tissues derived from a 3-day-old rat, incubated with [1-$^{14}$C]stearic acid, the uptake ranged from 67 000 to 240 000 c.p.m./mg protein. When fatty acids were added in the form of their albumin complexes a considerable proportion of the uptake remained unmetabolized, probably in the form of protein-bound free fatty acids. However, the relative amount of label incorporated into each of the lipid classes was nearly constant (Table 1). In the neutral lipid fraction triglycerides were the principal labelled lipid, with lesser amounts of radioactivity in diglycerides and cholesterol esters. Only a small amount of label was present in cholesterol. Cerebrosides were the principal labelled lipids identified in the glycolipid fraction. Fatty acids were incorporated into all major phospholipids, notably choline phosphoglycerides and ethanolamine phosphoglycerides, which together accounted for about 60% of the total phospholipid radioactivity (Table 1).

When the uptake of the various fatty acids into the phospholipid fraction was compared palmitic acid was found to be incorporated to the greatest extent, lignoceric the least.

Under the culture conditions employed a significant proportion of stearic,

TABLE 1

Distribution of radioactivity in lipids isolated from brain tissue explants after incubation with various lipid precursors

| *Fraction* | *Radioactivity* | | | |
|---|---|---|---|---|
| | *[1-$^{14}$C] sodium acetate* (5) | *[1-$^{14}$C] palmitic acid* (2) | *[1-$^{14}$C] stearic acid* (5) | *[1-$^{14}$C] lignoceric acid* (1) |
| Total radioactivity uptake (c.p.m. $\times$ $10^{-3}$/mg protein) | 5.4-62 | 104-177 | 67-241 | 5.6 |
| 'Neutral lipids' | 80.3 | 54.7 | 74.9 $\pm$ 7.4 | 90.7 |
| Triglycerides | 73.7 | 67.5 | 41.8 $\pm$ 10.9 | 10.9 |
| Diglycerides | 2.7 | 8.7 | 7.9 $\pm$ 2.6 | 3.2 |
| Cholesterol | 1.9 | 2.6 | 3.0 $\pm$ 1.3 | 2.0 |
| Free fatty acid | 6.0 | 12.3 | 39.2 $\pm$ 10.1 | 79.1 |
| Glycolipids | 0.7 | 0.6 | 1.9 $\pm$ 0.7 | 2.3 |
| Cerebrosides | 34.8 | 22.9 | 45.3 $\pm$ 8.5 | 58.5 |
| Sulphatides | 0 | 8.1 | 8.1 $\pm$ 2.6 | 23.4 |
| Phospholipids | 18.8 | 44.8 | 23.2 $\pm$ 7.8 | 6.9 |
| PE | 9.0 | 5.5 | 19.2 $\pm$ 1.0 | 5.5 |
| PI + PS | 4.1 | 23.4 | 15.6 $\pm$ 2.3 | 4.3 |
| PC | 53.0 | 26.3 | 40.7 $\pm$ 6.0 | 65.3 |
| Sphingomyelin | 15.7 | 21.2 | 5.5 $\pm$ 0.7 | 8.4 |

Figures are percentages of total radioactivity in principal subfractions and the percentage of subfraction found in each lipid species. Each value is the sum of 10 flasks. Values for stearic acid and sodium acetate were derived from five sets of experiments and represent means $\pm$ S.E.M.; values for palmitic acid are the mean of two sets of experiments. Figures in brackets indicate number of experiments. Experimental conditions are described in the body of the paper.

PE, phosphatidylethanolamine; PI, phosphatidylinositol; PS, phosphatidylserine; PC, phosphatidylcholine.

palmitic and lignoceric acids underwent desaturation (Table 2). Chain elongation of palmitic to stearic acid occurred in the explants, and proceeded more actively than the elongation of stearic acid to 20:0. Labelled acetate was incorporated into all fatty acids, including the polyunsaturated fraction.

### *Lipid metabolism of explants in various disease states*

*Metachromatic leucodystrophy.* In this progressive demyelinating disease the incorporation of [1-$^{14}$C]stearic acid was markedly reduced. The specific activity of the lipids in the biopsied brain tissue was 320 c.p.m./mg protein, contrasted with 3681 and 1555 c.p.m./mg protein for two age-adjusted rat

TABLE 2

Pattern of labelled fatty acids in tissue explants cultured from frontal lobes of 3-day-old rats in the presence of [1-$^{14}$C] stearic acid, [1-$^{14}$C]palmitic acid and [1-$^{14}$C]lignoceric acid

| *Fatty acid fraction* | *Radioactivity* | | | |
|---|---|---|---|---|
| | *Sodium acetate* % | *Palmitic acid* % | *Stearic acid* % ± S.E. | *Lignoceric acid* % |
| Non-hydroxy fatty acids (% total fatty acids) | 96.8 | 84.4 | 97.7 ± 1.3 | 96.8 |
| Saturated fatty acids (% non-hydroxy fatty acids) | 51.9 | 95.9 | 86.9 ± 2.8 | 88.9 |
| 16:0 | | 89.0 | 9.7 | |
| 18:0 | | 8.0 | 84.9 | |
| 20:0 | | 0.5 | 1.0 | |
| 22:0 | | 0.5 | 0.3 | |
| 23:0 | | 0.2 | 0.1 | |
| 24:0 | | 0.4 | 0.1 | |
| Mono-unsaturated fatty acids (% non-hydroxy fatty acids) | 13.0 | 4.7 | 10.2 ± 2.6 | 9.6 |
| 16:1 | | 51.8 | 1.1 | |
| 18:1 | | 43.6 | 89.4 | |
| 20:1 | | 2.4 | 1.7 | |
| Polyunsaturated fatty acids (% non-hydroxy fatty acids) | 35.0 | 0.1 | 1.1 ± 0.2 | 1.6 |

Radioactivities of the methyl esters of each fatty acid were measured as described in the text, and are expressed as percentages of the radioactivity in the principal fatty acid fractions.

[1-$^{14}$C]stearic acid (0.3 μCi, 4.1 × $10^{-9}$ M) and [1-$^{14}$C]palmitic acid (0.2 μCi, 2.0 × $10^{-8}$ M) were added with culture conditions as described in the text; growth was terminated after 48 hours. Lipids from 10 culture flasks were combined for fatty acid analysis. Values for stearic acid are the result of 5 experiments and represent means ± S.E.M.

explants run concurrently. Incorporation of label was reduced for all lipid fractions. Desaturation and chain elongation of stearic acid were impaired in this condition. Oleic acid (18:1) had a relative specific activity of 0.2 compared with a control value of 0.7; arachidic acid (20:0) had a relative specific activity of 0.1, compared with a control value of 1.5.

*Generalized $G_{M2}$ gangliosidosis, juvenile variant.* In this variant of Tay-Sachs disease (Menkes *et al.* 1971) the uptake of stearic acid and palmitic acid was normal (6130 c.p.m./mg protein and 23 090 c.p.m./mg protein respectively). A significant abnormality was noted in the distribution of label in the glycolipid fraction. Only 10.7% and 12.0% of the total radioactivity was found in the cerebroside fraction after incubation with stearic acid and palmitic acids respectively. The major amount of radioactivity was found in lipids whose chromatographic behaviour corresponded to ceramide di-and poly-hexosides.

### *Lipid biosynthesis in the presence of high concentrations of phenylalanine*

For this purpose a chemically defined incubating medium was prepared whose amino acid profile was identical to that of the usual patient with phenylketonuria (Perry *et al.* 1970). NCTC 109 medium (Grand Island Biological Company, Berkeley, Calif.) was used, but the concentration of L-phenylalanine was raised to 350 mg/litre ($2.1 \times 10^{3}$ M) of medium. In order to maintain the total amino acid concentration the concentrations of the other essential amino acids were reduced. For example, the concentration of L-tyrosine was 9.86 mg/litre, as compared with 16.4 mg/litre in the medium available commercially, and L-tryptophan was reduced from 17.5 mg/litre to 13.1 mg/litre.

Analysis of the amino acid composition at the beginning and end of a 48-hour incubation failed to show any significant reduction in the phenylalanine content, a finding to be expected in view of the absence from brain tissue of phenylalanine hydroxylase.

The uptake and incorporation of acetate, stearate and palmitate was studied, using concurrent controls, and incubating conditions identical with those employed for the other metabolic studies.

As shown in Table 3, no significant differences in uptake and distribution of incorporation in the presence of high phenylalanine are evident, even though stearic acid uptake was somewhat higher in the control cultures. When the amount of tissue-bound fatty acid was subtracted from the total uptake, no difference between the two groups of values was noted.

When the distribution of the labelled fatty acids was studied (Table 4), the proportion of label in the hydroxy fatty acids was slightly but not significantly increased in the presence of phenylalanine. Incorporation of stearate and acetate into saturated, mono- and polyunsaturated non-hydroxy fatty acids was unaffected by the presence of phenylalanine, and there were no consistent differences in the specific activity of the various fatty acids.

In two experiments sodium phenylpyruvate was added to NCTC 109 to a final concentration of 3.3 mg% ($1.8 \times 10^{-4}$ M). This did not affect the uptake or distribution of labelled stearate and acetate.

## DISCUSSION

The development of methods for routine cultivation of nervous tissue explants *in vitro* provides a new approach for the study of cerebral lipid

TABLE 3

Distribution of radioactivity in brain tissue explants incubated in the presence of high phenylalanine concentrations

| Fraction | *[1-$^{14}$C]sodium acetate* | | *[1-$^{14}$C]palmitic acid* | | *[1-$^{14}$C]stearic acid* | |
|---|---|---|---|---|---|---|
| | *Control* (4) | *High phenylalanine* (4) | *Control* (2) | *High phenylalanine* (2) | *Control* (4) | *High phenylalanine* (4) |
| Total lipids (c.p.m./mg protein $\times 10^{-3}$) | 30.2 ± 20.8 | 32.3 ± 21.8 | 140 | 186 | 124.7 ± 79.1 | 89.2 ± 38.2 |
| Neutral lipids (% total lipid radioactivity) | 80.3 | 77.6 | 54.6 | 57.0 | 69.5 ± 13.7 | 69.6 ± 17.0 |
| Glycolipids (% total lipid radioactivity) | 0.7 | 0.7 | 0.6 | 1.0 | 2.0 ± 1.3 | 2.5 ± 1.5 |
| Phospholipids (% total lipid radioactivity) | 10.8 | 21.7 | 44.8 | 42.0 | 28.4 ± 14.6 | 27.9 ± 17.8 |

Figures represent percentage of total radioactivity in the three principal subfractions. Incubation conditions as in text. Figures in brackets indicate number of experiments.

TABLE 4

Pattern of labelled fatty acids in tissue explants incubated in the presence of high phenylalanine

| *Fatty acid fraction* | *[1-$^{14}$C]sodium acetate* Control (1) | *[1-$^{14}$C]sodium acetate* High phenylalanine (1) | *[1-$^{14}$C]palmitic acid* Control (2) | *[1-$^{14}$C]palmitic acid* High phenylalanine (1) | *[1-$^{14}$C]stearic acid* Control (5) | *[1-$^{14}$C]stearic acid* High phenylalanine (3) |
|---|---|---|---|---|---|---|
| Non-hydroxy fatty acids (% total fatty acids) | 96.8 | 88.9 | 89.8 | 79.3 | 98.3 | 93.5 |
| Hydroxy fatty acids (% total fatty acids) | 3.2 | 11.1 | 10.2 | 18.6 | 1.3 | 5.5 |
| Saturated fatty acids (% non-hydroxy fatty acids) | 55.5 | 54.7 | 91.9 | — | 89.8 | 89.9 |
| Mono-unsaturated fatty acids (% non-hydroxy fatty acids) | 16.0 | 14.6 | 4.7 | — | 8.6 | 9.6 |
| Polyunsaturated fatty acids (% non-hydroxy fatty acids) | 28.5 | 30.7 | 3.0 | — | 1.3 | 0.7 |

Figures in brackets indicate number of experiments. Values are percentages of radioactivity in terms of incorporation into total fatty acids or into total non-hydroxy fatty acids. Incubation conditions as given in text.

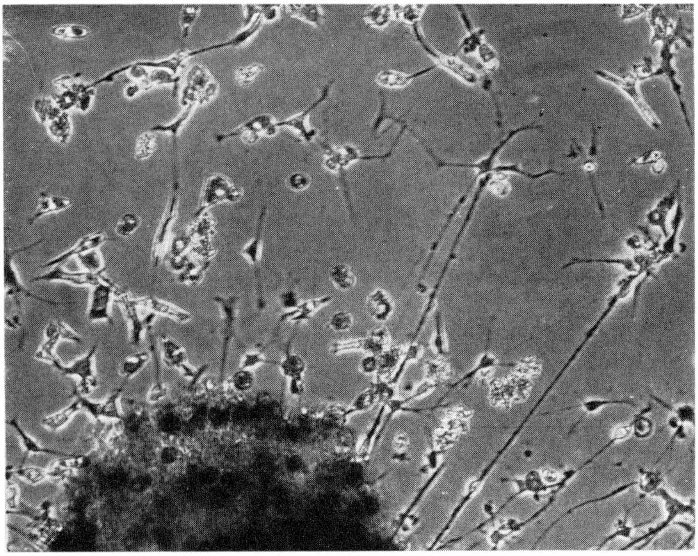

FIG. 1. Explant from frontal lobe of 1-day-old rat brain after 8 days of incubation in serum-enriched medium. Outgrowths include multipolar glial cells with a cytoplasm filled with refractile bodies. There was no conclusive evidence of neuronal outgrowth. The edge of the original explant is on the lower left. Phase-contrast microscopy × 100.

metabolism, particularly for the slower metabolic reactions relating to the synthesis and turnover of myelin components. Outgrowths from explants at the end of the incubation in enriched serum consisted of multipolar glial cells, principally fibrous astrocytes whose cytoplasm contained refractile bodies. A small number of bipolar fibroblasts, probably derived from the meninges and vasculature included in the explant, was also observed. No neuronal outgrowth was seen (Fig. 1). After subsequent incubation in a chemically defined medium there was little change in the appearance of the outgrowths. In interpreting data obtained from this study, several points must be emphasized.

The cellular environment during the metabolic studies is highly artificial; in the absence of serum the explant cannot be maintained indefinitely and there is considerable biochemical and morphological evidence that the metabolic processes begin to slow down after about 72 hours of incubation, as substrates are depleted and end-products accumulate. When the growth environment was enriched by the addition of serum, uptake of lipid precursors was reduced considerably (Menkes 1971), a finding consistent with the experience of Bailey (1966), who noted that incorporation of [1-$^{14}$C]acetate into L-strain mouse fibroblasts was almost completely inhibited by the addition of serum to growth medium. In view of the complexity of the cellular environment that is required for the maintenance of normal cerebral lipid metabolism, it seems unlikely that the chemically defined medium used in these experiments is adequate for optimal lipid biosynthesis. We have found significantly higher rates of fatty acid incorporation in lipids using cultured dissociated cells prepared by passage of brain tissue through a sterile nylon sieve (Yavin and Menkes 1972).

Our work indicates that fatty acids, when added to brain tissue explants in a lipid-free incubation medium, are in part incorporated into a variety of lipid fractions, notably triglycerides and phospholipids, and in part remain as tissue-bound free fatty acids. Since triglycerides constitute a minor fraction of brain lipids, this finding suggests that the acyl moiety of triglycerides is characterized by a more active uptake of radioactivity than the other lipid fractions, a suggestion consistent with *in vivo* observations of Sun and Horrocks (1969) and implying that in explants at least, triglyceride serves as a readily available source of acyl groups. Much less radioactivity was incorporated into cholesterol esters; apparently in the cellular environment of our experiments, cholesterol esters are of little importance as a source of fatty acids for phospholipid and glycolipid biosynthesis.

Examination of the fatty acid composition of lipids in the tissue explants indicates that a significant portion of the [1-$^{14}$C]stearic acid and [1-$^{14}$C]palmitic acid utilized by the cells underwent chain elongation or desaturation. This observation is compatible with our previous finding that brain, particularly at the stage of myelination or earlier, is capable of both metabolic processes (Aeberhard, Grippo and Menkes 1969). Our initial studies on pathological material indicate that incorporation of lipid precursors can be severely impaired, as in the demyelinating disorder, or can undergo a redistribution, as in the lipid storage disease. Our preliminary observation that incorporation of lipid precursors proceeds normally in the presence of high phenylalanine levels and at concentrations of phenylpyruvate comparable to those encountered in the blood of the usual untreated phenylketonuric patients (Jervis 1952) is at variance with the observations of a number of workers.

It would therefore appear that this method will aid in understanding the various metabolic disorders of the brain in which as yet no enzymic defect has been found.

Barbato, Barbato and Hamanaka (1968) found diminished uptake of [$^{14}$C]-acetate into myelin lipids, including cerebrosides, in 12-day-old rabbits in the presence of high levels of phenylalanine. However, phenylalanine concentrations between 68 and 115 mg% were required to demonstrate this effect, and at levels comparable to those established in our experiments no reduction in acetate incorporation was observed.

In the experiments of Weber, Glazer and Ross (1970), significant inhibition of incorporation of [6-$^{3}$H]glucose into lipids was observed at $2.5 \times 10^{-3}$ M-phenylpyruvate, a concentration much higher than occurs in serum in phenylketonuria.

Shah, Peterson and McKean (1970) found inhibition of *in vivo* incorporation of [U-$^{14}$C]glucose into rat brain lipids when the levels of phenylalanine in the brain were 0.15 to 0.21 μmol/g tissue. Inhibition was only 8% in 5-day-old animals, with the maximum effect, 26%, being observed in 13-day-old rats. However, these workers were unable to show any effect of phenylalanine on lipid biosynthesis in brain homogenates. Phenylpyruvic acid also impaired the incorporation of glucose into brain lipids, but concentrations of at least $5 \times 10^{-3}$ M were required to show any significant differences.

The experiments reported here are only preliminary, and need to be repeated on explants derived from animals at various stages of brain maturation. However, at present it is likely that the deleterious effects of phenylalanine cannot be demonstrated unless the blood-brain barrier remains intact.

## SUMMARY

Tissue explants from the frontal lobes of rats were used in the study of brain lipid metabolism over periods sufficiently extended to allow *in vitro* evaluation of the metabolism of lipid components with long half-lives. Tissues were maintained in serum-supplement medium until good glial outgrowth was evident. For explants derived from frontal lobes of 3-day-old rats this took about 10 days. A lipid-free medium was then substituted, and metabolic studies were made over the next 15 minutes to 120 hours. Under these conditions brain explants continued to take up lipid precursors for 48 to 72 hours, as judged by the incorporation of D, L-[2-$^{14}$C]mevalonic acid into cellular sterols. [1-$^{14}$C]-stearic acid, [1-$^{14}$C]palmitic acid and [1-$^{14}$C]lignoceric acid were bound to the cells in the form of the free fatty acid, or were incorporated into neutral lipids, notably triglycerides, and into phospholipids and glycolipids. In the glycolipid fraction cerebrosides were the major radioactive lipids. Choline phosphoglycerides, ethanolamine phosphoglycerides, inositol phosphoglycerides, and serine phosphoglycerides were the principal radioactive phospholipids. Fatty acids were incorporated into cellular lipids either unchanged or after desaturation, chain elongation, or both. Maximum incorporation of stearate occurred in tissues derived from 3-day-old animals. With increasing age the uptake of fatty acid dropped sharply.

When the time course of labelling was followed in 3-day-old animals, triglycerides and choline phosphoglycerides were the first fractions to take up stearate. Cerebroside synthesis occurred slowly, and first became evident after 24 hours.

In brain tissue from a patient with a demyelinating disease (metachromatic leucodystrophy), uptake of precursor was reduced, and chain elongation and desaturation of the fatty acids was diminished. In a patient with generalized $G_{M2}$ gangliosidosis, non-cerebroside glycolipids were labelled to a greater extent than normal. Increasing the phenylalanine concentrations of the medium or adding phenylpyruvate did not affect the incorporation of precursors into lipids.

These studies exemplify the usefulness of tissue explants for prolonged metabolic studies in normal and pathological specimens of brain.

ACKNOWLEDGEMENTS

The technical assistance of Mrs Natalie Stein and Mr Donald Harris is gratefully acknowledged.

This investigation was supported by grants from the U.S. Public Health Service, National Institutes of Health (NB 06938), National Genetics Foundation, and Childrens' Brain Diseases.

# References

Aeberhard, E., Grippo, J. and Menkes, J. H. (1969) *Pediatr. Res.* **3**, 590-596
Bailey, J. M. (1966) *Biochim. Biophys. Acta* **125**, 226
Barbato, L., Barbato, I. W. and Hamanaka, A. (1968) *Brain Res.* **7**, 399-406
Fillerup, D. L., Migliore, J. C. and Mead, J. F. (1958) *J. Biol. Chem.* **233**, 98
Gornall, A. G., Bardawill, C. J. and David, M. M. (1949) *J. Biol. Chem.* **177**, 751
Jervis, G. A. (1952) *Proc. Soc. Exp. Biol. Med.* **81**, 715
Menkes, J. H. (1971) *J. Neurochem.* **18**, 1433-1443
Menkes, J. H., O'Brien, J. S., Okada, S., Grippo, J., Andrews, J. M. and Cancilla, P. A. (1971) *Arch. Neurol. (Chic.)* **25**, 14
Morris, L. J. (1966) *J. Lipid Res.* **7**, 717
Morrison, W. R. and Smith, L. M. (1964) *J. Lipid Res.* **5**, 600
O'Brien, J. S. (1965) *Science* **147**, 1099
Perry, T. L., Hansen, S., Tischler, B., Bunting, R. and Diamond, S. (1970) *New Engl. J. Med.* **282**, 761-766
Shah, S. N., Peterson, N. A. and McKean, C. M. (1970) *J. Neurochem.* **17**, 279-284
Skipski, V. P., Peterson, R. F. and Barclay, M. (1964) *Biochem. J.* **90**, 374
Snyder, F. and Stephens, N. (1962) *Analyt. Biochem.* **4**, 128
Sun, G. Y. and Horrocks, L. A. (1969) *J. Neurochem.* **16**, 181
Weber, G., Glazer, R. I. and Ross, R. A. (1970) *Adv. Enzyme Regulat.* **8**, 13-36
Yavin, E. and Menkes, J. H. (1972) *Trans. Am. Soc. Neurochem.* 3, in press

# Discussion

*Davison:* The experiments on the effects of phenylalanine *in vivo* have been done in chronically treated animals given very high doses of phenylalanine. We find that if we give such high doses to rats, they become hypothermic and moribund. However, if we do an acute experiment *in vivo* with a level of phenylalanine comparable to that in a phenylketonuric infant, there is no effect on lipid synthesis, using acetate as a substrate. Your experiments therefore fit in very well with what we have found and it seems much more likely that in aminoacidurias, as in kwashiorkor, the primary effect, although slight, is on protein synthesis. The design of experiments to investigate whether protein synthesis is the primary biochemical effect is extremely difficult because of the problem of the competition of amino acids.

*Menkes:* I should add that total protein synthesis was unchanged in brain explants in the presence of high phenylalanine concentrations, as measured by incorporation of labelled leucine into protein. The addition of phenylpyruvic acid to the medium also failed to alter protein synthesis. The important point is that if the total amino acid level is increased the cells will tend to die.

*Winick:* Some experiments have been done by P. W. K. Wong, using a pure polysome system (unpublished results 1971). When the phenylalanine level of the medium is raised, there is disaggregation of polysomes with a profound reduction of protein synthesis, just as occurs if one *reduces* the phenylalanine content of the medium to a critical level. So there are data both *in vivo* and *in vitro* which show that protein synthesis can be affected by increased amounts of phenylalanine.

*Menkes:* There is one catch to this. In these experiments both the concentration of phenylalanine and the total α-amino nitrogen levels are raised. In our studies we reduced amino acids other than phenylalanine proportionately, in order to give a final total amino acid concentration like that reported for blood in phenylketonuric individuals (Perry *et al.* 1970). Tyrosine and tryptophan are therefore quite low and the total amino nitrogen is unchanged.

*Winick:* It's known from Munro's work (1964–1970) that tryptophan may be limiting and may affect protein synthesis, so by lowering the tryptophan concentration you may reach a level where tryptophan becomes critical. In your experiments you are not at a level where anything is critical, if you are getting normal protein synthesis.

*Ansell:* Did you examine the labelling of lipids in subcellular fractions?

*Menkes:* No. The total protein content per flask is only 25 mg.

*Aebi:* If your explants are incubated in a medium containing small amounts of fatty acids of different pattern, do they affect the rate of synthesis of lipid or the absolute amount accumulated in the cells at the end of the experiment? Rutstein and co-workers (1958) showed that the accumulation or formation of lipids in fibroblasts of human origin is profoundly influenced by adding small amounts of saturated or polyunsaturated fatty acids to the medium.

*Menkes:* I have not done this, but I have discussed doing it with Dr Mead. We should add increasing amounts of cold fatty acids to the medium in the presence of the labelled fatty acid.

*Mead:* In our liver cells, which are not fresh explants but have grown clonally for several generations, we also note first an uptake of the label into the cells into lipid droplets that are composed of triglyceride and phospholipid and then, after further incubation without additional substrate, the label is transferred to phospholipids which appear in the cell membranes.

*Herschkowitz:* Did you compare the synthetic capabilities of your explants with pure fibroblast lines?

*Menkes:* In only one respect; the incorporation of labelled linoleic acid into phospholipids was better in brain explants than in fibroblasts.

*Aebi:* I am a little worried by the generous extrapolation you made from your findings to the explanation of the mental defects in any inborn error of metabolism. There are at least 30 inborn errors which may ultimately lead to idiocy. Isn't it highly speculative to trace all those consequences back to a single alteration in amino acid metabolism?

*Menkes:* I certainly don't want to be understood as saying that. I don't even believe that in phenylketonuria this is the fact. In my opinion the mental defect in phenylketonuria is due to a number of factors. One is a potentially reversible defect, probably associated with impaired synthesis of serotonin or some other neural transmitter; secondly, there is a prenatal developmental defect, which may be recognized by the presence of microgyria and other developmental malformations; and finally there is a defect in the formation of myelin, with myelin being produced in diminished amounts and in a state where it is highly susceptible to demyelination.

With respect to the effects of high protein concentrations, we have investigated the results of high protein intake on the ultimate mental functioning of premature infants (Menkes *et al.* 1972). In 1962 we followed blood tyrosine concentrations from birth to discharge from the nursery in 71 premature infants who were being fed a high-protein formula (3.9% protein) supplemented by 60 mg/day of ascorbic acid. In 89% of the infants blood tyrosine concentrations were abnormal, and in 38% of the infants the maximum level observed was 15.0 mg% or higher (Menkes and Avery 1963). Maximum blood tyrosine levels correlated significantly with gestational age, but not with birth weight.

In the first follow-up study, made when the infants were on the average 15 months of age, those who had had high levels of tyrosine did not show any significant increase in the incidence of neurological abnormalities (Menkes, Chernick and Ringel 1966). Between 7 and 8 years of age a second follow-up study was made of 62 of these children. This included a Wechsler Intelligence Scale for Children (WISC), a Wide-Range Achievement Test (WRAT), and tests for psychomotor and language maturity. Two children had died in the interval and five of the 62 were too retarded for full testing.

The full-scale WISC I.Q. for all children correlated with birth weight at the 10% confidence level. The mean WISC I.Q. of subjects having high and low levels of tyrosine during their nursery stay was 82.9 and 81.6 respectively. When infants were grouped by birth weight, a significant difference was detected in those weighing 2000 g or more. In this group, high-tyrosine infants had a significantly lower I.Q. than low-tyrosine infants (82.4 and 97.8 respectively; $P<0.02$). Significant differences were also recorded in scores on Object Assembly, Picture Assembly, and Picture Completion subtests of the WISC. Significant differences were seen on the spelling subtests of the WRAT ($P<0.02$).

We did not observe any adverse effects of high levels of tyrosine on the intellectual performance of the smaller premature infants, who have a higher risk for the other complications of prematurity.

*Dobbing:* These children were born in 1962. Was there sufficient awareness then of the fact that one-third of low birth weight babies are 'small-for-dates'?

*Menkes:* We did not have this information then, but we had the data and have been able to look at those.

*Dobbing:* Retrospective analysis is a very imperfect way to investigate these things.

*Winick:* One of the most sensitive ways biochemically of differentiating small-for-dates infants from premature infants is by the excretion of tyrosine in the urine, as Rizzardini (1971) showed. Since you were measuring tyrosine, you could use these data to see if there was any difference between the high and low-tyrosine groups in the numbers of small-for-dates and premature babies.

*Menkes:* We did this, and it just exaggerates the differences, because small-for-dates babies who have low tyrosine levels and are known to fare poorly in terms of intellectual development tend to fall into the low-tyrosine group. Therefore if these infants were excluded from the study, the difference between high and low-tyrosine groups would become even more significant.

*Cobos:* Have you any data on the placentas of these babies?

*Menkes:* No.

*Cobos:* Is there any current evaluation of the metabolic status of the children? Are they excreting any amino acids, for example?

*Menkes:* I assume that as soon as the stress of the initial high-protein feeding went away and they were able to induce the enzymes, serum amino acids became normal. In fact, most infants were discharged with normal plasma levels of tyrosine and phenylalanine.

*Klein:* As I understand it, the only group that was significantly different in I.Q. performance from the other groups was the 'high tyrosine' and 2000 g birth weight group.

*Menkes:* Yes. If you take the entire group of infants, there is a fall in I.Q. with decreasing birth weight.

*Klein:* How was sex distributed?

*Menkes:* As in any other group of premature babies, the girls outnumbered the boys. The ratio between infants having high and low tyrosine was the same for boys and girls, also for black and white children.

*Klein:* Did you find that the girls performed differently from the boys on the spatial-perceptual tests?

*Menkes:* The girls did not tend to do as well as the boys on these kinds of test.

*Aebi:* Dr Menkes, would you accept the possibility that this special type of loading test which you obviously did, has simply revealed a new form of biochemical polymorphism? There are two groups behaving differently, but only feeding them proteins at a very high level makes this difference apparent.

*Menkes:* Yes. Possibly infants having high levels of tyrosine are more susceptible to brain damage for many different reasons.

*Winick:* It should be emphasized that this type of 'high-protein' formula was standard feeding practice in many places at that time; it is a half skim milk formula. So it is not a case of adding protein in this experiment; this is what was in use in many premature nurseries throughout the world.

These results are similar to observations in animals. Frankova (1970) has shown that in rats that were overfed during very early life, behaviour is abnormal and is much closer to the behaviour of her severely undernourished rats than to the normally fed control groups.

*Leathwood:* Frankova's (1970) results showed only that adult rats previously suckled in small litters were not superior to the controls. There is one publication at least which suggests that animals from small litters may be at an advantage. Bovet-Nitti, Oliverio and Bovet (1969) found that in mice of the BALB/c strain, adults originally reared as 'only children' acquired a conditioned avoidance response faster than controls reared in normal litters.

*Paoletti:* I am also interested in correlations between behaviour and biochemical changes. Recently, Shoemaker and Wurtman (1971) found that catecholamines (dopamine and noradrenaline) in brains of undernourished rats are decreased, but they did not give figures on turnover. Has anyone measured the levels and turnover of central nervous mediators in 'overfed' rats?

*Winick:* The data on noradrenaline have to be interpreted in the context of the other changes occurring in the brain. Sereni and co-workers (1966) originally found changes in noradrenaline *content*, but changes in *concentration* were either not present or very transient. The data reported by Shoemaker and Wurtman really indicate the same thing, an impaired accumulation of noradrenaline and dopamine in the brain. I don't think anybody has measured noradrenaline in the other direction, of 'superfed' animals. There are data on acetylcholinesterase in brain, showing some differences from noradrenaline, but this also has not been done in 'overfed' animals.

*von Muralt:* Professor Bovet commented earlier on the use of the word 'vulnerability' (p. 176). When one talks with officials, this term is clearly understood. There are millions of undernourished children, and the cases where there is overfeeding are so few that one should retain the term 'vulnerability'.

*Dobbing:* I welcome this comment. I can find little objection to the word 'vulnerability'. I have some sympathy for the use of 'sensitivity', but I am worried by expressions such as 'overfeeding' and the implication that there is some possibility of producing super-brains and super-people. What do we mean by these expressions? Unless we mean 'superfed' in the sense of malnutrition, that is, obesity, and the ills that are the consequence of this, are we entitled to talk about overfeeding and superfeeding? Would it be any more useful to talk about optimum feeding? I think we should avoid the implications that it is possible by overfeeding to produce a super-brain. Presumably there is a limiting rate at which the brain can grow. Have we any reason to believe that this is anything less than an optimum rate, and that any variance from that is a manifestation of vulnerability or sensitivity? I think it's a little more than a semantic question.

## References

Bovet-Nitti, F., Oliverio, A. and Bovet, D. (1969) *Life Sci. Part II Biochem. Gen. Mol. Biol.* **8**, 569-574

Frankova, S. (1970) *Nutr. Metab.* **12**, 228-239

Menkes, J. H. and Avery, M. E. (1963) *Bull. Johns Hopkins Hosp.* **113**, 301

Menkes, J. H., Chernick, V. and Ringel, B. (1966) *J. Pediatr.* **69**, 583

Menkes, J. H., Welcher, D. W., Levi, H. S., Dallas, J. and Gretsky, N. E. (1972) *Pediatrics*, **49**, 218-224

MUNRO, H. N. (1964-1970) *Mammalian Protein Metabolism*, vol. 1-4, ed. H. N. Munro and J. B. Allison. Academic Press, New York
PERRY, T. L., HANSEN, S., TISCHLER, B., BUNTING, R. and DIAMOND, S. (1970) *New Engl. J. Med.* **282**, 761-766
RIZZARDINI, M. (1971) *Am. J. Dis. Child.* **121**, 182-185
RUTSTEIN, D. D., INGENITO, E. F., CRAIG, J. M. and MARTINELLI, M. (1958) *Lancet* 1, 545-552
SERENI, F., PRINCIPI, N., PERLETTI, L. and SERENI, L. P. (1966) *Biol. Neonat.* **10**, 254-265
SHOEMAKER, W. J. and WURTMAN, R. J. (1971) *Science* **171**, 1017-1019

# Malnutrition and cellular growth in the brain: existence of critical periods

MYRON WINICK*, PEDRO ROSSO and JO ANNE BRASEL

*Department of Pediatrics, Cornell University Medical College, New York*

The development of the central nervous system may be viewed as a progression of biochemical, morphological and functional events which occur in a precise sequence and which depend to some extent on the orderly progression of the developmental processes which precede them. Cells proliferate during a specific period of brain growth in the rat (Mandel *et al.* 1964; Winick and Noble 1965) and in man (Winick 1968). Different brain regions show different rates of cellular proliferation (Fish and Winick 1969*a*). Various cell types divide at different rates and for different periods of time (Winick 1970; Dobbing and Sands 1970). Cells migrate from one area to another during specific periods (Altman and Das 1966). Enzyme activity appears sequentially in human brain (Duckett and Pearse 1966). The rate of myelin synthesis is maximum during specific periods in rat and pig brain (Davison and Dobbing 1968). The pathways of glucose metabolism shift during early development in rat brain (Winick 1970). Synthesis of certain neural hormones increases markedly during specific periods (Sereni *et al.* 1966). Concomitant with these and other biochemical and morphological changes a series of functional changes occur as the central nervous system develops. The relationship between these chemical and morphological changes and the functional changes is at present unknown, and represents one of the frontiers of developmental neurochemistry and neurophysiology.

Recently it has become apparent that interference with this orderly sequence of events will not only delay maturation but may impose irreversible changes. Thus not only is the nature of the insult important, but the time of the insult may be even more important. For example, undernutrition during proliferative growth will retard the rate of cell division and result in a permanent reduction in

---

* *Present address:* Institute of Human Nutrition, Faculty of Medicine, Columbia University, New York City.

brain cell number (Winick and Noble 1966). This retardation in cell division will affect any region where cells are dividing (Fish and Winick 1969*b*) and any cell type which is still proliferating (Winick 1970). The same degree of undernutrition imposed when cells are no longer dividing, but while they are still enlarging, will impede this hypertrophy, reducing the protein content per cell. However, this change is reversible (Winick and Noble 1966). Undernutrition occurring later, after brain growth is complete, will have little or no effect.

## ANIMAL STUDIES

The mechanisms regulating normal cell division also continue to pose a major unsolved problem. Although certain consequences of malnutrition for cellular growth can be demonstrated, it is not yet possible to elucidate the mechanisms involved. Thus a further understanding of how malnutrition affects cellular growth might not only allow us better to understand the nutritional consequences but could also provide a basic understanding of the factors controlling normal cellular growth.

Evidence from a number of sources demonstrates a curtailment of DNA synthesis and protein synthesis and a reduction in RNA content in malnutrition. Let us examine how these changes may occur. DNA synthesis could be impaired because of lack of substrate (nucleotides), because of reduced activity of enzymes necessary to accomplish synthesis, or because of a lack of energy (ATP) for synthetic polymerization. Recent observations (Culley 1971) would tend to rule out lack of ATP as a crucial factor, at least in brain. We have therefore investigated the other two possibilities.

The amount of free nucleotide per cell increases from birth to 21 days of life in the rat. Undernutrition during this period of life does not appear to affect the size of the total pool. However, since individual nucleotides have not been separated it is possible that specific nucleotide pools are reduced. The second possible mechanism by which DNA synthesis might be affected is by a reduction in activity of some of the enzymes involved in DNA synthesis. This could be either selective or secondary to the general reduction in protein synthesis which is known to occur.

In a previous report (Brasel, Ehrenkranz and Winick 1970) demonstrating that the activity of DNA polymerase parallels the rate of DNA synthesis in rat brain, we postulated that activity of this enzyme might serve as an *ad hoc* index of proliferative cell growth in normal tissues. Since individual brain regions have different rates of cell division and different times when maximum rates are attained, regional patterns of DNA polymerase activity have also been examined. Activity is always higher in cerebellum where the rate of DNA synthesis is rapid than it is in forebrain where cell division is slower. Activity in forebrain peaks between 10 and 12 days, precisely when the rate of DNA synthesis is maximal in this region. By contrast in cerebellum there are two peaks of DNA synthesis, at 7 and 13 days. DNA polymerase activity is also biphasic with peaks just preceding each of the peaks of synthesis. These data reinforce the concept that the activity of this enzyme parallels the rate of cell division during proliferative cell growth. As such it should provide a unique background against which to study the effects of malnutrition on DNA synthesis.

Preliminary experiments with malnutrition demonstrate a reduction in activity of this enzyme per cell in rat liver. Thus another mechanism by which malnutrition may impair cell division could be by limiting the amount of active DNA polymerase available for DNA synthesis. Moreover, this is only one protein involved in cell division and it is quite possible that other proteins, such as enzymes, histones or spindle proteins, may be selectively reduced in undernutrition.

Our interest in protein synthesis stems from the data of Munro and Drysdale (1970), Miller (1970) and others who have demonstrated profound quantitative and qualitative effects of undernutrition on general protein synthesis. For example, one of the earliest effects of amino acid restriction is a disaggregation of polysomes and a shift in the polysome profile which suggests a selective sparing of certain proteins. Thus protein synthesis which occurs on the polysome cannot really be separated from RNA metabolism. We do not yet know where the primary effect takes place. The disaggregated polysome does not synthesize protein as well as the intact polysome. In addition this, free ribosome is much more susceptible to the activity of alkaline ribonuclease and hence will be broken down more rapidly.

Thus, in malnutrition DNA synthesis is reduced and protein synthesis is reduced, either directly or secondary to changes in RNA metabolism. However, if one examines RNA metabolism, the rate of RNA synthesis is actually increased during malnutrition. How can we explain this seeming paradox, in view of the fact that the total amount of RNA per cell has been clearly demonstrated to be reduced? The answer must lie in enhanced catabolism. For this reason, a number of investigators have examined both the synthetic and catabolic rates of RNA metabolism during malnutrition. Studies in liver indicate an increased synthesis of RNA accompanied by a proportionally higher increase in RNA breakdown, resulting in a reduced content of RNA per cell. Thus the level of cellular RNA during malnutrition would appear to be

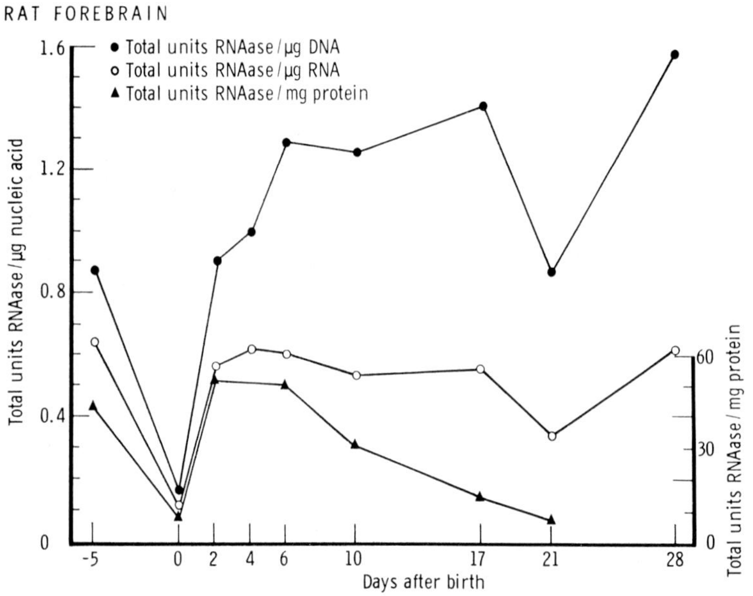


FIG. 1. Activity of alkaline ribonuclease during normal development in rat forebrain.

controlled by a balance between synthesis and breakdown with the regulation of this balance on the catabolic side. We therefore decided to study RNA turnover in brain and other organs during malnutrition. So far we can report on only one aspect of the problem: the activity of alkaline ribonuclease.

This enzyme has been described in most tissues; it exists in a free form and in a latent form in which the enzyme is bound to a protein inhibitor that can be released by substances interfering with SH groups, such as *p*-chloromercuribenzoate. We have measured total activity in rat brain during normal development and correlated this activity with changes in DNA, RNA and protein.

Fig. 1 demonstrates that ribonuclease activity per cell (µg DNA) increases with age except for two distinct drops at 0 and 21 days. This increase per cell is apparently not as great as the increase in other cellular proteins and hence the activity per mg of protein (specific activity) decreases. However, the increase exactly parallels the increase in cellular RNA content, resulting in no change in ribonuclease per mg of RNA during development. Thus a constant relationship is kept to substrate at the same time as an increase per cell is occurring, strongly suggesting a role for this enzyme in regulating the cellular content of RNA. Fig. 2 demonstrates that early undernutrition markedly elevates the activity of this enzyme per cell. Similarly, the activity per

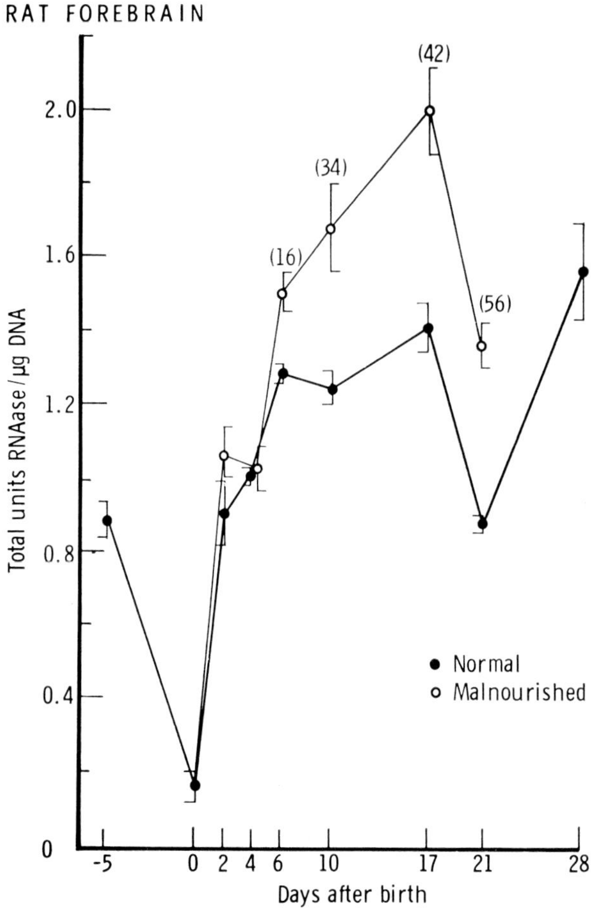


FIG. 2. The effect of undernutrition on ribonuclease activity in rat forebrain.

mg of RNA and of protein is also elevated. Preliminary data in liver suggest similar changes with malnutrition. Thus malnutrition, which is known to enhance RNA catabolism at least in liver, elevates the activity of alkaline ribonuclease in both liver and brain. Recently we have studied the synthetic phase of RNA metabolism by intracerebral pulse labelling with [$^{14}$C]orotic acid. Rats malnourished from birth to 14 days of age show an increased incorporation of label both into the total nucleotide pool and into RNA during the first 24 hours after injection.

Can we fit all the known data into a hypothesis which can interrelate the various aspects of normal cell growth and attempt to explain some of the mechanisms by which undernutrition affects this interrelation?

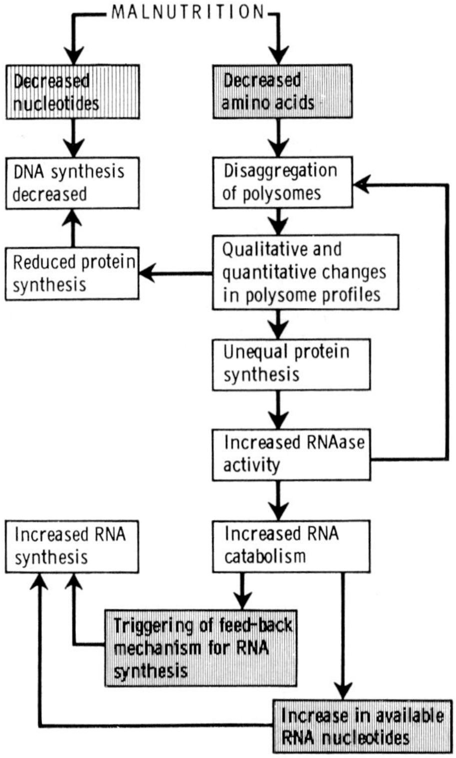


FIG. 3. Schematic representation of a hypothesis to explain some of the mechanisms by which undernutrition may affect brain growth. White areas are effects known to occur; shaded areas are hypothesized to occur.

In Fig. 3 the unshaded areas are effects of malnutrition proved to occur; the shaded areas are those hypothesized to occur. In malnutrition, the reduced substrates and co-factors may result in a reduction in specific nucleotide pool size which in turn limits DNA synthesis. This substrate reduction also results in polysome disaggregation which changes the polysome profile and leads to a quantitative and qualitative reduction in protein synthesis which may or may not secondarily retard DNA synthesis. The unequal protein synthesis results in an elevation of alkaline ribonuclease, which increases RNA catabolism. This increased catabolic rate could further decrease protein synthesis with all of its concomitant effects and at the same time trigger a feedback mechanism which would increase RNA synthesis. This in turn could be supported by the increased availability of nucleotides supplied by the increased catabolism.

## HUMAN STUDIES

The sequential changes in cellular growth of the human brain are not as clearly defined as in the animal studies. In addition, there are no studies in man which indicate the mechanisms by which these changes are produced. What is known, then, is strictly descriptive. We have previously demonstrated (Winick 1968) that DNA content increases linearly in whole human brain during the prenatal period, begins to taper off around birth and reaches a maximum around one year of life. More recent data (Dobbing and Sands 1970) have demonstrated two peaks of cell division in human brain, one from 15 to 20 weeks of gestation and a second beginning at about 25 weeks and continuing until around birth. Dobbing and Sands ascribe the first peak to neuronal division and the second to proliferation of glia. In two studies made at the Hospital Roberto Del Rio in Santiago, Chile (Winick and Rosso 1969*a*; Winick, Rosso and Waterlow 1970), it was shown that severe malnutrition during the first year of life, leading to the death of the infant, results in a reduced number of cells in the brain as well as a reduction in total lipid, cholesterol and phospholipid content. If the malnutrition is prolonged into the second year, then the lipid/DNA ratio or the amount of lipid per cell is also reduced. The rate of cell division in various regions of the human brain and the effect of malnutrition on those regions has also been studied (Rosso, Hormazabal and Winick 1970). The results indicate that the rate of cell division postnatally is about the same in cerebrum and cerebellum and that in both of these regions, as well as in brainstem, DNA synthesis stops at about the same time (approximately one year of age). Malnutrition reduces the number of cells in all three regions.

In addition to these studies, it has been demonstrated that head circumference is reduced in children who died of undernutrition during the first year of life and that this reduction reflects accurately the chemical changes just described (Winick and Rosso 1969*b*).

Thus the changes which have been demonstrated to occur in human brain are similar to those previously described in animal brain. Whether or not the mechanisms producing these changes are similar, and what the functional implications of these changes are, is still unknown.

## SUMMARY

Malnutrition during early brain development has been shown to curtail both protein synthesis and DNA synthesis. The result is a permanently stunted brain containing fewer cells of normal size. The same degree of malnutrition after cell division has stopped will retard net protein synthesis and result in a brain with a normal number of smaller cells. These changes are reversible with subsequent refeeding. Thus protein synthesis is curtailed and if DNA synthesis is occurring, it too is curtailed. Our data suggest that the regulation of RNA metabolism and hence protein synthesis may be affected by malnutrition in two ways: by elevation of alkaline ribonuclease activity and by limitation of the size of the nucleotide pool. In addition, during proliferative growth this limited pool size may retard DNA synthesis. Finally certain proteins, such as DNA polymerase, which are necessary for DNA synthesis, may also be reduced during early malnutrition.

In the human brain DNA synthesis and myelination are also curtailed by malnutrition occurring during the time that these processes are most active. The mechanisms for these changes as well as their functional significance are as yet unknown.

## References

ALTMAN, J. and DAS, G. (1966) *J.Comp. Neurol.* **126**, 337-360
BRASEL, J. A., EHRENKRANZ, R. A. and WINICK, M. (1970) *Dev. Biol.* **23**, 424-432
CULLEY, W. J. (1971) *Fed. Proc. Fed. Am. Soc. Exp. Biol.* **30**, 459
DAVISON, A. N. and DOBBING, J. (ed.) (1968) *Applied Neurochemistry*, pp. 253-257. Blackwell, Oxford
DOBBING, J. and SANDS, J. (1970) *Nature (Lond.)* **226**, 639-640
DUCKETT, S. and PEARSE, A. G. E. (1966) *Proc. 5th International Congress of Neuropathology.* (International Congress Series no. 100) pp. 738-739. Excerpta Medica, Amsterdam
FISH, I. and WINICK, M. (1969*a*) *Pediatr. Res.* **3**, 407-412
FISH, I. and WINICK, M. (1969*b*) *Exp. Neurol.* **25**, 534-540
MANDEL, P., REIN, H., HARTH-EDEL, S. and MARDELL, R. (1964) In *Comparative Neurochemistry*, pp. 153-158, ed. D. Richter. Pergamon Press, Oxford
MILLER, S. A. (1970) *Fed. Proc. Fed. Am. Soc. Exp. Biol.* **29**, 1497-1502
MUNRO, H. N. and DRYSDALE, J. W. (1970) *Fed. Proc. Fed.Am. Soc. Exp. Biol.* **29**, 1469-1473
ROSSO, P., HORMAZABAL, J. and WINICK, M. (1970) *Am. J. Clin. Nutr.* **23**, 1275-1279
SERENI, F., PRINCIPI, N., PERLETTI, L. and SERENI, L. P. (1966) *Biol. Neonat.* **10**, 254-256
WINICK, M. (1968) *Pediatr. Res.* **2**, 352-355
WINICK, M. (1970) *Fed. Proc. Fed. Am. Soc. Exp. Biol.* **29**, 1510-1515
WINICK, M. and NOBLE, A. (1965) *Dev. Biol.* **12**, 451-466
WINICK, M. and NOBLE, A. (1966) *J. Nutr.* **89**, 300-306
WINICK, M. and ROSSO, P. (1969*a*) *Pediatr. Res.* **3**, 181-184
WINICK, M. and ROSSO, P. (1969*b*) *J. Pediatr.* **74**, 774-778
WINICK, M., ROSSO, P. and WATERLOW, J. (1970) *Exp. Neurol.* **26**, 393-400

## Discussion

*Hollingsworth:* Dr Winick, when you talk about malnutrition, are you referring entirely to protein malnutrition or protein-calorie malnutrition, or does any other nutrient enter into this?

*Winick:* I wish I could answer this question for man; I can answer it for the rat. The kinds of malnutrition which have been produced in the rat during the first 21 days are either a total caloric and protein deprivation, as in most of the experiments mentioned, or a limitation of the protein intake of the mother, which limits the amount rather than the quality of the milk, and so we have again a total calorie deprivation. The kind of malnutrition imposed prenatally generally has been a severe reduction in the protein content of the diet of the mothers, keeping the calories normal. However, there is controversy about whether these animals are eating as much as they ordinarily would.

The human situation is much more complex. In the marasmic infants that we studied in Chile, the children are drinking flour and water. They are not breast fed. They are given milk, but then they get diarrhoea, because the hygienic conditions for preparing formula are totally impossible. The child is then simply put on flour and water, which is really total starvation, and he becomes marasmic very quickly.

*Menkes:* I have two clinical questions that I would like you to answer. I am often called to see a child who is less than one year of age, whose weight and height are under the third percentile, and whose head circumference is under the third percentile, and I'm asked: is this child microcephalic? I am also often asked to see a child under the first year of age, whose weight and height are under the third percentile and whose head is in the normal range. And I'm asked: is this child hydrocephalic? What are your answers to these questions?

*Winick:* Let me outline what is known about head circumference, height and weight in severely malnourished children, and then return to the questions. The head circumference in children who are malnourished is generally reduced. In the children who die of malnutrition, where we were able to measure the head circumference and at the same time to measure biochemical parameters, head circumference is appropriately reduced for the size of the brain, for the DNA content of the brain, and for the lipid content, since everything is reduced proportionately. So head circumference reflects the change in brain size. That is the situation with malnutrition severe enough to produce death. It has also been shown that changes in head circumference are relatively persistent after rehabilitation. Such children therefore tend to have smaller head circumferences, and it has been possible to correlate head circumference with subsequent development in these children. Height follows the same pattern but not as well, and weight doesn't follow this pattern at all. So that in severely malnourished populations, changes of this sort in head circumference indicate some kind of change in the brain.

When we talk about children under the third percentile in well-nourished populations, we're in a totally different situation. I think the small child under the third percentile with a head circumference under the third percentile but appropriate to the rest of his body, is a perfectly normal child. I think a child whose body is under the third percentile and whose head circumference is normal for his age, like many premature children, is a perfectly normal child as well. There's no evidence, at these ends of the spectrum, of any abnormality. But in severely malnourished children, head circumference could be an indication of brain size.

*Dobbing:* One thing that puzzles me about Dr Winick's original observations (not about his data, nor about his discovery that one can recover from food restriction at the time cells are growing in size, but not at the time when cells are dividing, which is one of the most significant contributions to the whole subject of 'catch-up'-potential), is the question of cellular enlargement in the brain. Because of the heterogeneity of the brain architecture, and the nature and shape of nerve cells, this must be quite a different idea from increasing cell size in the liver. For example, we know that the major features of neuronal growth are the extension and elongation of processes, the branching of dendrites, and the establishment of connections, and we suspect that these connections are functionally the most important aspects of neuronal development. These aspects would come into the category of cellular enlargement; they certainly are not in the category of cellular division. So the question must arise, and I think the neurochemists have to help us here, whether these very special sorts of cellular enlargement in the neuron are also, in our sense of the word, 'vulnerable', and whether in the brain there may be failure to catch up of other processes besides the multiplication of cells. Perhaps this is highlighted by the fact that in most experiments the retardation of growth has been imposed during the period of glial cell multiplication, and it must therefore be of these cells predominantly that there is an ultimate deficit. This is a major puzzle, and what we desperately require is a way of measuring effects on such non-mitotic events as neuronal growth and the establishment of connections, which must be much less laborious than quantitative histology.

My final puzzle concerns the finding of the reduction in brain size and cell number at birth in the rat born of an undernourished mother; for this would indicate a reduction in the number of neurons, since in this species there is no substantial glial multiplication before birth. We have a large series of animals who have been examined at birth following maternal undernutrition in which we can find distinct evidence of reduction of the body weight at birth but no evidence that stands up to statistical analysis over very large numbers of animals (200-300) of reduction in either brain weight or brain cell number. Possibly the answer is that Dr Zamenhof, who is the principal claimant that this can be achieved, has imposed a protein malnutrition on the mothers, whereas we impose an overall reduction, which you might call undernutrition. Unfortunately in no laboratory, as far as I know, have the two regimes been imposed simultaneously under the same roof, and I think this ought to be done.

*Winick:* It's quite clear that protein malnutrition will produce these changes. Zamenhof, Van Marthens and Margolis (1968) have done it a number of times; we have done it; so have B. Chow (unpublished observations 1967) and E. M. Widdowson. The fact that calorie restriction doesn't produce these changes is very interesting, and I agree that this has to be checked and worked out in terms of the mechanism involved.

As far as the increase in size of brain cells is concerned, I couldn't agree with you more. We are talking about averages, and in the brain or liver or any other organ there may be no single cell which really falls into this average, because we are making a calculation based on total protein and total DNA. But this kind of thought process has been useful in generating experiments. In the brain, when one asks what it is that retards function—is it an interference with the increase in size or of dendrites or other things?—I feel that correlative studies will never answer the question. Until we have some fundamental information about the control of function in the brain, and can then see what malnutrition does to such controls, we shall always be left simply with correlations. We may find that we can inhibit dendrites and that the animals then don't function properly, but to say that the inhibition of dendrites is causing the functional abnormality will be just as difficult, if not impossible, as to say that the reduction of cells is doing this. Probably most of the changes we are describing are not the reason for the functional changes we see. We really don't know what the controls of function are, and that will be one of the exciting areas in the future.

*Menkes:* In answer to Dr Dobbing, if you wish to estimate the number of glial cells and neuronal cells in a given population, would it not be simple to measure glutamic decarboxylase, which is a specific neuronal enzyme, and express the values in terms of DNA?

*Dobbing:* Fortunately, this has been suggested to us already, and we have begun to do this, but it's not possible at this stage to say more. We hope this will be productive.

*Herschkowitz:* Dr Winick has discussed mechanisms which are affected by malnutrition, and in particular the effect on DNA polymerase. We also have evidence that under certain circumstances, neuroblast proliferation can be affected by malnutrition. That brings me to the question of the vulnerable periods, and I would like to ask Dr Dobbing: have we any evidence from experimental data that one period of brain development, namely neuronal proliferation, is *not* vulnerable, which would imply that the first months of pregnancy in humans is not a vulnerable period?

*Dobbing:* No. I suspect that in human pregnancy for various physiological reasons of supply and demand and availability, the second trimester is not usually open to the influences of malnutrition. But this is far from saying that the process of neuroblast multiplication is invulnerable. Indeed, as you say, if we accept the evidence of Zamenhof and others, neuroblast proliferation in the rat *is* vulnerable. We haven't been able to show this, but we may not have been trying in the right way. I wouldn't say that neuroblast proliferation appears not to be vulnerable. This is another thing from suggesting that the second human trimester is ever exposed to malnutrition. It may be, but we're brought up in the belief that it isn't, and without any demonstration that it is.

*von Muralt:* Is this not a body weight relationship between mother and foetus? Even if the mother is malnourished, there are some reserves on which the small foetus can be nourished.

*Dobbing:* I would put it even more specifically; it's not simply a body weight relationship, but an imbalance which we know develops in later pregnancy between the declining placenta and the growing foetus, which leads to foetal demands more closely approaching the limits of placental supply.

*Winick:* There is a piece of information which makes us worry whether or not the second trimester is invulnerable. If one looks at the rate of cell division in human placentas, one finds that DNA synthesis occurs at first in a linear fashion, but DNA content begins to level out at around 34 weeks of gestation. This allows us to examine the placenta retrospectively, and to see whether cell number is affected, whether cell size is affected, and to attempt to time the insult. One would assume that if there is a reduction in the number of cells, the insult occurred before 34 weeks. If one looks at the placentas of malnourished women, one finds a reduced number of cells, which would indicate that at least at the level of the placenta, malnutrition has been occurring before 34 weeks of gestation. We don't know whether this gets through to the foetus or whether it occurs as early as the second trimester of pregnancy, but it means we have to look critically at the whole period of pregnancy.

*Dobbing:* The placenta is an organ in which cells are lost during the course of its lifetime, so an estimate of cell number in later pregnancy showing a reduction in cell number could equally indicate loss of cells, as failure to produce them.

*Winick:* In the rat, this curve has been worked out both with total DNA and with studies using [$^{3}$H]thymidine incorporation, and in fact the amount of cell loss occurring in the rat placenta during this phase is not significant, either in the normal rat or in the malnourished rat (Jollie 1964). But in the human, where incorporation studies have not been done, what you say is certainly possible.

*Aebi:* Dr Winick, your plea 'to sharpen our tools' obviously deserves special attention, and in this respect you have a lot to offer. Your data clearly show that measurement of ribonuclease activity in serum is another valuable tool which should be included in the generally accepted battery of tests. This is specially so since in man active cells are normally not available, except leucocytes. On the other hand, I wonder what in your experience is the value of the tests accepted by the Committee on Procedures for Appraisal of Protein-Calorie Malnutrition of the International Union of Nutritional Sciences? What test (tests) has (or have) proved to be in your hands the most interesting and informative in the study of malnutrition?

*Winick:* I am not an expert on this, but I think that the use of the creatinine index and of hydroxyproline determinations has, at least in some hands, been very fruitful. Another determination which is a variant of hydroxyproline determination, namely the use of non-dialysable hydroxyproline, has been shown to affect the excretory product, during rapid collagen synthesis, and we have recently finished a study in which we measured the non-dialysable hydroxyproline content of human amniotic fluid throughout gestation. This proves to be a very good indicator of the gestational age of the baby. Whether it is really indicating, as we hope it is, the growth rate of the baby, and whether in the malnourished baby it is reduced I can't say, but it would appear that it may be better than measuring total hydroxyproline. As far as some of the other indicators go, it depends on the kind of malnutrition; plasma protein or albumin is reduced in kwashiorkor but is little affected in marasmus. At the present time, I'm not sure that in children the biochemical data are much sharper than the anthropometric data. In children at least we have growth to measure, which we don't have in the adult.

*Cobos:* I would agree entirely with Dr Winick's statement about biochemical data, and I would go a little further on the use of even the hydroxyproline or total proteins or protein fractions or amino acids in epidemiological studies. The correlations with weight are even poorer than with other well-known measures such as skin-fold or head circumference.

*von Muralt:* Knowing how careful one must be in making determinations of hydroxyproline, I can recommend a method which we use in the Ivory Coast with very good results. Dr J.-P. Habicht (at I.N.C.A.P.) has developed a new technique for hydroxyproline which is more complicated but much safer than the classical one. Has his thesis, where he describes the method, been published, Dr Klein?

*Klein:* We have a copy of the thesis at I.N.C.A.P., and there is a copy in the M.I.T. library, but to my knowledge he hasn't published the thesis.

## References

JOLLIE, W. P. (1964) *Am. J. Anat.* **114**, 161-167
ZAMENHOF, S., VAN MARTHENS, E. and MARGOLIS, F. L. (1968) *Science* **160**, 322-323

# Evaluation of modern foods as sources of lipids

U. M. T. HOUTSMULLER

*Unilever Research, Vlaardingen/Duiven, The Netherlands*

Extensive investigations in recent years have revealed many potential sources of lipids for the production of modern foods. Since these oils and fats diverge widely in composition, it seems relevant to evaluate them periodically on the basis of our rapidly expanding insight into the role of fats in human health.

In this paper I shall attempt to appraise the minimal requirements in the lipid fraction of the maternal and infant diet necessary to ensure adequate brain development. Three main questions arise:

(1) Which lipids are essential for brain development?
(2) In which period and to what extent are they needed?
(3) Does the diet contain factors affecting the need for the essential components?

## WHICH LIPIDS ARE ESSENTIAL FOR BRAIN DEVELOPMENT?

With respect to the first question, it appears that the lipid fraction of the diet must contain as essential components certain fatty acids (EFA) and the fat-soluble vitamins.

### *n–6 fatty acids*

Of the fatty acids, linoleic acid is of course of vital importance. Absence of the *n*-6 fatty acids from the diet gives rise to many deficiency symptoms, such as retarded growth, increased skin permeability, sterility, and malfunctions in many organs. But the *n*–6 fatty acids seem to play an important role in brain development also:

(1) Churchill, Ayers and Caldwell (1967) in a retrospective study found a

negative correlation between the severity of biliary tract disease of expectant mothers and the I.Q. of their children ($r = -0.77$). This connection is ascribed to the low fat intake of patients with biliary diseases. To provide additional evidence for this observation in man, Caldwell and Churchill (1966) compared the offspring of rats fed a fat-free diet during pregnancy with the offspring of females fed a standard diet throughout pregnancy. After parturition all rats were placed on the standard diet. Performance on the Lashley III maze for food reward was significantly poorer for the young of the fat-deprived mothers.

(2) Paoletti and his co-workers (Galli, White and Paoletti 1971; White, Galli and Paoletti 1971; Paoletti and Galli 1972) have found decreased brain weight, lower phospholipid content and abnormal fatty acid composition concomitant with decreased learning ability in rats deficient in essential fatty acids.

### *n–3 fatty acids*

An essential function is often ascribed also to the fatty acids of the linolenic acid family. These *n*–3 fatty acids can prevent some but not all of the symptoms of EFA deficiency. For example, in the restoration of body weight or the normalization of the swelling of liver mitochondria they display about the same activity as linoleic acid. However, the degeneration of the testes or the infertility of females is not prevented by *n*–3 fatty acids, while they show about 10% of the activity of linoleic acid in curing the skin permeability. The linolenic acid family is also said to have a specific function in the brain, which cannot be performed by linoleic acid: Bernsohn and Stephanides (1967) have summarized the arguments for their hypothesis that multiple sclerosis is the result of a deficiency in *n*–3 fatty acids during brain maturation. The arguments are indirect and based partly on aetiological considerations: when individuals move from a region of high risk to a region of low risk, they carry the higher susceptibility for multiple sclerosis with them, indicating that the development of this disease stems from the early phases of brain maturation. Moreover, chemical analyses of brain lipids reveal a decreased content in *n*–3 fatty acids in brain tissue of multiple sclerosis patients. However, the latter argument seems to be of little consequence: first, it has been shown that brain tissue is able to incorporate fatty acids at any age and second, a decrease in *n*–3 fatty acids has also been shown in other circumstances, such as vitamin E deficiency.

To rats the absence of *n*–3 fatty acids seems to be of little consequence:

(1) Churchill, Ayers and Caldwell (1967) state that if linoleic acid is given as the sole fatty acid to pregnant rats, it completely prevents the decrease in learning ability exhibited by the young of fat-deprived mothers.

(2) Recently Tinoco and co-workers (1971) described the raising of three generations of rats on a diet free of *n*–3 fatty acids. In the third generation only very small amounts of *n*–3 fatty acids were found, but still no abnormalities were observed, although as the authors state 'the rats may have experienced subtle changes in behaviour, which we did not investigate'.

Thus a specific function for *n*–3 fatty acids in brain maturation, although not excluded, seems improbable, leaving the linoleic acid family as the only essential group of fatty acids. The relatively high concentrations of *n*–3 fatty acids in brain matter are caused by the virtually unavoidable presence of linolenic acid in the diet and the high affinity for the more unsaturated fatty acid of the enzymes concerned with unsaturation and chain elongation.

## WHEN AND TO WHAT EXTENT ARE THE ESSENTIAL LIPIDS REQUIRED?

### *Critical periods*

On the question of the period of brain maturation at which linoleic acid is needed, it appears that the foetus in particular needs adequate amounts. When the maternal diet is low in linoleic acid, the offspring have decreased learning ability (Caldwell and Churchill 1966; Churchill, Ayers and Caldwell 1967), although the alterations in brain lipids can be reversed by giving linoleic acid in subsequent periods (Galli, White and Paoletti 1971). In the lactation period the lipid composition of the brain is less susceptible to diets lacking in linoleic acid, but deficiency symptoms in the fatty acid pattern do occur. No information is available on changes in brain function due to EFA-deficient feeding in this period, so it is not known whether such a diet might cause irreversible retardation in brain development.

### *Requirement for n–6 fatty acids*

Quantitative information on the requirement for linoleic acid for optimal brain development is lacking, because of the difficulty in properly assessing brain function. The use of a biochemical criterion for EFA deficiency, such as the percentage of eicosatrienoic acid, 20:3 (*n*-9), can be misleading, as many polyunsaturated fatty acids cause a decrease in this compound without curing all the symptoms of EFA deficiency. For example, feeding linolenic acid to deficient rats lowers the content of 20:3 (*n*–9) even more than linoleic acid, whereas it has hardly any effect on the skin. On the other hand, the content of *n*–6 fatty acids in an organ is not necessarily a parameter of the functional status of that tissue either; one has to establish in addition the fatty acid composition at which the organ functions optimally. For the brain, intelligence tests may be applicable. However, extrapolation to man of results obtained with animals seems to be disputable, as only learning ability can be tested in animals.

In the prenatal period a complicating factor is the selectivity of the placenta towards individual fatty acids. Very little lipid passes through this barrier, and therefore the fatty acid composition of maternal and foetal plasma may differ considerably. The amount of linoleic acid is lower in the newborn than in the mother (Hansen *et al.* 1964; Holman *et al.* 1965; Pikaar and Fernandes 1966) but the reverse is true for arachidonic acid (Pikaar and Fernandes 1966). As a result it has been impossible to find a correlation between serum lipids of the newborn and the diet of their mothers (Hansen *et al.* 1964).

Thus, lacking pertinent information on the optimal amount of linoleic acid in the diet of expectant mothers, it seems advisable to keep this level on the safe side. For man, Söderhjelm, Wiese and Holman (1970) calculated an optimal level of 2% of calories. Therefore at least this amount but preferably more should be incorporated in the diet of pregnant women.

After birth the serum lipids of the infant depend largely on the composition of the formula (Hansen *et al.* 1964; Holman *et al.* 1965; Pikaar and Fernandes 1966). Babies fed cow's milk were found to have increased levels of 20:3 (*n*–9) which returned to normal on changing to feeding breast milk (Pikaar and Fernandes 1966). However, breast milk may vary widely in linoleic acid content with the diet of the mother (Söderhjelm 1953; Insull *et al.* 1959).

At low levels of linoleic acid, deficiency symptoms are observed. A dry, scaly skin develops (Hansen *et al.* 1963; Warwick *et al.* 1959) and the caloric efficiency decreases (Adam, Hansen and Wiese 1958; Combes, Pratt and Wiese 1962; Hansen *et al.* 1963) concomitant with a poor gain in weight. The changes in the skin disappear upon administration of 1 cal% of linoleic acid, but the caloric utilization increases at least up to 4 or 5% of calories. Therefore baby food should contain a minimum of 5 cal% of linoleic acid.

## FACTORS AFFECTING THE NEED FOR ESSENTIAL COMPONENTS

### *Vitamin E*

If the diet is to contain substantial amounts of linoleic acid, autoxidation must be prevented. Also, the anti-oxidation potential has to be adequate within the organism. In this respect vitamin E seems to have an important function, especially in protecting the highly unsaturated fatty acids derived in the body from linoleic and linolenic acid.

Symptoms of vitamin E deficiency—oedema, skin lesions and changes in blood cells—have been observed in children (Hassan *et al.* 1966), which could be cured by the administration of 60 mg tocopherol per day. The actual requirement of vitamin E has been investigated mainly in animals, using as criteria creatinuria, myopathy and haemolysis *in vitro*. F. C. Jager, feeding a diet containing 35 cal % fat to ducklings and using myopathy as a criterion, has established a requirement of 3 mg D-α-tocopherol per 1000 kcal when the linoleic acid content of the oil or fat used is below 20 % (to be published). For a higher content of linoleic acid, the requirement is doubled.

A requirement for vitamin E in brain has only been observed in chickens. Deficiency leads to encephalomalacia and a decrease of pentaenoic and hexaenoic acids in the brain, while the content of arachidonic acid increases (Witting 1969). Analogous observations were made in various tissues of the rat (Witting 1967; Witting and Horwitt 1967; Witting, Likhite and Horwitt 1967; Witting, Theron and Horwitt 1967). This indicates that when the anti-oxidant potential of a cell is lowered as a consequence of a vitamin E deficiency, the most highly unsaturated fatty acids (pentaenes and hexaenes) are primarily oxidized and replaced by the less readily oxidizable arachidonic acid, in order to compensate for the loss in unsaturation. Clearly the function of vitamin E as anti-oxidant is to protect not only the fatty acids of the *n*–6 family but particularly the pentaenes and hexaenes of the linolenic type. However, the requirement for vitamin E is usually established as a function of dietary linoleic acid. It is therefore conceivable that the actual requirement is higher than found in these experiments, especially for the developing brain, which is relatively abundant in the highly unsaturated *n*–3 fatty acids and low in vitamin E compared with other organs (Table 1).

TABLE 1

Tocopherol content in various tissues of infants

| *Tissue* | *Content mg/100 g tissue* |
|---|---|
| Adipose tissue | 2.8 |
| Liver | 1.4 |
| Blood | 1.0 |
| Lung | 0.7 |
| Muscle | 0.6 |
| Brain | 0.25 |

(From Dju, Mason and Filer 1958.)

*Other factors*

Apart from the essential compounds the lipid fraction of the diet may also contain factors that affect the growing child adversely.

It is now widely accepted that the dietary level of cholesterol should be kept low. Although as yet no effect of cholesterol on brain maturation is known, lipid sources rich in this compound—such as animal fats—should not be selected as oils for infant foods, in order to prevent the development of fatty streaks in arterial tissue—the first signs of atherosclerosis.

Saturated fatty acids are reported to increase the cholesterol content in blood. Both cholesterol and saturated fatty acids may accelerate the development of EFA deficiency. Therefore high levels of saturated fatty acids in the diets should be avoided.

The question whether *trans* fatty acids increase the demand for linoleic acid has not yet been answered, but it has been demonstrated that elaidic acid passes through the placental barrier to the same extent as oleic acid and can subsequently be found in brain tissue (Billek 1968). In the absence of definite information on possible harmful effects, the *trans* fatty acids have to be regarded with some reserve.

Monoenoic fatty acids containing 20 or more carbon atoms cause lipidosis in the hearts of various animal species (Abdellatif and Vles 1970*a*, *b*). The triglyceride content of the hearts increased tenfold (Houtsmuller, Struijk and Van der Beek 1970), while the rate of oxidation of various substrates by isolated mitochondria was decreased to about 50% of controls. Since young animals are especially susceptible to these effects of very long-chain fatty acids, they should be excluded from baby food.

Summarizing, it seems that oils high in linoleic acid and containing adequate amounts of vitamin E are especially suited for the preparation of modern foods for mothers and children. In Table 2 a few commonly used oils and fats are listed with their contents of linoleic and linolenic acid and the vitamin E equivalents (i.e. the sum of the various tocopherols in the oil, each multiplied by the respective 'biological activity factor'). If the optimal level of 5% of calories for linoleic acid (see p. 216) is to be attained in a diet containing 40 cal % fat, then only the oils in the first half of the list are of interest.

With respect to vitamin E it is noticeable that the highly unsaturated oils are especially rich sources of vitamin E, with the exception of soyabean oil and peanut oil. In the former this is of some concern, as this oil also contains substantial amounts of linolenic acid. A possible shortage in antioxidant in foods prepared with soyabean oil has to be avoided.

TABLE 2

Linoleic and linolenic acid content and vitamin E 'adequacy' of several oils and fats

| | *Linoleic acid 18:2(n–6) %* | *Linolenic acid 18:3(n–3) %* | *Equivalents* D-*α-tocopherol mg/kg* | *Vitamin E 'adequacy'* |
|---|---|---|---|---|
| Safflower seed | 73 | 0.5 | 400 | ++ |
| Sunflower seed | 60 | 0.5 | 650 | ++ |
| Maize | 54 | 1 | 500 | ++ |
| Soyabean | 53 | 8 | 230 | + |
| Cotton seed | 51 | 0.5 | 650 | ++ |
| Peanut | 20 | 0.5 | 270 | + |
| Palm | 10 | 0.5 | 420 | ++ |
| Olive | 10 | 1.5 | 85 | ± |
| Lard | 8 | 1 | 7 | — |
| Butter | 4 | — | 18 | — |
| Cocoabutter | 3 | — | 45 | — |
| Coconut | 2 | — | 14 | — |
| Beef tallow | 2 | — | 7 | — |

(F. C. Jager, to be published.)

# References


ABDELLATIF, A. M. M. and VLES, R. O. (1970*a*) *Nutr. Metab.* **12**, 285-295

ABDELLATIF, A. M. M. and VLES, R. O. (1970*b*) *Nutr. Metab.* **12**, 296-305

ADAM, D. J. D., HANSEN, A. E. and WIESE, H. F. (1958) *J. Nutr.* **66**, 555-564

BERNSOHN, J. and STEPHANIDES, L. M. (1967) *Nature (Lond.)* **215**, 821-823

BILLEK, G. V. (1968) *Proceedings of the 9th Congress of the International Society for Fat Research*, I, 15

CALDWELL, D. F. and CHURCHILL, J. A. (1966) *Psychol. Rep.* **19**, 99-102

CHURCHILL, J. A., AYERS, M. A. and CALDWELL, D. F. (1967) *J. Am. Med. Assoc.* **201**, 482-484

COMBES, M., PRATT, E. L. and WIESE, H. F. (1962) *Pediatrics* **30**, 136-144

DJU, M. Y., MASON, K. E. and FILER, J. (1958) *Am. J. Clin. Nutr.* **6**, 50-60

GALLI, C., WHITE, H. B., JR and PAOLETTI, R. (1971) *Lipids* **6**, 378-387

HANSEN, A. E., WIESE, H. F., BOELSCHE, A. N., HAGGARD, M. E., ADAM, D. J. D. and DAVIS, H. (1963) *Pediatrics* **31** (suppl. 1, pt. 2), 171-192

HANSEN, A. E., WIESE, H. F., ADAM, D. J. D., BOELSCHE, A. N., HAGGARD, M. E. and DAVIS, H. (1964) *Am. J. Clin. Nutr.* **15**, 11-19

HASSAN, H., HASHIM, S. A., VAN ITALLIE, T. B. and SEBRELL, W. H. (1966) *Am. J. Clin. Nutr.* **19**, 147-157

HOLMAN, R. T., HAYES, H., RINNE, A. and SÖDERHJELM, L. (1965) *Acta Pediat. Scand.* **54**, 573-577

HOUTSMULLER, U. M. T., STRUIJK, C. B. and VAN DER BEEK, A. (1970) *Biochim. Biophys. Acta* **218**, 564-566

INSULL, W. J., JR, HIRSCH, J., JAMES, T. and AHRENS, E. H., JR (1959) *J. Clin. Invest.* **38**, 443-450

PAOLETTI, R. and GALLI, C. (1972) This volume, pp. 121-132.

PIKAAR, N. A. and FERNANDES, J. (1966) *Am. J. Clin. Nutr.* **19**, 194-204

SÖDERHJELM, L. (1953) *Acta Soc. Med. Upsalien* **58**, 239-251

Söderhjelm, L., Wiese, H. F. and Holman, R. T. (1970) In *Progress in the Chemistry of Fats and other Lipids*, vol. 9, pt. 4, pp. 557-585, ed. R. T. Holman. Pergamon Press, Oxford
Tinoco, J., Williams, M. A., Hincenbergs, I. and Lyman, R. L. (1971) *J. Nutr.* **101**, 937-946
Warwick, W. J., Holman, R. T., Quie, P. G. and Good, R. A. (1959) *Am. J. Dis. Child.* **98**, 317-329
White, H. B., Jr, Galli, C. and Paoletti, R. (1971) *J. Neurochem.* **18**, 869-882
Witting, L. A. (1967) *Lipids* **2**, 109-113
Witting, L. A. (1969) *J. Neurochem.* **16**, 1253-1256
Witting, L. A. and Horwitt, M. K. (1967) *Lipids* **2**, 89-96
Witting, L. A., Likhite, V. N. and Horwitt, M. K. (1967) *Lipids* **2**, 103-108
Witting, L. A., Theron, J. J. and Horwitt, M. K. (1967) *Lipids* **2**, 97-102

# Discussion

*Young:* Dr Houtsmuller, I think you implied that the properties of erucic acid, 22:1(*n*–9), in regard to ATP synthesis might be shared with other monoenoic acids?

*Houtsmuller:* Yes, the quality of isolated heart mitochondria is inferior after feeding 20:1(*n*–9), 22:1(*n*–9) and 24:1(*n*–9) to rats. The rate of oxygen consumption ($QO_2$) is substantially decreased, but the ADP/O ratio and Respiratory Control Index (RCI) are also adversely affected. Therefore the rate of ATP synthesis, being a product of $QO_2$ and the ADP/O ratio, shows the largest decrease.

*Young:* Does the position of the double bond have an effect?

*Houtsmuller:* Yes, but as these are only preliminary results I would not like to go into details.

*Young*: You also mentioned that *trans* unsaturated fatty acids can be incorporated in the brain. Is this possible with acids with two or three double bonds in the *trans* position? Or more?

*Houtsmuller:* The *trans* isomer of oleic acid, elaidic acid, with one double bond, passes the placental barrier and is incorporated into phospholipids but mainly in the $\alpha$ position, not the $\beta$ position.

*Young:* Is there any evidence of antagonism between the *trans* and the *cis* isomers?

*Houtsmuller:* There is some indication that *trans* fatty acids enhance the demand for linoleic acid.

*Young:* It's a rather important matter, presumably, since *trans* compounds can be formed by the hydrogenation of more unsaturated fats.

*Ansell:* Dr Houtsmuller, am I right in thinking that the *n*–6 fatty acids do not normally pass through the placenta?

*Houtsmuller:* The placental barrier is selective to the fatty acids; for example, erucic acid does not pass, but *n*–6 fatty acids do pass. But the placental barrier is a membrane. Probably it takes up linoleic acid from the mother's blood, synthesizes arachidonic acid from it and releases this to the infant. That is probably why the infant has a higher content of arachidonic acid than the mother but a lower content of linoleic acid. As I said, little lipid passes through the placental barrier, and therefore the infant has very little lipid available, which is why almost no lipid oxidation takes place in the foetus.

*Davison:* Dr Houtsmuller, are you not ignoring Dr Svennerholm's data on EFA deficiency, which seems contradictory? I also wonder whether it isn't wrong to conclude that vitamin E is necessary in foodstuffs of human infants, when as far as I am aware vitamin E has not been shown to have any effect in human nutrition?

*Houtsmuller:* As I mentioned, it has been established by Hassan and others that lack of vitamin E causes deficiency in young infants. Several investigators have suggested that feeding high amounts of linoleic acid could be harmful, because of auto-oxidation *in vivo*.

*Crawford:* Losowsky and Leonard (1967; Leonard and Losowsky 1971) have produced information on vitamin E deficiency in both adults and children, particularly red cell fragility, where they are specifically using vitamin E to restore normal red cell fragility.

*Houtsmuller:* I don't think that the test for red cell fragility *in vitro* is an indication of vitamin E deficiency. It is just an indirect way of measuring the amount of vitamin E in the red cells.

*Crawford:* The red cell fragility was corrected by vitamin E.

*Mead:* Matsuo (1954) and Kaneda, Sakai and Ishii (1955) did experiments in which, instead of using vegetable oil as a source of polyunsaturates, they used fish oil, which has almost no tocopherol but very high amounts of polyunsaturated fatty acids. When this was fed at 5-10% by weight of the diet, the rats died. This is a very dramatic effect, leading to some reluctance even to try these experiments on children.

*Houtsmuller:* The effects in vitamin E deficiency of *n*–3 fatty acids—which are the main fatty acids in fish oil—seem to be more complex: linolenic acid (*n*–3) does not affect encephalomalacia in chickens, whereas linoleic acid (*n*–6) does.

*Lloyd:* I share Professor Davison's scepticism about the evidence for the function of vitamin E in humans. There are only very few reports of symptomatic vitamin E deficiency in babies. We have been studying both serum vitamin E and tests of red cell haemolysis, in children with various malabsorptive disorders (Harries and Muller 1969, 1971) including abetalipoproteinaemia (in which the most severe degree of vitamin E deficiency is found: Lloyd and

Muller 1972), and remain open-minded about the functions of vitamin E in man.

On another point, in Table 2 (p. 219) in which you summarized the linoleic and linolenic acid contents of various oils, where would you put breast milk?

*Houtsmuller:* Breast milk may vary considerably in composition (Söderhjelm 1953; Insull *et al.* 1959), depending on the mother's diet. The lipid content and the fatty acid composition may vary. Therefore it is difficult to put mother's milk into this table. However, babies fed cow's milk were found to have increased levels of 20:3(*n*–9)—a symptom of EFA deficiency— and these levels returned to 'normal' upon switching to breast milk (Pikaar and Fernandes 1966). This means that in that experiment breast milk contained adequate amounts of linoleic acid. Let us assume that this was 3-5 cal %. If a formula containing 40 cal % of fat is prepared from the oils listed in Table 2, then the linoleic acid content of this formula would be 0.4 times the figures given in the table. This would put breast milk at the same level as palm oil or olive oil.

*Bernsohn:* We obtained some data on the milk of Japanese mothers (Saito *et al.* 1965). The linoleic and linolenic acid composition of the total lipids was 13.0% and 2.5% respectively. Published values by the National Research Council (1953) for American women were 8.3% and 0.4% for the comparable fatty acids. At 3.8% lipids in human milk, the National Research Council's figures for the fatty acids fall below the 1% of calories level found by Mohrhauer and Holman (1963) to be required for optimal growth in rats, as well as the values reported by Pudelkiewicz, Seufert and Holman (1968). The low level of linolenic acid in the American milk is particularly striking, and if it is an essential dietary component during early development it may be a limiting factor.

*Svennerholm:* In Sweden pooled breast milk contained 3.5 cal % of linoleic acid, 1.2% of linolenic acid, and 0.5% of arachidonic acid (Olegård and Svennerholm 1971). Infants fed breast milk showed a diminished concentration of fatty acids of the linoleic acid series in blood lecithin, as compared with formula-fed infants or with older infants and children. We consider breast milk to give a suboptimal level of essential fatty acids in Sweden. Hansen and co-workers (1963) found a large variation between individuals in the fatty acid composition of human breast milk. We have, however, not been able to corroborate this statement in Sweden. On the contrary, we have found the range of variation to be very narrow, which is also evident from the small standard deviations of the fatty acid composition of the blood phosphoglycerides (Olegård and Svennerholm 1971). The constancy of the breast milk composition may perhaps be explained by the small differences in dietary habits with regard to fat, calorie consumption and the use of fat for cooking.

*Crawford:* We have recently been separating phospholipids from breast milk. Largely what people mean by 'animal fat' is adipose tissue and they forget that cells are built from a highly complex structural lipid which is of a completely different composition. Adipose tissue is largely triglyceride, and I think that when people analyse human milk they separate the cream, or extract the whole milk in which they are analysing what is predominantly a triglyceride pattern. The triglyceride is to a large extent a calorie source. If you separate the protein it has lipid attached to it, predominantly phospholipid, which has quite different fatty acid patterns from the triglycerides. Within the phospholipids you find not just linoleic and linolenic acids, but also the long-chain products, arachidonic and docosahexaenoic acids. We have recently completed a sequential study on breast milk in three people. We looked predominantly at phospholipids and found that in the first week of lactation, the phospholipids exhibited what might be called a classical deficiency pattern in the sense that 20:3($n$–9) was present and there were only small amounts of the long-chain acids in the ethanolamine phosphoglycerides. We thought this must be wrong, because if human breast milk is meant to be good for babies to eat one might have expected something more appropriate to what is used in cell construction. When we followed these lactations, we discovered that in the 2nd and 3rd week there was a recovery with respect to the long-chain acids. This is interesting in view of the time-scales of development that we have been talking about. Certainly you cannot just talk about breast milk in terms of linoleic and linolenic acids because it's immensely more complex than that; quite apart from the phospholipids, there must be other considerations, like the hormonal influence. But as a general point it's surprising that we know much more about cow's milk than we do about human milk.

*Aebi:* Dr Crawford, from your results one might conclude that there is no such thing as average mother's milk. Bearing in mind Dr Svennerholm's finding of a significant difference in linoleic acid content in the serum of 3-month-old babies, comparing breast milk-fed and formula-fed babies, it seems to me that we have to abandon the sacred belief that mother's milk is the optimal food for babies. Or might it be that with the recommendation of a high essential fatty acid intake at this early stage, we are overshooting the target?

*Winick:* Are we establishing that a large population is getting a mother's milk which would be considered inadequate in essential fatty acid content in terms of the ranking given in Dr Houtsmuller's Table 2?

*Houtsmuller:* What is 'deficient'? If the caloric efficiency is not optimal, it does not mean that a deficiency exists. The absorption of fatty acids also depends on the composition of the triglycerides. It could be that mother's milk contains the fatty acids in a more adequate way than other lipid sources, as Dr Crawford pointed out. There have been hardly any investigations of this.

*Crawford:* Human breast milk contains only 1.4% protein and I don't think the figure for EFA of 3 or 5% of calories is really relevant; the balance with protein must be considered. Secondly, the availability of long-chain acids is important. Mohrhauer and Holman (1963) have shown that they are incorporated into tissue lipids with greater efficiency than the $C_{18}$ vegetable acids. As Dr Houtsmuller suggests, the 'arrangement' is more adequate in human milk; the balance with protein may also be better for man than the balance found in cow's milk.

*Winick:* Cow's milk has even more protein per gramme, so why not give cow's milk, which was what was done before?

*Crawford:* For the reason that cow's milk has much more protein in it than human breast milk but much less of the essential lipids, and if you accept Dr Menkes' findings on the effects of formulas containing 3.9% protein (p. 193), there is another good reason for not using cow's milk. The comparison in Dr Houtsmuller's Table 2 is relevant to a much higher protein intake.

*Svennerholm:* Dr Dobbing said earlier (p. 196) that it would be better to talk about optimal or not optimal rather than of deficient EFA intake. I agree completely. I would then say that human breast milk will not give the optimal concentration of linoleic acid, but it might be sufficient, because at 6 months of age breast-fed infants reach the same level as the formula-fed infants. We have recommendations for vitamins, which give figures for a minimal and an optimal supply, and I think such a recommendation for essential fatty acids, which were previously considered vitamins, would also be useful.

*Houtsmuller:* Professor Svennerholm, you found that mother's milk in Sweden contains 3.5 cal% linoleic acid. Hansen calculated that for optimal caloric efficiency about 5 cal% is required, so human milk may not be optimal, but this does not mean that the children show deficiency symptoms.

*Cobos:* Enormous numbers of children in the world are being fed on skim milk alone, probably enriched by sugar; are we making them fatty acid deficient? Should we modify the terms of that diet? This is an essential question.

*Houtsmuller:* In children with kwashiorkor the fatty acid composition is normal (low 20:3(*n*–9)), but as soon as a diet with high protein content but low in linoleic acid is fed to the children, deficiency symptoms appear (e.g. increase in 20:3(*n*–9)). The explanation of this phenomenon most probably is, as Professor Mead said earlier (p. 155), that for deficiency symptoms to appear cells must divide. In kwashiorkor all growth stops and therefore no deficiency symptoms appear. But upon refeeding of protein, growth resumes and consequently the deficiency symptoms appear.

*Cobos:* Thousands of children are being fed with the aim of supplementing the low intake of proteins and thus preventing protein-calorie malnutrition.

However, in view of these findings, it seems that EFA deficiencies must also be taken into consideration.

*Winick:* In half the population in Chile, this is the standard way of feeding children.

*Houtsmuller:* You should add an adequate amount of essential fatty acids, I am certain.

*Hollingsworth:* What are the signs of EFA deficiency that Dr Cobos ought to be looking for among the children?

*Houtsmuller:* The most demanding criterion is the food efficiency (the caloric efficiency); that is, growth as a function of caloric intake: measure the caloric value of what is eaten, subtract what is excreted, and see how much the children grow on it. It is often easier to establish the fatty acid pattern of serum and calculate the triene/tetraene ratio; according to Holman this is a measure of EFA deficiency. However, as I pointed out, this can be misleading when a non-essential polyunsaturated fatty acid depresses the 20:3($n$–9) content.

## References

HANSEN, A. E., WIESE, H. F., BOELSCHE, A. N., HAGGARD, M. E., ADAM, D. J. D. and DAVIS, H. (1963) *Pediatrics* **31** (suppl.), 171-192

HARRIES, J. T. and MULLER, D. P. R. (1969) *Proc. 5th International Cystic Fibrosis Conference*, pp. 298-306, ed. D. Lawson. Cystic Fibrosis Research Trust, London

HARRIES, J. T. and MULLER, D. P. R. (1971) *Gut* **12**, 579-584

INSULL, W. J., JR, HIRCH, J., JAMES, T. and AHRENS, E. H., JR (1959) *J. Clin. Invest.* **38**, 443-450

KANEDA, T. P., SAKAI, H. and ISHII, S. (1955) *J. Biochem. (Japan)* **42**, 561-573

LEONARD, P. J. and LOSOWSKY, M. S. (1971) *Am. J. Clin. Nutr.* **24**, 388

LLOYD, J. K. and MULLER, D. P. R. (1972) *Proc. XIXth Colloquium on Protides of the Biological Fluids*, pp. 331-335, ed. H. Peeters. Pergamon Press, Oxford

LOSOWSKY, M. S. and LEONARD, P. J. (1967) *Gut* **8**, 539

MATSUO, N. (1954) *J. Biochem. (Japan)* **41**, 647-652

MOHRHAUER, H. and HOLMAN, R. T. (1963) *J. Lipid Res.* **4**, 151-159

NATIONAL RESEARCH COUNCIL (1953) *The Composition of Milks*. Publ. No. 254. Washington D.C.

OLEGÅRD, R. and SVENNERHOLM, L. (1971) *Acta Paediatr. Scand.* **60**, 505-511

PIKAAR, N. A. and FERNANDES, J. (1966) *Am. J. Clin. Nutr.* **19**, 194-204

PUDELKIEWICZ, C., SEUFERT, J. and HOLMAN, R. T. (1968) *J. Nutr.* **94**, 138-146

SAITO, K., FURVICHI, E., KONDO, S., KAWANISHI, G., NISHIKAWA, I., NAKAZATO, H., NOGUCHI, Y., DOI, T., NOGUCHI, A. and SHINGO, S. (1965) *Report of Research Laboratory*, No. 69. Snow Brand Milk Prod. Co. Ltd, Kitako, Tokyo

SÖDERHJELM, L. (1953) *Acta Soc. Med. Upsalien* **58**, 239-251

# Malnutrition and mental retardation: conceptual issues

FRANCISCO COBOS

*Department of Nutrition, Harvard School of Public Health, Boston*

The evidence that malnutrition causes mental retardation is not conclusive, but it is suggestive, particularly under certain specific conditions, as pointed out by a recent review of the pertinent literature (Klein, Habicht and Yarbrough 1971). The need to clarify the nature of the relationship between these two entities is dramatized by the example of Colombia.

Colombia, a prototypical developing country, has a calculated population for 1971 of 21 791 818, of whom 14.0% are children under 5 years of age, according to the Departamento Nacional de Estadística. The Dirección de Nutrición, I.C.B.F., recognizes that, using the Gómez Classification of Nutritional Status (modified by Bengoa) (Gómez *et al.* 1954), the prevalence of malnutrition in children under 5 years of age is as follows:

| | |
|---|---|
| First degree malnutrition: | 45.6% |
| Second degree malnutrition: | 19.3% |
| Third degree malnutrition: | 1.7% |
| All degrees of malnutrition: | 66.6% |

If we accept these data, the fact that 2 014 223 Colombians under 5 years of age are malnourished is in itself staggering. Figures gathered by the Harvard-I.C.B.F.-Cornell Research Project in Bogota among children under 5 years of age from poverty areas of the city suggest that the prevalence is still higher among urban children.

Among this urban population, measurements of mental performance using the Griffiths Scale of Mental Measurement (Griffiths 1954, 1970), standardized for Bogota subjects, suggest a clear-cut difference between the scores of properly nourished and malnourished subjects, as shown in Table 1. These differences would suggest, at the most superficial level of analysis, that around 2 million Colombian children of less than 5 years of age are mentally retarded, if the assumption of a causal linkage between the deficits in nutrition and psycho-

TABLE 1

Comparisons between scores obtained in the Griffiths Scale of Mental Measurement in well-nourished and malnourished children from a poverty area of Bogota, Colombia

| *Sub-scale* | *Well-nourished subjects (n = 100)* | | *Malnourished subjects (n = 118)* | |
|---|---|---|---|---|
| | *Mean* | *S.D.* | *Mean* | *S.D.* |
| Locomotor | 102.0 | 17.8 | 84.7 | 20.7 |
| Personal-social | 96.3 | 13.4 | 86.7 | 16.5 |
| Hearing and language | 90.4 | 15.5 | 78.4 | 17.9 |
| Eye-hand coordination | 97.6 | 15.5 | 85.6 | 17.9 |
| General performance | 93.4 | 16.7 | 80.2 | 16.8 |
| Practical reasoning | 94.0 | 14.3 | 87.1 | 16.8 |
| General quotient | 94.0 | 14.6 | 82.1 | 16.5 |

Differences of 3.5 are significant at the $P = 0.05$ level on the assumption that S.D. = 15, using the $Z$ test. For the average mean and average S.D. on the $t$ test for $P = 0.05$, differences of 4.0 are significant. For $P = 0.01$ the significant difference is 5.75.

logical performance is accepted. Under these conditions a similar massive prevalence of mental retardation would be found in underdeveloped countries generally.

Apart from humanitarian reasons, the presence of such a large number of psychologically handicapped subjects is of the greatest national significance for developing countries and for underdeveloped areas of advanced nations. If malnutrition causes mental retardation, the recognition of this fact and of the need for appropriate intervention to prevent or to reverse the effects would probably radically change both the theory and implementation of national development.

As an example of the importance of this problem for nations undergoing development, Berg (1967) raised the question of 'what would be the cost/benefit ratio of a $10 million investment in food enrichment, as compared with other forms of development expenditures, e.g. spending the $10 million for fertilizers, dams, roads or schools?' This question dramatizes the impact that the clarification of the question might have. The problem, however, remains unsolved because a number of theoretical and methodological issues make the clarification of the relationships between malnutrition and mental functioning extremely difficult. If not faced and solved, these issues condemn the outcome of relevant investigations and studies to being very limited views of small areas of the problem.

Among these issues at least three deserve special consideration.

### *(1) Lack of precision in the definition of malnutrition*

In studies of malnutrition and mental functioning there is a tendency to overlook the fact that the term malnutrition may cover deficits in one or more nutrients. The presence or absence of these nutrients may have different impacts on the functioning of the psychological apparatus. Protein-calorie malnutrition, for example, is usually the only type blamed for deficits in psychometric scores, although it is recognized that it is extremely difficult to isolate pure forms of protein deficit without associated deficits in other nutrients. It has been demonstrated that deficiencies of vitamins (Coursin 1968) as well as of other trace nutrients (Dumont, Delange and Ermano 1969) may lead through specific mechanisms to psychological deficit.

In addition, the age at which the subject is deprived of food intake, the severity, the repetition of the food deprivation and the concomitance of the episode with other deprivations of a non-nutritional character, all distort the picture of psychological functioning.

In the absence of a definition of malnutrition, nutritional status is generally established by measuring deficits in physical growth—that is, anthropometrically. However, the variations in anthropometric measurements and their relation to the effects of nutrition are not fully understood. Probably a more accurate way of assessing nutritional status would be to measure food intake, but unfortunately this is unreliable.

When anthropometric measurements are used, the isolated use of weight, which is recognized to fluctuate rapidly, introduces the need to consider a measure of the duration of the nutritional deficit. This is done by taking height into consideration, which basically reflects the chronic impact. It is worth noting that most reports dealing with protein-calorie malnutrition and mental development take into account only variations in weight, as reflected in classifications like that of Gómez, modified by Bengoa (Gómez *et al.* 1954).

In summary, studies relating malnutrition to mental retardation should be very precise in defining malnutrition beyond the clinical level. Operational definitions should include an appreciation of the chronicity of the deficit and should specify the normal values with which the comparisons are made.

### *(2) Occurrence of malnutrition within the context of massive deprivation*

This is a fact that although not exhaustively documented is generally accepted. A classical example of the presence of confounding variables in evaluations of the impact of malnutrition on psychological scores is the study by Chase and

Martin (1970) in which differences in the Yale Revised Developmental Examination scores were found between groups of 19 malnourished and 19 control subjects. However, although the experimental and control groups were matched for race, birth weight and sex, came from similar socio-economic levels, and had been born in the same hospital, there were marked differences in other areas: scores on a parent–child interaction scale, total number of siblings,

TABLE 2

Prevalence of malnutrition in subjects under 5 years of age, by levels of socio-economic indicators and significance of the differences, in children from 150 families in poverty areas of Bogota, Colombia

| *Socio-economic indicator* | *Number of families* | *Number of subjects* | *Number of malnourished subjects* | *% of malnourished subjects* | $\chi^2$ |
|---|---|---|---|---|---|
| 1. Number of persons per family | | | | | |
| 4 or less | 13 | 26 | 13 | 50 | |
| 5 to 9 | 105 | 262 | 134 | 51 | |
| 10 or more | 32 | 83 | 55 | 66 | $P = 0.015$* |
| 2. Number of persons per room | | | | | |
| 1 to 3 | 79 | 194 | 86 | 44 | |
| 4 to 6 | 53 | 128 | 83 | 65 | |
| 7 or more | 18 | 49 | 33 | 67 | $P = 0.01$ |
| 3. Family income | | | | | |
| Over Col $ 1000 | 52 | 128 | 55 | 43 | |
| Col $999 and less | 98 | 243 | 147 | 60 | $P = 0.001$ |
| 4. Food expenditure/person/month | | | | | |
| Over Col $ 100 | 37 | 89 | 30 | 34 | |
| Col $ 99 and less | 98 | 260 | 159 | 61 | $P = 0.001$ |
| 5. Schooling of father | | | | | |
| 6 and more years | 22 | 52 | 20 | 38 | |
| One to 5 years | 13 | 34 | 15 | 44 | |
| None | 100 | 247 | 143 | 54 | $P = 0.01$ |
| 6. Schooling of mother | | | | | |
| 6 and more years | 16 | 36 | 14 | 39 | |
| One to 5 years | 114 | 285 | 156 | 55 | |
| None | 19 | 48 | 32 | 67 | $P = 0.020$ |
| 7. Working condition of mother | | | | | |
| Working mother | 30 | 72 | 24 | 33 | |
| Mother at home | 120 | 299 | 154 | 51 | $P = 0.018$ |

* Comparison between extremes.

number of siblings under 2 years of age at the time of birth, number of marital separations at the time of birth, and the probability that the subjects were the product of unwanted pregnancies. This suggests that factors usually associated with conditions of multiple deprivation were also present.

In our own work, differences in the prevalence of malnutrition have always been correlated with indices of deprivatory conditions. When groups of malnourished children are compared with well-nourished subjects from the same socio-economic class, those affected by malnutrition are also found to have higher indications of deprivation, as shown in Table 2.

These findings make it impossible, at present, to distinguish the effects that malnutrition alone may have on the psychological function of subjects.

### *(3) Lack of precision in the measurement of psychological deficit*

This lack of precision is derived from two main sources. On one hand, it is probable that malnutrition affects differentially several areas of psychological function. This differential impact may be further complicated by the possibility that the age at which the deprivation occurs, in relation to the critical periods of development of the brain, as well as the intensity and severity of the insult, may determine not only the importance and reversibility of the psychological deficit but also the area predominantly affected. For example, it is known that acute starvation in the adult affects mainly the affective area while cognition is preserved, and when they occur, the cognitive deficits are reversible.

Furthermore, whichever the areas affected, and whichever the areas that are taken into consideration, the actual measurement of psychological function is extremely difficult. The well-known controversy over the definition of intelligence, the recognized intricacies of the methodology of measurement, and the complicated issues related to the genetic and environmental components of psychological performance, all preclude the desired clarity.

The design or selection of instruments for psychological measurement must be based on a theoretical perspective of the areas of functioning that may be affected by nutritional deficits. This naturally leads to the measurement problems of cultural congruence, validity and reliability. Frequently compromises in one or more of these criteria must be made for the sake of another.

The object of this paper is to discuss some of the theoretical considerations related to the issues presented so far, and to describe a research project designed to answer some of the questions implicit in the relationship between malnutrition and psychological functioning.

## A COMPREHENSIVE MODEL FOR MALNUTRITION

Because of the imprecision of the definition of malnutrition, which is traditionally detected as a retardation of physical growth, a comprehensive functional model of malnutrition is a prerequisite for the exploration of its relationship to mental retardation.

Traditionally protein-calorie malnutrition, the most important type of food deficit today, has been associated with limited availability of food, and indirectly with the inability of the subjects to obtain it, mainly because of poverty.

The association of ecological, general sociological and familial dynamic factors with malnutrition has been studied for some time (Benedict, Miles and Smith 1919; Blanton 1919), although their precise role in determining psychological retardation, either independently, in association with malnutrition, or by association with each other, has not been elucidated. Apart from malnutrition, however, it is accepted that cultural deprivation affects negatively the usual measures of psychological performance. In the last decade emphasis has been placed on other, non-nutritional factors associated with a poor nutritional state, namely the general health of the subjects (Scrimshaw, Taylor and Gordon 1967).

Furthermore, human behavioural scientists have traditionally stressed the importance of psychological factors, particularly motivational ones, in the feeding behaviour and resulting nutritional status of children (Cobos 1968). On the other hand, complex psychological and familial dynamic factors have been recognized as capable of inducing severe malnutrition in young children (Powell, Brasel and Blizzard 1967; Powell *et al.* 1967).

The multifactorial causation of an unbalanced food intake, that leads to the identifiable alterations in body measurements by which malnutrition is diagnosed, should therefore be thought of as a complex system of interactions or a network of subsystems, that can be represented in a simplified manner as:

Nutritional status (Food needs/food intake) $= f$[(FA), (H), (PS.F), (F.F), (S.F)]. This indicates that the perceived nutritional status is the outcome of biological processes depending on the equilibrium between food needs and food intake, the latter being a function of, at least, food availability (FA), physical health (H), and psychological (PS.F), familial (F.F.), and sociological (S.F) factors.

The elements in this system are related to each other and to the total system in ways not yet well specified. Furthermore, each element is itself a subsystem, although the exact composition of the subsystem is, generally speaking, unknown. For example, the availability of food is obviously linked to factors such as economic status, family size, and food habits.

This conceptual model suggests that malnutrition is the result of the mutual interaction of several factors, some or all of which are present at suboptimal levels or in disequilibrium. It will rarely be present as an alteration of a single factor; rather, in each specific situation, it will respond to differential alterations of the subsystems.

The refinement of a conceptual model such as this may be useful in demonstrating that changes in any one area may affect, in varying degree, any or all of the others, leading in any case to a disequilibrium in the relation between food needs and food intake, and thus generating conditions of malnutrition, through different pathways.

The model should also allow the problem of malnutrition to be examined within the framework of the concept of general deprivation. This situation is usually described as a continuous flow of interacting events related to the conditions of life of the individual, his family or his social group, reflecting the lack or inappropriateness of physical, psychological or social elements that are essential for an individual to achieve optimal development.

Bearing this in mind, it is conceivable that only when the total system is taken into consideration will it be possible to gain insight into the relationship between malnutrition and mental retardation.

## HYPOTHETICAL BASIS OF A RELATIONSHIP BETWEEN MALNUTRITION AND MENTAL RETARDATION

Any attempt to discover relationships between malnutrition and mental retardation implies some hypothesis about possible mechanisms of such relationships. The difficulty in building a hypothesis of this nature is greatly increased by the fact that malnutrition is usually conceived of only in terms of its reflection upon physical development. When a model of malnutrition such as the one presented above is used, and the interaction between food and the resulting nutritional status is taken into account, the task of postulating hypothetical relationships is made easier.

Without such a working hypothesis as a frame of reference the selection of psychometric instruments to assess the possible impact of malnutrition on psychological functioning becomes a matter of individual preference, as evident in the use of tests in the past.

Table 3 lists the most obvious functions of food, as well as some of the biological conditions that generate such functions, and the effect of decreasing the functions listed. This table suggests that deficits in the functions of food may lead to psychological deficit in several ways, for example:

*Text continued p. 236*

TABLE 3

Example of hypothetical functions of food and effects of decrease in such functions

| *Type of function* | *Food function* | *Effects of a reduction in function* |
|---|---|---|
| Mechanical | Stimulation of perception (mainly taste, smell) | *Poor development of perception* related to food |
| | Stimulation of maturation of gastrointestinal tract | Poor development and function of gastrointestinal tract |
| Biochemical | Calorie needs: supplying energy (movement) | Low energy levels *may affect psychological function;* storage affects body weight |
| | Proteins: building of tissue structures and chemical components (hormones, neurohormones, enzymes, etc.) | May affect CNS development as well as body height |
| | Lipids and fats: high-energy elements: important constituent of CNS functional and structural elements | *May affect biochemistry* of CNS and therefore development or function<br>*May affect CNS function and structure* |
| | Vitamins: mediators in chemical processes, affecting CNS | *Some known to impair CNS function leading to mental retardation or illness* (beri-beri) |
| | Trace elements: mainly catalysts in metabolic processes | Deficit will eventually *alter CNS functioning* |
| | | Extreme deficits of the biochemical function of food will result in starvation and death |

| | | |
|---|---|---|
| Physiological | The biochemical elements of food are needed to maintain an optimal level of health through immunological and other defensive systems<br>Illness in increasing metabolic needs increases the need for food | High risk of infection, leading to altered psychological function<br>High risk of illness |
| Psychological | Intra-individual: satisfaction of 'hunger', allows concentration on psychological events | Activation of mechanisms to increase survival possibilities with heightened attention to the 'self' and less attention to extra-individual factors *leading to distorted psychological function* |
| | Inter-individual:<br>*Mother-child* – at this developmental level, feeding is, after breathing, the activity with the highest survival value. It cannot be accomplished without interaction with the mother. An important part of the function of the mother-child dyad is mediated through feeding | Maternal deprivation syndrome *leading to damage to all areas of psychological development* (cognitive, affective, primary socialization) |
| | Intra-family: food as 'currency' for intra-family transactions, as element of the reward and punishment system | Syndrome of family deprivation *leading to damage of several areas of psychosocial development* including secondary socialization |
| Sociological | As measurement of social competence<br>As indicator of specific social role<br>As indicator of affiliation to class or specific group | Self-definition as member of 'marginal' group<br>*Impoverishment of psychological and social performance* |

1. Due to deficits in the development of perception.
2. Due to low levels of energy that may impair not only reception of stimuli but also integration processes and behavioural output.
3. Due to intense hunger that may impair the subject's ability to free himself from the internal stimulation of the unsatisfied drive.
4. Due to organic illness caused directly or fostered by the effects of food deficit on other organic systems.
5. Due to damage or alteration of functions or structures of the central nervous system, at any age. This process may be irreversible and accompanied by other manifestations of the damage, or temporary and reversible and reflected only in retardation of maturational processes essential to development.
6. In extreme cases, due to impoverishment of central nervous system function, as part of total, progressive biological impairment, resulting in fatal starvation.
7. Due to damage to psychological developmental processes occurring within the mother–child interaction. The maternal function, which requires the satisfaction of basic drives of the child, is impaired as a result of food deprivation. This syndrome of maternal deprivation, that may take the form of partial deprivation (Bowlby 1966, 1969; Glaser and Eisenberg 1956), or be masked (Prugh and Harlow 1966), clearly leads not only to deficits in non-cognitive areas, but also and principally to emotional malfunction.
8. Due to impairment of the maturational stimulation supplied by interaction with a normally functioning family group. The inability of the family to protect the child from lack of food implies some degree of impairment of the function of the family. This will affect the developmental processes of the child. Traditionally recognized situations such as 'familial mental retardation' or 'psycho-social mental retardation' refer to this specific situation.
9. Due to impairment of proper social stimulation, as a result of malfunction of the social group, as occurs when the subject belongs to a 'disadvantaged' group.

A general overview of the effects on psychological function of deficits in food, accompanied or not by deficits in physical growth, suggests that they may be divided into the following groups: (*a*) effects mainly on the central nervous system, resulting in organic impairment of its functions (reflected in deficits in neurological and psychological functions); (*b*) transient effects on the central nervous system that are reflected not in neurological or psychological changes but in consequences manifested as delayed development; (*c*) damage to psychological mechanisms without an organic component.

It is clear that in most cases all areas of psychological functioning will be involved and that their involvement will vary in intensity, severity and reversibility. All possible combinations may appear whenever there is lack of food. If the psychological deficit is accompanied by alteration in physical growth, then it will be recognized that malnutrition is accompanied by manifestations of psychological impairment, in those areas that have been tested.

This suggests that in order to refine our appreciation of the effects of malnutrition on psychological functioning the minimal instrument to measure changes in the latter should ideally include the widest possible testing of non-cognitive as well as cognitive areas. This is best done by measuring the presence or absence of central nervous system damage, the speed of developmental processes and the performance of culturally dependent behaviours.

## MODEL OF A BATTERY OF INSTRUMENTS TO ASSESS PSYCHOLOGICAL CHANGES INDUCED BY MALNUTRITION

The previous considerations offer a theoretical framework for devising a battery to assess the most important changes in psychological function, involving the following components:

1. Cognitive instruments:
   (*a*) Measurement of neurological proficiency.
   (*b*) Tests of intellectual performance.
   (*c*) Tests of cognitive development.
2. Non-cognitive instruments:
   (*a*) Tests of situational interaction.
   (*b*) Tests of family interaction.

The main criteria for selecting or building such a battery of tests should be:

(*a*) The feasibility of their administration.
(*b*) The cultural congruency for the area in which they will be used.
(*c*) Their reflection of the theoretical needs presented above (validity).
(*d*) Their applicability to the total population under scrutiny and therefore the possibility of establishing normative values (reliability).
(*e*) If possible, their ability to permit transcultural comparisons.

## THE HARVARD-I.C.B.F.-CORNELL PROJECT

This project aims both to explore the question whether malnutrition, under local conditions, causes deficits in defined psychological areas, and also, if possible, to clarify the extent to which the psychological deficit may be prevented or reversed by food supplementation. The project is attempting to discover whether the possible nutritional causes of psychological deficit can be distinguished from other causes, by determining the nature of the interaction between nutritional and other non-nutritional factors affecting psychological function.

The research approach was based on the known fact that siblings have highly correlated psychological scores (Burt 1958; McCall 1970), a result which was also found in our target population (see Table 4). This correlation reflects the notion that siblings belong to the same genetic pool, have been exposed to similar physical and psychological stimulation, and have been exposed to similar epidemiological risks.

TABLE 4

Intra-class correlation coefficients for 48 pairs of siblings from Bogota, Colombia, in scores of the Griffiths Scale of Mental Measurement

| *Sub-scale* | *Intra-class coefficients* | *Significance levels* |
|---|---|---|
| Locomotor | 0.41 | 0.002 |
| Personal-social | 0.23 | 0.054 |
| Hearing and speech | 0.22 | 0.063 |
| Eye-hand coordination | 0.55 | 0.001 |
| General performance | 0.22 | 0.061 |
| General quotient | 0.47 | 0.001 |

The research design is also based on the fact that in areas where malnutrition is frequent it is common to find a child who is malnourished and has one well-nourished sibling. Food supplementation of the family should lead to the recovery of the malnourished child and the prevention of malnutrition in the well-nourished child. This allows a comparison to be made between the sibs, in order to identify the effect of a history of malnutrition.

In order to separate effects of birth order from the nutritional effects, different groups of siblings must be studied, which requires a number of groups (see Table 5). This basic research approach requires not only the baseline measurements of pertinent parameters but also their longitudinal assessment, as illustrated in Table 6.

The project's main hypothesis, in its longitudinal phase, will be tested primarily through classical analysis of variance and covariance procedures. An extensive effort has been made to assure statistical control through the paired-sibling model. In fact, the attempt to eliminate confounding variables from the main effect will allow us to detect nutritional effects acting alone, if they

TABLE 5

Distribution of siblings in cells by birth order, nutritional status and food supplementation, in the Harvard-I.C.B.F.-Cornell Research Project on Malnutrition and Mental Development

| *Birth order* | *Food supplementation* | | |
|---|---|---|---|
| | *Supplemented* | | *Not supplemented* |
| | Cell I | Cell III | Cell V |
| Older sibling | Well-nourished | Well-nourished | Well-nourished |
| Younger sibling | Well-nourished | Malnourished | Well-nourished |
| | Cell II | Cell IV | |
| Older sibling | Malnourished | Malnourished | — |
| Younger sibling | Well-nourished | Malnourished | — |

TABLE 6

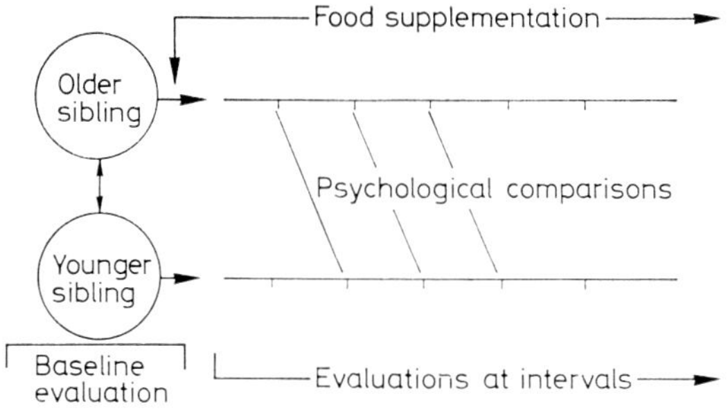


exist. This will answer the question whether malnutrition has any effect upon psychological scores, other things being equal. It is, however, recognized that the dynamics of the functions of food, health, social, family factors, and so on, are extremely important. Thus, there is a definite need for supportive methodologies to investigate the dynamics of all the variables studied, acting singly and in combination. The static effects of the totality of variables will be approached using multiple regression correlation, while the interaction of nutrition with other factors will require the use of techniques such as discriminate functions to create separate 'social populations'.

Furthermore, the dynamics of all variables, acting singly and jointly, will be elicited by applying techniques using structural models, causal models, and system models, which may yield simulations to guide further experimental efforts.

*Implementation*

In order to implement this project in Bogota, Colombia, a working structure was created which included nutritional, medical, sociological and psychological working teams. A time-table was made in which a period of one year was to be spent in confirming the feasibility of the research, under the local conditions. Instruments were developed during a two-year period, and the project is now making a pilot study, simulating on a small scale the longitudinal definitive study.

In what follows, the psychometric instruments are discussed that will be used to measure changes in the dependent variable, according to the theoretical model proposed.

*The psychological battery*

The selected battery includes a neurological evaluation, limited to a careful but routine clinical evaluation of the neurological status of the subject, including an assessment of the medical history and a complete neurological examination. These procedures are carried out by a paediatric neurologist and yield scores on a three-point scale (normal, doubtful and deficient neurological status).

The non-cognitive instrument, still being developed, consists mainly of observation of the mother–child interaction under standardized conditions, and of the reaction to maternal separation, the scoring of exploratory behaviours, and observation of the reaction to social contact with the observer.

The Griffiths Scale of Mental Measurement was selected for assessment of performance within the cognitive area. This is an I.Q. type of psychometric scale, developed in England by Dr R. Griffiths and widely used in several countries. It provides subquotients for the locomotor, personal–social, eye and hand coordination, hearing and speech, general performance, and practical reasoning areas, as well as a general quotient, which is an average of the values of the subquotients. This scale has been standardized for the population of Bogota. Cultural congruency has been assured through a limited number of small changes. It has proved to be able to discriminate nutritional status (see Table 1) and socio-economic level. The reliability correlation between testing and retesting, using Mosier's formula (Guilford 1954), was 0.84, which indicates that the test can be used for differential prediction, as contemplated by the project.

The developmental instrument has been based on the theories of the development of cognition proposed by Jean Piaget, and based on the work of A. Pinard in Montreal and S. K. Escalona and H. H. Corman in New York. A continuous ordinal scaling has been achieved to diagnose the level of cognitive development that the subject has attained, according to Piaget's theory, as reflected in each answer within the scale. The scaling procedure follows the suggestions of Pinard and Laurendeau (1964). An example of the results is shown in Table 7.

TABLE 7

Scalogram analysis for Einstein scales: Bogota standardization sample ($n = 500$)

| *Prehension* | | | *Object* | | | *Space* | | |
|---|---|---|---|---|---|---|---|---|
| *Stage* | *Passed all preceding stages* | *Passed some* | *Stage* | *Passed all preceding stages* | *Passed some* | *Stage* | *Passed all preceding stages* | *Passed some* |
| II-1 | 14 | — | III | 13 | — | III | 2 | — |
| II-2 | 8 | — | IV | 11 | — | IV | 9 | 1 |
| II-3 | 25 | — | V | 20 | — | V | 34 | 1 |
| II-4 | 10 | — | VI | 135 | 1 | VI | 130 | 3 |
| III | 212 | 51 | — | — | — | — | — | — |
| Total subjects | 269 | 51 | | 179 | 1 | | 175 | 5 |
| 12 months or younger | $n = 320$ | | | 1 year $n = 180$ | | | 1 year $n = 180$ | |
| Green's index of consistency | | 0.81 | | 0.99 | | | 0.97 | |

Results of Corman and Escalona (1966) are shown below for comparison:

| | | | | | | | | |
|---|---|---|---|---|---|---|---|---|
| II-1 | — | — | III | — | — | III | — | — |
| II-2 | 6 | 0 | IV | 24 | 0 | IV | 23 | 0 |
| II-3 | 19 | 3 | V | 19 | 0 | V | 17 | 0 |
| III | 5 | 7 | VI | 56 | 0 | VI | 33 | 1 |
| Total subjects | 30 | 10 | | 113 | 0 | | 83 | 1 |
| Green's index of consistency | | 0.66 | | 1.00 | | | 0.98 | |

A factorial analysis of these scales was made, yielding nearly a one-factor solution, as would be expected from an instrument based on theories of 'genetic psychology'. To arrive at a 'Cognitive Developmental Quotient' the scales are first scored by assigning the highest age value attained by each subject within each scale; the scales are then averaged to compute a cognitive developmental age. The quotient is computed in the conventional way for the I.Q. To preserve the diagnostic value the developmental stage attained by subjects is maintained and displayed as needed.

A preliminary estimate of reliability has been calculated using Mosier's formula (Guilford 1954), yielding a value of 0.77. As part of the standardization study these scales were compared to the Griffiths I.Q. and to true age: the Pearson Product Moment Correlations were 0.85 and 0.87 respectively.

As an example of the ability of these scales to discriminate nutritional status, Table 8 shows values for children under 2 years of age.

TABLE 8

Mean Cognitive Developmental Quotients by nutritional status of two areas of cognitive development (development of the concepts of the object and of space) from the sensorimotor scale, administered to pairs of siblings from Bogota, Colombia

| *Nutritional cell* | *Object scale* | | *Spatial scale* | |
|---|---|---|---|---|
| | *General score* | *S.D.* | *General score* | *S.D.* |
| Cell I (WW)* ($n = 45$) | 105.4 | 22.6 | 101.9 | 18.9 |
| Cell II (MW) ($n = 44$) | 93.2 | 31.8 | 103.6 | 30.8 |
| Cell III (WM) ($n = 48$) | 91.1 | 29.9 | 96.2 | 20.0 |
| Cell IV (MM) ($n = 52$) | 89.0 | 31.1 | 89.3 | 27.2 |

* See Table 5. W, well-nourished. M, malnourished.
Differences of 10 points are statistically significant at the 5% level.

In addition, a limited sample of performance items from the psychological tests in use at the Human Development Division, Instituto de Nutrición de Centro America y Panama, in Guatemala is being used in order to be able to compare populations in a transcultural framework. Table 9 suggests that scores from these items are able to discriminate nutritional status. This also reinforces the notion that psychological deficits are correlated with nutritional deficits.

TABLE 9

Mean score values and standard deviations of well-nourished and malnourished children from poverty areas of Bogota in six general items of performance ($n = 45$ in each group)

| *Nutritional status* | *Embedded figures* | | *Digit span* | | *Sentence completion* | | *Naming objects* | | *Recognizing objects* | | *Verbal inference* | |
|---|---|---|---|---|---|---|---|---|---|---|---|---|
| | *Value* | *S.D.* | *Value* | *S.D.* | *Value* | *S.D.* | *Value* | *S.D.* | *Value* | *S.D.* | *Value* | *S.D.* |
| Well-nourished | 2.4 | 3.1 | 3.7 | 4.4 | 26.9 | 15.4 | 42.6 | 27.2 | 15.8 | 6.3 | 26.9 | 9.1 |
| Mal-nourished | 1.2 | 2.3 | 2.0 | 3.6 | 20.0 | 15.0 | 30.1 | 25.5 | 8.6 | 6.5 | 22.8 | 10.0 |
| $t$ value: | 2.16 | | 2.60 | | 2.16 | | 2.29 | | 2.30 | | 2.01 | |
| Significance: | $P < 0.05$ | | $P < 0.01$ | | $P < 0.05$ | | $P < 0.05$ | | $P < 0.05$ | | $P < 0.05$ | |

## DISCUSSION

So far the progress made in the Harvard-I.C.B.F.-Cornell Project on Malnutrition and Mental Development has shown that in the populations studied it is possible to demonstrate that malnutrition is correlated with deficits in psychological scores and deficits in sociological variables. In order to further explore the conjunction of malnutrition with psychological and other deficits, the psychological tests were administered to a population of 69 families, randomly chosen from the poverty areas of the city of Bogota, and the sociological scales of the nutritional evaluation of paired siblings were also applied.

In this sample, scores of psychological performance (Griffiths Scale) were regressed on the social variables. The resultant multiple correlations indicate that various linear combinations of the social variables significantly account for a considerable part of the variance in the individual psychology scores.

Nutritional measures were also regressed on the social variables. The $R^2$ values are large, indicating a considerable overlap between the nutritional scales and linear combinations of sociological variables.

The social variables that entered the regressions predicting the psychological scores were 'forced' into new multiple equations, after which the nutritional items were allowed to 'vie' with one another to see which, if any, could make a significant additional contribution to predicting the psychological residuals. In most instances a number of nutritional items did enter the equation. Some of these entries considerably increased the squared multiple correlation coefficients. Thus, even after the social variables measured have been accounted for, nutritional factors had an impact on the psychological scores. Table 10 presents some of these data.

TABLE 10

Multiple correlations of the Griffiths scores on nutrition, with social factors first 'stepped in', on children from the poverty areas of Bogota ($n = 69$ pairs of siblings)

| *Sub-scales* | *$R^2$ with social factors only* | *$R^2$ with nutritional factors added* | *Increase in $R^2$ with nutritional factors* | *Significance level of multiple correlation with nutritional variables* |
|---|---|---|---|---|
| Locomotor | 0.28 | 0.40 | 0.12 | 0.001 |
| Personal-social | 0.39 | 0.44 | 0.05 | 0.001 |
| Hearing and speech | 0.27 | — | — | — |
| Eye-hand coordination | 0.36 | 0.41 | 0.05 | 0.001 |
| General performance | 0.35 | 0.46 | 0.10 | 0.001 |
| General quotient | 0.31 | 0.40 | 0.08 | 0.001 |

So far, the concomitance of deficits in psychological scores with malnutrition and of this with conditions of deprivation has been established. However, no definite causal linkage can yet be made between malnutrition and the psychological deficits since their effect may still be mediated through unknown mechanisms, such as, for example, unexplored sociological factors. However, the information available suggests that the theoretical framework used, and upon which the instruments have been devised, is appropriate. It is obvious that further evaluation of the efficiency of the instruments is desirable before an attempt is made to explore the interactional effects of the several sets of variables that must be taken into account in order to understand the mental retardation or psychological deficits possibly generated by malnutrition.

## SUMMARY

The evidence that malnutrition causes mental retardation is so far suggestive but not conclusive. It is important to clarify the relationship between these two entities, particularly in view of the prevalence of malnutrition in some areas of the world.

Certain factors complicate the investigation of this problem: the lack of precision of the definition of malnutrition; the fact that the clinical picture of malnutrition almost always occurs within a context of massive deprivation; and the fact that the assessment of mental retardation is in itself a complex issue. Any approach to the problem requires theoretical models to be devised that must be tested before they can be profitably used in research projects.

This paper discusses some of these issues and describes a project designed to answer some of the questions related to the interaction between malnutrition and mental development. The conception of malnutrition as a complex system is presented and it is suggested that only by considering the different subsystems involved is it possible to have an operative view of the entity. The bases for the definition of methodology to assess the psychological variable are derived from the previous notions, and considerations for its use are presented. Preliminary results from the pilot study are outlined.

ACKNOWLEDGEMENTS

This paper and the research reported in it has been supported by a contract from the National Institute of Child Health and Human Development, Bethesda, Md. and in part by funds from the Department of Nutrition, Harvard School of Public Health, and from the Dirección de Nutrición, I.C.B.F., Bogotá. Thanks are given to all members of the Harvard-I.C.B.F.-Cornell Project on Malnutrition and Mental Development, and especially to Dr D. Franklin. It is their work that is reported here.

# References

BERG, A. D. (1967) *Foreign Affairs* **46**, 1
BENEDICT, P. G., MILES, W. R. and SMITH, H. M. (1919) *Human vitality and efficiency under prolonged restricted diet.* Carnegie Inst. Wash. publication no. 20.
BLANTON, S. (1919) *Ment. Hyg.* **3**, 343
BOWLBY, J. (ed.) (1966) *Maternal Care and Mental Health – Deprivation of Maternal Care: A Reassessment of its Effects.* Schocken Books, New York
BOWLBY, J. (1969) *Attachment and Loss*, vol. 1. *Attachment.* Basic Books, New York
BURT, C. (1958) *Am. Psychol.* **13**, 1-15
COBOS, F. (1968) *Interam. J. Psychol.* **2**, 3
CORMAN, H. H. and ESCALONA, S. K. (1966) *Merrill-Palmer Quarterly* **15**, 4
COURSIN, D. B. (1968) In *Malnutrition, Learning and Behavior*, ed. N. S. Scrimshaw and J. E. Gordon. The M.I.T. Press, Cambridge, Mass.
CHASE, H. P. and MARTIN, H. P. (1970) *New Engl. J. Med.* **282**, 933-939
DUMONT, J. E., DELANGE, F. and ERMANO, A. M. (1969) In *Endemic Goiter*, pp. 151-158, ed. J. B. Stanbury. Pan American Health Organization Publication no. 193, Washington, D.C.
GLASER, K. and EISENBERG, L. (1956) *Pediatrics* **18**, 626
GÓMEZ, F., RAMOS GALVÁN, R., CRAVIOTO, J. and FRENK, S. (1954) *Acta Pediatr.* **43**, 336-357
GRIFFITHS, R. (1954) *The Abilities of Babies.* University of London Press, London
GRIFFITHS, R. (1970) *The Abilities of Young Children.* Young, London
GUILFORD, J. P. (1954) *The Psychometric Method.* McGraw-Hill, New York
KLEIN, R. E., HABICHT, J.-P. and YARBROUGH, C. (1971) *Adv. Pediatr.* **18**, 75-91
MCCALL, R. B.(1970) *Science* **170**, 644-648
PINARD, A. and LAURENDEAU, M. (1964) *J. Res. Sci. Teach.* **2**, 253
POWELL, G. F., BRASEL, J. A. and BLIZZARD, R. M. (1967) *New Engl. J. Med.* **276**, 1271-1278

Powell, G. F., Brasel, J. A., Raiti, B. and Blizzard, R. M. (1967) *New Engl. J. Med.* **276**, 1279-1283
Prugh, D. and Harlow, R. G. (1966) In *Maternal Care and Mental Health – Deprivation of Maternal Care: A Reassessment of its Effects*, ed. J. Bowlby. Schocken Books, New York
Scrimshaw, N. S., Taylor, C. E. and Gordon, J. E. (1967) *Interactions of Nutrition and Infection.* WHO Monograph Series, Geneva

# Discussion

*Rossi:* Dr Cobos, have you separated your children into borderline cases and very severe cases for the analysis, or are they all very severe cases?

*Cobos:* We have not divided them up; we select them randomly. Most of them are, therefore, mildly malnourished. This is another reason why we work in the outskirts of the city and not in the rural area; we think that these are the realities of life, and we want to study the problem as it occurs under natural conditions.

*Chapman:* What is the measurement of malnourishment that you use?

*Cobos:* Efforts have been made for many years to find an efficient definition of clinical malnutrition. In our project we have been dissatisfied with those classifications that only reflect changes in weight. We have combined changes in weight with changes in height. There are, however, a number of complex issues involved in this approach; for example, figures for the prevalence of malnutrition are usually comparisons between a given population and a standard for that population. The norms frequently applied are the mean values for weight and height for the high class of the locality. Since weight and height are strongly correlated with social class, one cannot expect lower-class people to reach the height and weight of the high class just by providing them with food, because social class affiliation also implies other things. Therefore issues such as the role played by sociological factors have to be dealt with before a satisfactory definition of malnutrition is found.

*Rossi:* What about bone age and thickness of the skin in the evaluation of the nutritional state?

*Cobos:* Skin-fold thickness yields quite good correlations with anthropometric criteria for nutritional status. We do not use bone age, because the methodologies available are still too complicated for field use.

*Klein:* We find that head circumference, total height and bone age correlate very differently with performance in psychological tests. Bone age is not a particularly useful measure. A simple count of the number of ossification centres is faster, gives the same amount of information, and requires less standardization. However, we don't know why the appearance of ossification centres is more poorly related to psychological test performance than are head circumference and total height.

*von Muralt:* In our work, McLaren's method of determining the ratio of head circumference to mid-arm circumference has proved to be very useful in detecting even mild forms of protein-calorie malnutrition in preschool children (Kanawati and McLaren 1970).

*Cobos:* The leader of the nutrition team in our project, Dr F. Pardo, looked at anthropometric values statistically, and he arrived at a very simple classification in which he identifies as well-nourished children those whose weight is 85% or more of the expected value for age, simultaneously with 95% or more of the value for height. He defines as malnourished all those children under 80% of the expected weight for age and below 95% of the expected height. That leaves a no-man's land which would seem at first glance to be a small one. However, the no-man's land corresponds to 33% of the population. This no-man's land represents a large number of people whose nutritional status is undefined.

*Chapman:* Dr Cobos, if we accept that there is something in your selection of the malnourished group, do you do any tests which are more objective than, say, the recognition of objects; for example, do you test sensitivity to pain, or make any measurements which reflect automatic responses of the nervous system?

*Cobos:* The objectivity of psychological measurements is a very complex problem. Physiological measures, for example the response of the heart rate to a loud sound, may be quite consistent and reliable but their explanatory value is usually low within the psychological framework. On the other hand, another physiological measurement such as the peripheral nerve conduction rate may be very important in determining the sensorimotor abilities of the child under 3 years of age, which are the building blocks for further psychological activity. Therefore, the use of 'objective' physiological measurements in relation to psychological function depends greatly on their ability to explain psychological phenomena.

*Dobbing:* Five or six years ago great prominence was given to a field finding that there is a difference in the ultimate behavioural development of underfed children according to whether they are underfed before or after the age of 2 years. Clearly, this is not only of academic interest. If it could be substantiated, it would have immense political significance. My own very small acquaintance with such field-work makes me suspect that this would be extremely difficult to establish. What is the current standing of this idea, and do you feel that for purposes of arranging priorities in giving aid, it would be possible to establish it more closely?

*Cobos:* One of the reasons that led us to select a psychological assessment based on Piaget's work in order to appreciate psychological changes possibly produced by malnutrition is the fact that he postulates well-defined stages of cognitive development, sensorimotor development under 2 years, and representational after that. This type of notion is therefore closely related to other maturational events and may help to clarify the question whether nutritional aid should be preferentially channelled to a given age group.

## Reference

KANAWATI, A. A. and MCLAREN, D. S. (1970) *Nature (Lond.)* **228**, 573-574

# Cross-cultural evaluation of human intelligence

ROBERT E. KLEIN, BARRY M. LESTER, CHARLES YARBROUGH and JEAN-PIERRE HABICHT

*Division of Human Development, Instituto de Nutrición de Centro América y Panama, Guatemala City*

The cross-cultural evaluation of intellectual function is simultaneously a most exciting and difficult task, for it promises insight into man's basic capacities that it will not deliver until both intelligence and culture are more clearly understood. Since Westerners view mental phenomena as derived from biological forces, many scientists have been attracted to the role of nutrition in cognitive function. After a brief introduction to the concept of intelligence and its cross-cultural evaluation, we shall consider data that lend support to the view that research into malnutrition cannot afford to avoid socio-cultural variables.

Although most people believe they understand the meaning of 'intelligence', it appears that it is difficult to obtain agreement on its definition. The atheoretical approach of Alfred Binet continues to be the most prominent. This view of performance on culturally appropriate problems, which began with Binet and was extended by L. Terman and D. Wechsler, assumes that the human intellect consists of a general mental ability which can be accurately measured by scoring correct answers to questions of fact and inference. The basic goal of the I.Q. test is the estimation of a hypothetical capacity to which separate abilities may be attached. The ability of the I.Q. to predict school performance in many populations is well documented, and this index is widely used in job and educational placement. Its predictive power is so good that its proponents have been almost exclusively interested in the prediction of quality of performance in a particular context. Analysis of the cognitive processes that relate to performance in tests of intellectual ability and the development of these underlying capacities has been of minor concern.

An alternative view focuses on a set of relatively independent cognitive processes, and is due to J. Guilford and L. Thurstone. A central difference between the two orientations lies in the fact that this 'separate process' approach attempts to understand the basic thought processes that contribute to the development of cognitive functioning.

Both views acknowledge that performance depends intimately upon the culture of the person being studied. If one views intelligence largely as the internalization of tools provided by the culture (Greenfield and Bruner 1969), the necessity of accounting for the impact of culture on I.Q. scores is obvious. But culture may also be seen as a naturally occurring experimental treatment which illuminates the processes of development. Incisive experiments become possible by comparing aspects of intellectual development across disparate cultures. Although not always explicitly stated, this is an approach which has animated much of the existing cross-cultural research in intellectual development (Le Vine 1970).

Our research group is interested in the *sequelae* of malnutrition. In the context of understanding the relations between malnutrition and human intellectual development, cross-cultural studies allow independent replications of significant findings. For example, children in the United States do a little better on a short-term memory task than children from rural Guatemalan villages. Is this memory impairment the result of undernutrition? Perhaps, but we think that a more important factor may be motivation. The United States children try a lot harder to please the examiner; moreover, differences within these rural villages also seem to be motivational. Nutrition may be a false or relatively unimportant issue. Only the repeated observation of powerful relationships across cultures can solve this issue.

For the rest of the paper we shall focus on three general areas: the measurement of prenatal and perinatal factors which may affect the course of intellectual development; the assessment of cognitive development during infancy; and the evaluation of intelligence in preschool-age children. Where appropriate, we shall use specific examples from the study of the relations between malnutrition and intellectual development.

## PRENATAL FACTORS IN INTELLECTUAL DEVELOPMENT

Among the prenatal factors that may affect intellectual development, the nutritional status of the mother during pregnancy has frequently been mentioned as an important early determinant. Although there is no *direct* evidence of a relation between maternal diet and later intelligence, some data are suggestive. These data derive from a study we are conducting in rural villages in eastern Guatemala (Lechtig *et al.* 1971*b*).

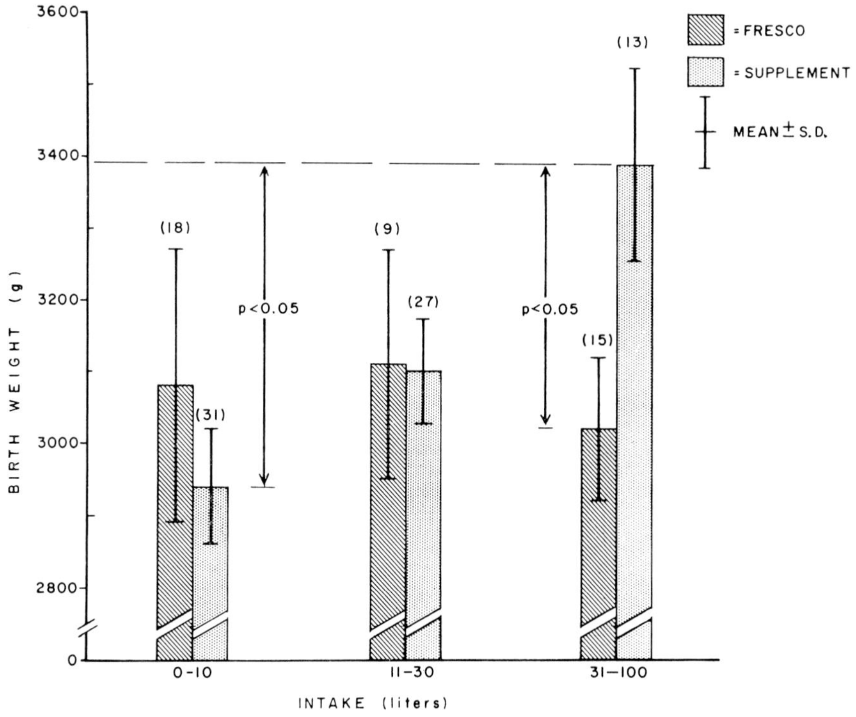


FIG. 1. Relation between intake of supplement or 'Fresco' (a low-calorie soft drink containing no protein) by mothers and the birth weight of infants.

Fig. 1 presents the birth weights of children born to mothers with varying levels of nutritional supplementation (Lechtig *et al.* 1971*a*). There is a positive and statistically significant relationship between the mother's diet during pregnancy and the birth weight of the child. Although there is no known direct relationship between birth weight and later psychological performance, the correlates of low birth weight are well known. They include hyperkinetic behaviour, lower scores on achievement and intelligence tests, and poorer school performance (Caputo and Mandell 1970; Birch and Gussow 1970). These correlates are sufficiently consistent to imply that maternal nutrition should be considered in any model which seeks to characterize the course of intellectual development.

An additional prenatal factor which may complicate the course of human intellectual development and about which relatively little is known is intrauterine infection. Some types of intrauterine infection, such as toxoplasmosis, cytomegalovirus, rubella and herpes virus, have been definitely implicated in retarded intellectual development (Eichenwald 1957; Lundstrom 1962; Nahmias, Josey and Naib 1971; Weller and Hanshaw 1962; Weller, Alford and Neva 1965). For other types of infections, the relation is still unclear. In general, however, we do know that rates of infection as estimated by immunoglobulin antibodies in cord blood vary directly with estimates of social class. Thus, Alford estimates the incidence of intrauterine infection to be about 1.4% among poor blacks in Alabama (Alford *et al.* 1969). This is the highest reported for the United States. In Guatemala and Peru (Lechtig and Mata 1971*a*, *b*) the rates among native populations have been estimated to be at least ten times higher than those found by Alford.

In our village study, analyses of the cord blood immunoglobulin antibodies reveal that 60% of the sample have high levels of IgM and approximately 11% have positive IgM antitoxoplasma antibodies. These antibodies are probably produced by the foetus, since the human placenta cannot transport IgM from the mother to the foetus. On the relation between toxoplasmosis and the risk of mental retardation, intrauterine infection presents especially troublesome problems of interpretation because mentally retarded infants may have a much higher risk of becoming malnourished. We feel that intrauterine infection should be added to maternal nutrition as an important environmental factor in human intellectual development in depressed areas.

## EVALUATION OF COGNITIVE DEVELOPMENT DURING INFANCY

Research on cognitive development in infants has expanded dramatically during the last decade. At present, there is no adequate theory to relate the experience and behaviour of an infant to its cognitive development. Further, there is general agreement that traditional ways of conceptualizing and measuring infant intelligence are relatively uninformative. Kagan (1971) points out that the measurement of emerging behavioural response systems (like reaching, standing and walking) as valid indices of intelligence, an assumption on which traditional psychomotor tests for infants are based, has essentially no predictive validity for future intelligence. Further, Piaget's assumption (1952) that cognitive structures are necessarily derived from sensorimotor actions does not receive systematic support from empirical data (Kagan 1971). Hence, there is no theoretical coherence to the discussion of early intellectual development.

In spite of the absence of theory to guide the study of cognitive development in infancy, there are (at an empirical level) several variables that seem to co-vary with factors which we believe to reflect basic cognitive development.

The line of research to be described grows out of the study of information-processing in animals. Beginning with Pavlov's identification of the orienting reflex, Sokolov (1960) proposed a neural model which seeks to explain attentional responses to novel stimuli and the decrease in these responses upon repeated presentation of the stimuli. Within this model, an orienting response is elicited when there is a mismatch between an incoming stimulus and the existing neural model. Stimulus information from the environment is constantly being coded and stored and with repeated presentation of the novel stimulus a new model is formed and the orienting response disappears. The progressive decrease in the orienting reflex upon repeated presentation of an event is referred to as *habituation.*

Using this model, one can study information-processing in infants by measuring components of the orienting response obtained when novel stimuli are presented. Thus habituation can be studied by repeated presentations of novel stimuli, and rudimentary memory or recognition would be indicated by recovery (dishabituation) of the habituated response when the stimulus is changed. There is some evidence that absence of habituation and dishabituation may, on occasion, be sensitive indices of damage to the central nervous system. For example, Eisenberg, Coursin and Rupp (1966) demonstrated dramatic differences in habituation between normal children and those suspected of brain damage. We are beginning to apply similar techniques to the study of severely malnourished infants seen before and after nutritional rehabilitation.

In a recent study, four children ranging from 8 months to 3½ years of age who were rehabilitated after severe nutritional marasmus were compared with four age and sex-matched controls for responses to repeated presentations of pure tones, with heart rate as the dependent variable. Twenty presentations of a 400 Hz pure tone were followed by ten presentations of a 750 Hz pure tone; these were followed by 15 presentations of the original, 400 Hz pure tone. All tones were presented at 63 decibels for 5 seconds with a randomized inter-stimulus interval which had a mean of 15 seconds and a range of 10 to 18 seconds.

Three indices of heart rate activity were computed across blocks of 5 presentations: heart rate deceleration, heart rate acceleration and range of heart rate activity. Heart rate deceleration was calculated as the mean of the lowest two beats during the 5-second pre-stimulus period, minus the mean of the lowest two beats during presentation of the stimulus. Heart rate acceleration was the difference between the mean of the two highest beats during the pre-stimulus period minus the mean of the two highest beats during presentation of the stimulus. To calculate the range of heart rate activity, the range for the stimulus presentation period (mean of two highs minus mean of two lows during stimulus presentation) was subtracted from the baseline range (mean of two highs minus mean of two lows for the pre-stimulus period).

TABLE 1

Heart rate deceleration, acceleration and range changes by blocks of five trials in malnourished and well-nourished children

| | *Mean number of heart rate decelerations* | | | | | | | | | | | |
|---|---|---|---|---|---|---|---|---|---|---|---|---|
| | *S1* | *S2* | *S3* | *S4* | $\bar{x}$ | *T1* | *T2* | $\bar{x}$ | *R1* | *R2* | *R3* | $\bar{x}$ |
| Experimental (malnourished) ($n$=4) | 3.70 | 2.35 | 2.40 | 2.90 | 2.81 | 2.45 | 3.15 | 2.80 | 1.70 | 1.70 | 2.80 | 2.07 |
| Control (well-nourished) ($n$=4) | 8.45 | 3.75 | 4.30 | 1.05 | 4.39 | 2.75 | 2.45 | 2.60 | 1.85 | 2.30 | 3.35 | 2.50 |
| | *Mean number of heart rate accelerations* | | | | | | | | | | | |
| | *S1* | *S2* | *S3* | *S4* | $\bar{x}$ | *T1* | *T2* | $\bar{x}$ | *R1* | *R2* | *R3* | $\bar{x}$ |
| Experimental | 1.40 | 2.40 | 1.00 | 1.90 | 1.67 | 2.85 | 2.35 | 2.60 | 2.50 | 2.30 | 0.90 | 1.90 |
| Control | 0.40 | 1.35 | 3.80 | 1.95 | 1.87 | 2.70 | 4.05 | 3.37 | 3.30 | 1.20 | 2.45 | 2.32 |
| | *Mean of change in range of heart rate* | | | | | | | | | | | |
| | *S1* | *S2* | *S3* | *S4* | $\bar{x}$ | *T1* | *T2* | $\bar{x}$ | *R1* | *R2* | *R3* | $\bar{x}$ |
| Experimental | 3.50 | 3.05 | 2.85 | 4.05 | 3.36 | 3.70 | 3.65 | 3.67 | 3.60 | 2.80 | 3.60 | 3.33 |
| Control | 4.85 | 1.90 | 6.40 | 3.25 | 4.10 | 3.95 | 5.60 | 4.77 | 3.25 | 3.60 | 6.50 | 4.45 |

S1 – S4, blocks of five presentations of 400 Hz tone.
T1, T2, blocks of five presentations of 750 Hz tone.
R1 – R3, blocks of five presentations of 400 Hz tone.

Table 1 presents heart rate deceleration, acceleration and range of heart rate activity by blocks of trials for the previously malnourished and control children. The control subjects show a classic habituation pattern for the first 20 presentations of the standard tone (400 Hz). The magnitudes of the decelerations are substantial during the first block of trials (S1) and gradually level off by the final block (S4). In contrast, the malnourished subjects show no such habituation pattern. Their slight deceleration of heart rate remains stable across all the presentations of the standard tone.

During the ten presentations of the transformation (750 Hz), the control subjects show a significant increase in the number of heart rate accelerations compared to the previously malnourished children. These data suggest that the transformation had a disquieting effect on the control children, and that in contrast to the previously malnourished children, the control subjects recognized the change in tone and responded to the tone as if it violated an expectation.

Similarly, for the last three blocks of trials (R1-R3), heart rate accelerations were higher for the control than for the previously malnourished subjects. This difference was particularly strong for the first block of trials (R1) and suggests again that the control subjects recognized the change in stimulus. These findings are also supported by the data on the heart rate range. The changes in heart rate range reflect substantially more heart rate activity during the entire experimental procedure for the controls than for the previously malnourished children. Indeed, the three heart rate measures, taken together, show greater stability for the malnourished subjects, whereas for the control subjects both accelerations and decelerations vary with stimulus presentation and are accompanied by consistent and marked increases in the range of heart rate activity.

These data on four malnourished children and their controls suggest that the technique of studying attention to a transformation of a habituated event will be useful in elaborating relationships between early, severe malnutrition and subsequent cognitive development. Ultimately, we plan to combine the use of behavioural and physiological measures of attention in our study of the effects of severe marasmic malnutrition on cognitive development.

Psychologists are currently extending these techniques to include more complex stimuli appropriate for older infants. Kagan (1971) has demonstrated a direct relation between age and duration of attention to transformation of a human face among middle-class American children and we have replicated this finding in children aged 4 to 36 months living in isolated rural villages in Guatemala (Sellers *et al.* 1972).

## EVALUATION OF COGNITIVE DEVELOPMENT IN PRESCHOOL-AGE CHILDREN

When working at the preschool level, the investigator has a wider variety of techniques and a richer set of hypotheses to guide him in his evaluation of cognitive development. In the specific case of evaluating the effects of malnutrition cross-culturally, investigators have little choice but to cast a moderately wide net in terms of methodology and focus hard on the basic cognitive processes that underlie thought and action. This orientation is necessary because there are only very general models of how malnutrition might interact with mental development. Neither are there replicable results which can be interpreted clearly to suggest that malnutrition in fact *is* causally related to depressed mental development (Klein, Habicht and Yarbrough 1971).

Modes of operation and specific techniques for addressing the problem of the cultural appropriateness of the tests employed have been discussed in detail elsewhere (Klein 1971; LeVine 1970) and will not be dealt with here. However, a related issue is the degree of correspondence between formal measures of cognitive development and indigenous or naive conceptions of intelligence in the culture where the study is being made.

In a study comparing the performance of preschool children in psychological tests with estimates by the village adults of these children's intelligence, we find good correspondence for several types of measures. Table 2 shows the Kendall

TABLE 2

Kendall Rank Order correlation coefficients between judged order of 'smartness' and psychological test performance

| | *TAU* | *Significance level* |
|---|---|---|
| Embedded figures: correct responses to first presentation | 0.60 | $P < 0.02$ |
| Response time, first presentation | 0.42 | $P < 0.05$ |
| Verbal analogies | 0.51 | $P < 0.02$ |
| Picture naming | 0.24 | $P < 0.19$ |
| Picture recognition | 0.11 | $P < 0.36$ |
| Memory for designs | | |
| Trial 1 | 0.33 | $P < 0.11$ |
| Trial 2 | 0.38 | $P < 0.08$ |
| Trial 3 | 0.47 | $P < 0.04$ |

Rank Order coefficients between judged 'smartness' and psychological test performance for ten 7-year-old boys. Judged 'smartness' predicts memory and language performance and some of the more subtle qualities of performance, such as speed of response.

Related to the issue of the concordance between test performance and naive estimates of intelligence is the relationship of test performance to the social-structural position of the family in the community. Here we try to identify parental attitudes and behaviour as well as physical characteristics of the environment which relate to our measures of cognitive development. Included in this analysis are four measures of psychological performance, two measures of the social and physical environment and one measure of physical growth. The psychological measures included Memory for Digits; Draw a Line slowly (a measure of the child's willingness and ability to follow instructions and to control his motor behaviour); and two measures of verbal ability, Verbal

Analogies and Picture Vocabulary naming. The two measures of the social and physical environmental characteristics are Housing, which is a composite score based on the quality of the interior of the house and its construction, and Teaching, a summary of the number of different tasks systematically taught to the preschool child by his mother, father and older siblings, reflecting the degree of family involvement in the child's upbringing. Finally, Head Circumference is included as the index of physical growth.

TABLE 3

Correlations between housing, teaching, psychological performance and head circumference for boys and girls

| | *Girls* | | *Boys* | |
|---|---|---|---|---|
| | *Housing* | *Teaching* | *Housing* | *Teaching* |
| Digits | 0.23** | 0.23** | 0.15* | 0.10 |
| Line | –0.22** | –0.22** | –0.11 | –0.05 |
| Analogies | 0.21** | 0.33** | 0.13 | 0.07 |
| Vocabulary | 0.29** | 0.31** | 0.16* | 0.17* |
| Head circumference | 0.26** | 0.34** | 0.24** | 0.31** |
| Teaching | 0.24** | — | 0.18* | — |
| Housing | — | 0.24** | — | 0.18* |
| | | *Partialled on housing* | | |
| Digits | 0.00 | 0.18* | 0.00 | 0.07 |
| Line | 0.00 | –0.17* | 0.00 | –0.03 |
| Analogies | 0.00 | 0.29** | 0.00 | 0.04 |
| Vocabulary | 0.00 | 0.25** | 0.00 | 0.14 |
| Head circumference | 0.00 | 0.29** | 0.00 | 0.27* |
| Teaching | 0.00 | — | 0.00 | — |
| Housing | 0.00 | 0.00 | 0.00 | 0.00 |
| | | *Partialled on teaching* | | |
| Digits | 0.18* | 0.00 | 0.13 | 0.00 |
| Line | –0.17* | 0.00 | –0.10 | 0.00 |
| Analogies | 0.14 | 0.00 | 0.11 | 0.00 |
| Vocabulary | 0.23** | 0.00 | 0.13 | 0.00 |
| Head circumference | 0.19* | 0.00 | 0.19* | 0.00 |
| Teaching | 0.00 | 0.00 | — | 0.00 |
| Housing | — | 0.00 | 0.00 | 0.00 |
| | | *Partialled on head circumference* | | |
| Digits | 0.16* | 0.13 | 0.11 | 0.05 |
| Line | –0.18* | –0.17* | –0.10 | –0.04 |
| Analogies | 0.15* | 0.27** | 0.10 | 0.03 |
| Vocabulary | 0.22** | 0.21** | 0.10 | 0.09 |
| Head circumference | 0.00 | 0.00 | 0.00 | 0.00 |
| Teaching | 0.16* | — | 0.11 | — |
| Housing | — | 0.16* | — | 0.11 |

* $P < 0.05$  ** $P < 0.01$.

Table 3 shows the correlation matrix for the four psychological variables and head circumference for each of the socio-cultural variables, separately for boys and girls. It can be seen that head circumference and the four psychological variables are significantly related to both housing and teaching for girls. In contrast, only Digits and Vocabulary are correlated with housing for boys and only Vocabulary with teaching for boys.

Also presented in Table 3 are the matrices partialled respectively on Housing, Teaching and Head Circumference. In general, the relationships noted in the simple correlation matrix still obtain for the partialled matrices. Psychological performance and Head Circumference remain significantly related to Housing and teaching for girls, with the exception of the correlation between Housing and Verbal Analogies, when the matrix is partialled on Teaching. In contrast, only Head Circumference remains significantly correlated with Housing and Teaching for boys across the respective partialled matrices. There are two points of major interest in these correlation matrices. First, there are the powerful sex differences in the relation between measures of socio-cultural status and psychological performance. The finding that psychological performance is more strongly predicted by environmental factors for girls than for boys has been reported elsewhere (Hess *et al.* 1968, 1969; Kagan 1971) for technologically advanced societies.

The second point of interest is that our three major dimensions, psychological performance, environmental characteristics and physical growth, are strongly interrelated for girls and moderately linked for boys.

Another useful way to consider these data is to examine the multiple correlations between socio-cultural measures, physical growth and psychological performance.

TABLE 4

Multiple correlations between socio-cultural variables, head circumference and psychological performance

| | *Boys* | | | | *Girls* | | | |
|---|---|---|---|---|---|---|---|---|
| | *Housing & teaching* | | *Head, housing & teaching* | | *Housing & teaching* | | *Head, housing & teaching* | |
| | *r* | $r^2 \times 100$ | *r* | $r^2 \times 100$ | *r* | $r^2 \times 100$ | *r* | $r^2 \times 100$ |
| Head circumference | 0.39 | 14.8 | — | — | 0.39 | 15.5 | — | — |
| Digits | 0.15 | 2.3 | 0.23 | 5.2 | 0.32 | 10.5 | 0.41 | 17.0 |
| Line | 0.12 | 1.5 | 0.12 | 1.5 | 0.29 | 8.2 | 0.32 | 10.3 |
| Analogies | 0.16 | 2.6 | 0.19 | 3.8 | 0.38 | 14.4 | 0.38 | 14.4 |
| Vocabulary | 0.23 | 5.4 | 0.32 | 10.2 | 0.41 | 16.6 | 0.44 | 19.2 |

Table 4 shows the multiple correlation matrices for Housing and Teaching combined, against Head Circumference and the four psychological variables. Also presented are the multiple correlations for the combination of Head Circumference, Housing and Teaching against psychological performance. Here again we note that when combined, Housing and Teaching are similarly related to Head Circumference for both sexes and that they continue to predict psychological performance more strongly for girls than for boys. When Head Circumference is added to the socio-cultural factors, multiple correlations improve somewhat, with the exception of Draw-a-Line slowly for boys and Verbal Analogies for girls.

In order to demonstrate the predictive power of environmental measures, even in relatively homogeneous subsistence farming communities, three additional indices are included among the independent variables. These are the quality of the mother's clothing; the mother's hygienic practices with respect to herself and her child; and an index of family sociability based on a total number of social contacts the family maintains with people outside the home.

TABLE 5

Multiple correlations between five socio-cultural variables, head circumference and psychological performance

| | *Correlations with five socio-cultural variables* | | | |
|---|---|---|---|---|
| | *Boys* | | *Girls* | |
| | $r$ | $r^2 \times 100$ | $r$ | $r^2 \times 100$ |
| Head Circumference | 0.46 | 21.4 | 0.53 | 28.3 |
| Digits | 0.21 | 4.2 | 0.37 | 13.6 |
| Line | 0.17 | 3.0 | 0.33 | 10.6 |
| Analogies | 0.15 | 2.4 | 0.39 | 15.3 |
| Vocabulary | 0.34 | 11.5 | 0.44 | 20.0 |

Table 5 shows the multiple correlations for the five socio-cultural factors against Head Circumference and psychological performance, separately for boys and girls. Head Circumference is better predicted than psychological performance for both boys and girls. Psychological performance, on the other hand, is still more strongly predicted for girls than for boys by these five socio-cultural indices.

These data reflect the uncommonly complicated relationships which exist between head circumference, socio-cultural indices and psychological performance of preschool children in isolated rural villages in Guatemala. Moreover, when nutritional status is placed in such matrices, they will undoubtedly become more complicated. For this reason, the simple demonstrations of relations between indices of socio-cultural status, cognitive development and physical growth are in themselves relatively uninformative. Rather, these relationships simply underline the necessity to search out systematically the mechanisms which mediate these provocative relationships.

## SUMMARY

We have discussed some considerations in the cross-cultural evaluation of human intelligence. Two general approaches to the definition of human intelligence were noted.

Important prenatal factors which may affect subsequent intellectual development are the nutritional status of the mother during pregnancy and intrauterine infection. Data were presented to suggest that the evaluation of intellectual development of subjects living in depressed areas cannot afford to neglect these factors.

Data from a preliminary study comparing previously malnourished with well-nourished infants indicated that one of the immediate effects of early severe malnutrition may be an inability to process incoming stimuli. Our findings showed that when malnourished infants were given repeated presentations of a novel stimulus, they failed both to habituate to the novel stimulus and to recognize a transformation of that stimulus. The study of habituation and dishabituation promises to be a useful technique for elaborating subtle differences in information-processing between well-nourished and poorly nourished children.

Finally, the powerful role of socio-economic factors in intellectual development was demonstrated. The complicated relationships found between indices of cognitive development, physical growth and socio-cultural status suggest that much work needs to be done in systematically mapping the mechanisms which mediate these relationships.

The study of the relations between malnutrition and mental development is a research problem of sufficient complexity to warrant attempts to validate such preliminary research findings in diverse cultural contexts.

## ACKNOWLEDGEMENTS

This research was supported by Contract PH 43-65-640 from the National Institute of Child Health and Human Development, Bethesda. It was also supported in part by the Association for the Aid of Crippled Children, New York.

# References

ALFORD, C. A., FOFT, J. W., BLANKENSHIP, W. J., CASSADY, G. and BENTON, J. W. (1969) *J. Pediatr.* **75**, 1287-1291

BIRCH, H. G. and GUSSOW, J. D. (1970) *Disadvantaged Children. Health, Nutrition, and School Failure.* Harcourt, Brace & World, New York

CAPUTO, D. V. and MANDELL, W. (1970) *Dev. Psychol.* **3**, 363-383

EICHENWALD, H. F. (1957) *Am. J. Dis. Child.* **94**, 411-412

EISENBERG, R. B., COURSIN, D. B. and RUPP, N. R. (1966) *J. Aud. Res.* **6**, 239-248

GREENFIELD, P. M. and BRUNER, J. S. (1969) In *Handbook of Socialization Theory and Research*, pp. 633-657, ed. D. A. Goslin. Rand McNally, Chicago

HESS, R. D., SHIPMAN, V. C., BROPHY, J. E. and BEAR, R. M. (1968) *The Cognitive Environments of Urban Preschool Children. Report to the Graduate School of Education.* University of Chicago

HESS, R. D., SHIPMAN, V. C., BROPHY, J. E. and BEAR, R. M. (1969) *The Cognitive Environments of Urban Preschool Children: Follow-up Phase.* The Graduate School of Education, University of Chicago

KAGAN, J. (1971) *Change & Continuity in Infancy.* Wiley, New York

KLEIN, R. E., HABICHT, J-P. and YARBROUGH, C. (1971) *Adv. Pediatr.* **18**, 75-91

KLEIN, R. E. (1971) In *Proceedings of the International Conference on Amino Acid Fortification of Protein Foods*, ed. N. S. Scrimshaw and J. E. Gordon. The M.I.T. Press, Cambridge, Mass. In press

LECHTIG, A., ARROYAVE, G., HABICHT, J-P. and BÉHAR, M. (1971*a*) *Arch. Latinoam. Nutr.* **21**, 505-530

LECHTIG, A., KLEIN, R. E., MATA, L. J. and BÉHAR, M. (1971*b*) Influencia de la infección intrauterina sobre el crecimiento físico y desarrollo mental. (INCAP)

LECHTIG, A. and MATA, L. J. (1971*a*) *J. Pediatr.* **78**, 909-910

LECHTIG, A. and MATA, L. J. (1971*b*) *Fed. Proc. Fed. Am. Soc. Exp. Biol.* **30**, 300

LEVINE, R. A. (1970) In *Carmichael's Manual of Child Psychology*, vol. 2, pp. 559-612, ed. P. H. Mussen. Wiley, New York

LUNDSTROM, R. (1962) *Acta Paediatr.* **51**, 1-110

NAHMIAS, A. J., JOSEY, W. E. and NAIB, Z. M. (1971) In *Prenatal Infections*, pp. 44-52, ed. O. Thalhammer. Georg Thieme Verlag, Stuttgart

PIAGET, J. (1952) *The Origins of Intelligence in Children*, pp. 23-46. International Universities Press, New York

SELLERS, M. J., KLEIN, R. E., KAGAN, J. and MINTON, C. (1972) *Dev. Psychol.* **6** (1)

SOKOLOV, E. N. (1960) *Perception and the Conditioned Reflex.* Macmillan, New York

WELLER, T. H. and HANSHAW, J. B. (1962) *New Engl. J. Med.* **266**, 1233-1244

WELLER, T. H., ALFORD, C. A. and NEVA, F. A. (1965) *Yale J. Biol. Med.* **37**, 455-472

# Discussion

*Chapman:* Dr Klein, are you saying that there is a correlation between head size and these measures of intelligence within the social group studied, and also that this correlation extends to all social groups?

*Klein:* We find a correlation between head circumference and test performance for children between 3 and 7 years of age in four villages in rural Guatemala. Other investigations, in other geographical locations, report similar relationships between psychological test performance and head circumference as well as the measure of physical development (Stoch and Smythe 1968).

*Chapman:* Do you assume that there is a difference between intelligence and the ability for intellectual abstraction? Or are they the same?

*Klein:* I would have to answer that in the context of a specific task. For example, in a verbal analogies test, we ask the child: 'the skin of a banana is smooth, and the skin of a pineapple is .........?' That's an abstraction; it is also a problem that is frequently included in intelligence tests and it seems to correlate with social class in our rural preschool sample.

*Cobos:* I would beg people to discard the term 'intelligence'. It is so extremely confusing that it is doing harm. We can talk about cognitive development, and then we know a little more, in the sense that we understand that certain intellectual accomplishments are correlated with age; we can explore notions such, as for example, that children learn to classify at a given age. Then we can see whether this is true across social class or whether the age at which children achieve such a cognitive event is influenced by nutritional factors, for example. That provides us with a closer grasp of reality.

*Bovet:* Do you think that the differences between male and female performance are mainly constitutional, or are they a reflection of cultural differences?

*Klein:* Sex differences in psychological test performance such as those I described are frequently encountered (Kagan and Moss 1962; Kagan 1971). It's my opinion that systematically different child-rearing practices for the two sexes will account for more of the variance than will biological differences between the sexes. However, this is an empirical question which could be studied cross-culturally. One could find cultures with systematically different child-rearing practices for the two sexes and put this opinion to test.

*Dobbing:* There is a big sex difference in the facility for catching up bodily growth after food deprivation. Male mammals or birds don't catch up after nutritional restriction anything like as well as females, many of which apparently catch up totally, as far as we can measure. In the rats raised in small and large litters, for example, our figures were obtained entirely on males. In female rats we find great difficulty in detecting an ultimate difference in bodily growth. These sex differences have also been shown for cockerels and hens (Lister, Cowen and McCance 1966) and for sows and boars (Lister and McCance 1967).

*Leathwood:* This observation that females are less vulnerable to early malnutrition seems to be reflected in the results of behavioural studies as well.

*Winick:* The data on cellular changes are different for boys and girls. Cheek (1968) has reported that the slopes of the curves for muscle cell division, which accounts for a good bit of somatic growth, are quite different in boys and girls. Also cell division proceeds for longer in boys.

*Menkes:* What was your experience with auditory-visual integration tests, which have been used in Mexico?

*Klein:* We spent some time investigating the utility of auditory-visual and haptic-visual integration ('cross-modal' matching) tests. We have given up these tests because we don't find them particularly useful or reliable for children between 3 and 7 years of age. Moreover, Dr Wagner Bridger, in a paper entitled 'Cognitive factors in perceptual dysfunction' (Bridger 1970), has shown that poor performance on cross-modal integration tests is related to an inability to employ abstract verbal labels rather than to perceptual deficits.

*Cobos:* From the point of view of developmental psychology *à la* Piaget, it is now well recognized that the acquisition of spatial notions, of a topological, projective and euclidean nature, is not simultaneous. This fact has a tremendous impact on this kind of testing, that had not been recognized before. The stimuli used in these tests do not differentiate these different lines of development and the results are frequently very confusing.

*Menkes:* One thing that disturbs me is whether we are not overestimating the influence of nutrition on 'intelligence'. Is it not the same in Guatemala as in the United States, that a nutritionally deprived child is also an emotionally deprived child, and that, unless extremes of malnutrition are reached, the effect of malnutrition on I.Q. is mainly due to a concomitant emotional deprivation?

*Cobos:* This is obviously a very important field that we should consider in greater detail in the future. It is necessary that we know about the emotional development of the children studied and how it affects the impact of malnutrition on psychological functioning. Dr Bovet made a comment earlier about appetite. We have found in our project in Colombia that there is a decrease in appetite among malnourished children, while simultaneously the prevalence of pica is increased (the craving to eat substances not fit for food). These findings suggest that emotional factors may be strongly linked, as would be expected, with other components of the malnutrition-psychological function unit.

*Menkes:* Emotional deprivation affects the growth hormone secretion (Powell *et al.* 1967; Krieger and Mellinger 1971). The children who have strange appetites have depressed output of growth hormone.

*Cobos:* The technology for measuring 'affect' is really very primitive. We have done two things in an attempt to understand the part played by these factors. First, a simple three-point scale of emotional adjustment is applied at the time of the administration of the formal tests. The general feeling, based on these low-reliability, low-validity data, is that there is a direct correlation between adjustment, intellectual performance and nutritional status. I have also examined mothers of malnourished children, in a traditional, non-structured psychiatric interview of 2 hours, with the main aim of exploring aggressive fantasies. There is as yet no way of formally reporting these findings except perhaps as anecdotes, but most of these mothers are what a psychiatrist would call 'primitive', narcissistic characters, unable to love anyone but themselves.

*Menkes:* They are not depressed?

*Cobos:* They are full of anger. Their discussions of their children's health or nutrition are just a demonstration of their ongoing dissatisfaction with their children. It reflects a permanent 'state of war' between the members of the mother–child unit. Frequently the aggressive fantasies come into the open in expressions such as: 'This child is crucifying me. He will kill me. I have to get up three or four times a night to see if he has already died'.

The behaviour of these people is full of emotions that are not present in well-nourished individuals.

On the other hand, we have collected a small number of cases of malnutrition among high-class people. Most of the parents of these malnourished high-class children were obviously mentally ill.

*Rossi:* Dr Klein, you mentioned that you found an increase of IgM immunoglobulins in 60% of cord blood samples, and of IgM antitoxoplasma antibodies. Have you checked whether there is evidence of intrauterine cytomegalovirus infection, which might also be important from the point of view of mental retardation and nutrition? Since you find this change in the immunoglobulins in cord blood, it is likely that you have an increase of cytomegalic virus infection. This might be an important co-factor influencing brain development and leading to mental retardation.

*Klein:* Dr Lechtig is preparing to look at five or six specific infectious agents, and this is one of them. If our first tentative data are confirmed and our suspicion about intrauterine infection is true, and if there is evidence of central nervous system damage due to infection, one can begin to speculate on the probability of this child becoming malnourished, as opposed to a sibling or a member of his group outside his family. There will obviously be some very complicated interpretative problems.

*Herschkowitz:* You mentioned among prenatal factors the nutritional status of the mother during pregnancy. Placental metabolism is also of great importance. There are now possibilities of assessing placental metabolism. Have you any experience with measurements of this kind?

*Klein:* No, we are not studying placental metabolism at present. It is possible that we will attempt to do so in the future.

# *Discussion*

BRIDGER, W. H. (1970) In *Perception and its Disorders* (Research Publication of the Association for Research in Nervous and Mental Disease, U.S.A. vol. 48), pp. 255-265

CHEEK, D. B. (1968) *Human Growth: Body Composition, Cell, Growth, Energy, and Intelligence*, chapter 24. Lea & Febiger, Philadelphia

KAGAN, J. (1971) *Change and Continuity in Infancy.* Wiley, New York

KAGAN, J. and MOSS, H. A. (1962) *Birth to Maturity. A Study in Psychological Development.* Wiley, New York

KRIEGER, I. and MELLINGER, R. C. (1971) *J. Pediatr.* **79**, 216

LISTER, D., COWEN, T. and MCCANCE, R. A. (1966) *Br. J. Nutr.* **20**, 633

LISTER, D. and MCCANCE, R. A. (1967) *Br. J. Nutr.* **21**, 787

POWELL, G. F., BRASEL, J. A., RAITI, S. and BLIZZARD, R. M. (1967) *New Engl. J. Med.* **276**, 1279

STOCH, M. B. and SMYTHE, P. M. (1968) In *Malnutrition, Learning and Behavior*, pp. 278-289, ed. N. S. Scrimshaw and J. E. Gordon. M.I.T. Press, Cambridge, Mass.

# Nutritional influences in the evolution of mammalian brain

M. A. CRAWFORD and A. J. SINCLAIR

*Nuffield Institute of Comparative Medicine,*
*Zoological Society of London*

Cell construction is generally considered only in terms of protein biosynthesis; this restriction in outlook arises from the convention of investigating the isolated cell, the bacterium and the virus. Bacteria and viruses are in close contact with the external environment from which they withdraw nutrients; the cells of a differentiated system may be some distance from their external environment. The coordinated functioning of a complex system such as we see in mammals depends upon quite new factors not found in unicellular life. These new factors are control of action and distribution of nutrients. The control of action is dependent upon the nervous system and the distribution of nutrients on the vascular system. The integrity of both systems is known to be dependent on lipids, since distortion of oil-soluble nutrients is associated with the degeneration of the nervous and the vascular systems.

More than 60% of the nervous tissue is lipid and as Dr Bernsohn commented earlier (p. 56), there is not enough protein to match all the lipid in nervous tissue. Hence the important new factor associated with the transition from the single cell to integrated, differentiated life forms is the lipids.

We should like to present evidence to suggest that the availability of lipid nutrients is correlated closely with the development of the attributes of the nervous system in land mammals. It is first necessary to comment on some of the points raised during the symposium that have a direct bearing upon the interpretation of recent knowledge on lipid function and nutrition.

## COMPOSITION OF LIPIDS

It is important to establish what we are concerned with in discussions on lipids since 'guests' to the field of lipids may not be familiar with lipid chemistry and how it relates to nutrition.

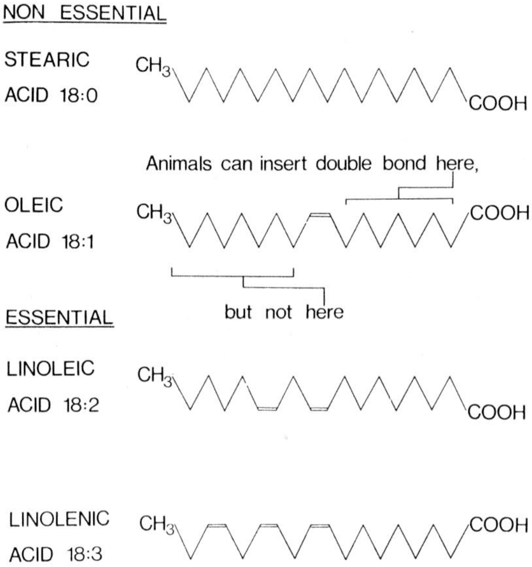


FIG. 1. Structures of 18-carbon fatty acids.

The structures of every cell in advanced life forms are made up of protein, lipid and polyhydric alcohols. Quantitatively the two most important are the proteins and lipids, but the balance between them varies specifically depending upon cell type and cell structure. Lipid may make up as much as 15% of the dry weight of a muscle cell, 25% of mitochondria, 30% of succinic oxidase, and 50% of the grey matter of the brain and 70% of the white matter. The lipids found in mammalian cells consist of phospholipids, sterols and their esters, triglycerides and glycolipids; quantitatively the phospholipids and sterols are the most important components. The phospholipids can be further subdivided into choline, ethanolamine, serine and inositol phosphoglycerides and the sphingolipids (sphingomyelin, cerebrosides, sulphatides and gangliosides). In most mammalian cells the ethanolamine and choline phosphoglycerides together with sphingomyelin are the major components and each accounts for one-quarter to one-third of the total phospholipid. The whole group of these lipids is referred to as the structural lipids because they are found in cell structures.

The phosphoglycerides are constructed from a glycerol backbone with saturated or mono-unsaturated fatty acids esterified in the α-position, mono- or polyunsaturated acids in the β-position, and phosphate and ethanolamine or one of the other three radicals in the third position. The phospholipid content is remarkably similar in similar cell types, regardless of species (Rouser, Simon

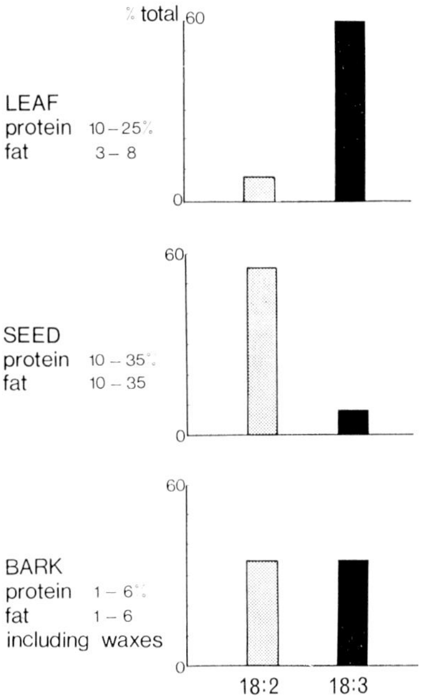


FIG. 2. Complementary distribution of the parent polyunsaturated fatty acids (18:2, linoleic acid and 18:3, linolenic acid) in different parts of plants. The results are expressed as the percentage of the total fatty acids.

and Kritchevsky 1969; Simon and Rouser 1969); however, we have found clear species differences in the phosphoglyceride fatty acids. Consequently much of our interest is in the fatty acids.

The notion of essential and non-essential amino acids is familiar and there is a similarity between the amino acids of proteins and the fatty acids of phospholipids in that there are fatty acids that animals can make and those that they cannot. In general, animal systems possess enzymes for both the degradation and synthesis of fatty acids. Mammalian systems can synthesize fatty acids and introduce at least one double bond between the carboxyl group and the 9 position in a $C_{18}$ fatty acid. Plants can introduce double bonds beyond the 9 position. Two 18-carbon acids which occur in plants, linoleic and linolenic acids, have two and three double bonds respectively, in position 9, 12 (and 15) distal to the carboxyl group. These two polyunsaturated fatty acids are similar to the essential amino acids of proteins in that they cannot be made by animal systems but are found in the structural lipids. Being polyunsaturated acids they occur in the β-position of the phospholipids.

Our own analyses and those of others (Hitchcock and Nichols 1971) indicate a complementary pattern of distribution of these two polyunsaturated acids in plants. Linoleic acid is most frequently found in seeds and linolenic acid in leaf material, and they are found together in the young growing points and buds of plants.

Animals which feed on vegetation obtain both acids. Although the food selection patterns of some herbivorous species may include more leaf or alternatively more seed material, most mammals will obtain both acids from their food. After absorption the liver metabolizes these parent vegetable acids, increasing the chain length and degree of unsaturation by adding extra double bonds close to the carboxyl group; this process results in two families of fatty acids with 20 and 22 carbons and four, five or six double bonds. Both parent fatty acids, together with their long-chain derivatives, are found in phospholipids and may make up approximately a third to a half of the fatty acids in the structural lipids. The parent linoleic acid has a six-carbon saturated chain between the double bonds and the methyl end; linolenic acid has a three-carbon saturated chain at the methyl end. As these saturated end chains are inaccessible to mammalian desaturating enzyme systems, any long-chain acid can be identified as being derived from linoleic acid if it has a six-carbon saturated end chain (*n*–6) and from linolenic acid if it has a three-carbon end chain (*n*–3). For example:

18:1 (*n*–9) → 20:3 (*n*–9) → 22:3 (*n*–9)
18:2 (*n*–6) → 20:4 (*n*–6) → 22:4 (*n*–6) → 22:5 (*n*–6)
18:3 (*n*–3) → 20:5 (*n*–3) → 22:5 (*n*–3) → 22:6 (*n*–3)

In acute deficiency of polyunsaturated acids animals may desaturate and elongate oleic acid to eicosatrienoic acid and 22:3 (*n*–9), but the enzyme systems are unable to introduce double bonds between the 9 position and the methyl end of the oleic acid. Since animals fail to breed when they are fed diets lacking polyunsaturated fatty acids (Holman 1968), it is clear that the position of the double bonds and the degree of unsaturation in fatty acids is biologically important.

## STRUCTURAL LIPIDS AND MEMBRANE PROPERTIES

If we examine the structural lipids of mammals we find that the ability to elongate and desaturate the parent polyenoic acids provides the animal with a remarkable diversity of fatty acids. In the α-position of phosphoglycerides we can have 16:0, 16:1, 18:0 or 18:1 and a polyenoic acid in the β-position. The different permutations of acids in the α and β positions together with variations of the radical attached to the phosphate provide a theoretical possibility of about 200 molecular species within the structural lipids; in practice, certain acids occur with greater frequency, such as 16:0, 18:0 and 18:1 in the α-position and in the β-position, *18:2 (n–6)*, 18:3 (*n*–3), 20:3 (*n*–6), *20:4 (n–6)*, 20:5 (*n*–3) and *22:5 (n–3)* or *22:6 (n–3)*; the underlined acids occur most commonly and give rise to about 70 different molecular species in the phosphoglycerides alone.

There is also diversity in the sphingolipids, but they primarily contain saturated and mono-unsaturated acids, particularly 18:0, 18:1, 24:0 and 24:1. Professor Mead has evidence that there may be acids of even longer chain length (see p. 84).

This diversity of structure associated with the differing electrical properties of the basic group, ranging from a quaternary to a primary ammonium compound and a polyhydric alcohol, provides for a wide range of different stereochemical structures with different polarities, varying from a strong to a weak electrophilic force in association with the powerful electrophobic phosphate. These electro-active constituents provide the appropriate physical properties for interaction within this chemical family and for physical interaction within the matrix of a protein molecule. On this basis, a degree of specificity in protein-lipid complexes would be predicted and indeed this has been demonstrated (Coppock and Daniels 1962).

An important conclusion can be drawn from the diversity of structure in the lipids. The Davson–Danielli concept of the membrane may be incorrect, or at least is incomplete (Danielli and Davson 1935). This concept of the membrane appears in most textbooks as two protein surfaces facing each other, separated by lipid. The lipids are represented by rods of identical length with their polar ends in the protein surface and the non-polar tails towards each other. However, this is a static concept of the membrane which is encouraged by pictures of fixed tissue seen with the electron microscope. On the contrary, living systems by definition are in a constant dynamic state of flux. Professor Chapman has discussed ideas of fluidity in membranes and in particular the relationship of the degree of unsaturation to liquidity (pp. 31-50). If one considers the diversity of chain length and the different degrees of unsaturation in the fatty acids it is immediately apparent that the membrane lipids are regular neither in their three-dimensional nor in their liquidity characteristics.

Some time ago we constructed a model of the membrane based on the Davson-Danielli idea of a regular protein surface but introduced the fact of differing chain lengths in the lipid (Fig. 3). By taking into account the simple chemistry of the lipids, we obtain a membrane system which has at least two properties not found in the Davson-Danielli model.

1. The differing chain lengths allow for interlocking of the lipid, whereas a regular chain length allows slipping. Interlocking permits stability in the juxtaposition of functions on opposite sides of the membrane; slipping allows relative movement of the functions to occur.

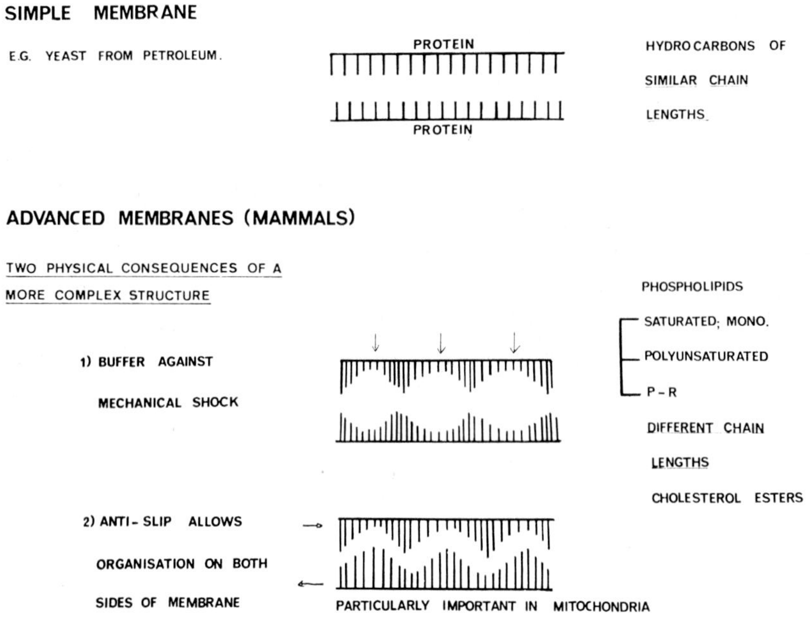


FIG. 3. Schematic illustration of the difference between membranes built with regular as opposed to irregular components. In practice, the physical considerations are likely to be more complex than is illustrated here.

2. The differing chain lengths and degree of unsaturation allow for a buffering action to shock waves on one side of the membrane. Any movement creates a shock wave and as the living system is in continuous motion, shock waves will be a regular feature of cellular activity. Such movements will be particularly important to the endothelial cells lining the heart and the arteries, and it is interesting that the endothelial cell has a high ratio of membrane to cytoplasm.

If we consider that the protein surface of a membrane cannot be flat, that a proportion of the lipid is inside the protein matrix, and that the liquidity of the system depends on the degree of unsaturation and on temperature, we have a very different picture of the membrane from that represented by either the Davson-Danielli model or our own model. The nearest approach to the Davson-Danielli model might be the myelin sheath, but even here the model breaks down because of the diversity of acids in sphingolipids and also the simple fact that in myelin there is about three times as much lipid as protein. Professor Chapman's concepts of liquidity give us a clearer idea than that offered by the static models. If we introduce the diversity of the lipids, the possibility of protein-lipid and lipid-lipid interactions gives a more realistic and complex picture of the membrane. The membrane, if such a feature exists at all in a living cell, is evidently not like a polythene bilayer but is a system of aggregates in which the properties of movement and stability are both critical to the homeostatic relationships between the intracellular and extracellular environments.

We have discussed this question at some length because this new conception of fluidity and stability of membrane systems leads to an important conclusion: the function of protein-lipid interactions in cell structures is qualitatively dependent on the balance of chain length and degree of unsaturation in the fatty acids.

## GENERAL NUTRITIONAL IMPLICATIONS

Much of our current nutritional thinking is conditioned by quantitative ideas of 'essential' biochemicals, 'vitamins' and 'daily requirements'. Nutritional diseases consequently become classified as specific entities such as 'protein malnutrition' or 'vitamin C deficiency'. Dobbing (pp. 9-20) has been concerned with a broad nutritional challenge in which many factors are changing simultaneously, and we would agree that in practice, isolated 'protein' or 'vitamin' deficiency seldom occurs. Vitamin C was discovered because sailors lacked fresh food on long voyages. Certainly the accounts of scurvy on, for example, Anson's voyage suggest a more profound nutritional deficiency than of vitamin C alone and the method adopted for prevention by the mariners, once it was accepted as a nutritional problem, was of course not to use crystalline vitamin C but to improve the general standard of nourishment. In pernicious anaemia there is never a complete deficiency of vitamin $B_{12}$; the vitamin is always present in the blood and is only deficient relative to commonly accepted standards. The practice of feeding liver to patients would have contributed a much broader spectrum of nutrients than simply $B_{12}$, since liver provides a range of oil-soluble nutrients, including the structural lipids.

If we consider 'protein' malnutrition in Africa and the fact that protein, in plant and animal products, is consistently associated with lipid, it is clear that a diet low in protein will also be low in lipid. Dr Houtsmuller has reminded us (p. 224) of Hansen's work in South Africa, where children suffering from kwashiorkor were fed on high-protein diets which precipitated a gross lipid deficiency (Schendel and Hansen 1959). This is an important demonstration of the requirement for lipid in man, which has also been demonstrated in adults (Collins *et al.* 1970). It also illustrates that 'protein malnutrition' is not only a function of protein and demonstrates the practical consequences of the fact that both protein and lipid are involved in cell construction. This practical implication is indicated by Cravioto's studies showing that kwashiorkor may be associated with permanent intellectual impairment (see Cravioto *et al.* 1969). In experimental fatty acid deficiency 20:3 (*n*–9) (eicosatrienoic acid, derived from oleic acid), accumulates in response to the lack of linoleic and arachidonic acids. This acid was not present in significant quantities in the children with kwashiorkor but appeared when they were given high-protein diets. This suggests that the responsibility for the impairment of brain function could rest more with the refeeding of protein-rich regimes than with the malnutrition itself. Dr Menkes' observations on the subsequent intellectual performance of premature infants who were given high-protein (3.9%) substitutes for breast milk (p. 193) underline this possibility, and suggest that high-protein nutrition might accelerate protein synthesis to the point where it becomes out of phase with lipid synthesis, which leads to qualitative changes in the development of the nervous system. Such examples also illustrate how nutrition has been concerned more with quantitative than with qualitative factors.

## APPEARANCE OF POLYUNSATURATED FATTY ACIDS IN THE DEVELOPING RAT BRAIN

A requirement for lipid has been demonstrated in man (Collins *et al.* 1970) and other mammals (Holman 1968). Our evidence indicates that whereas muscle tissue protein has a similar composition regardless of species or of pattern of food selection (Crawford *et al.* 1970), the fatty acids differ. We have found that group specificity occurs in the mammals (Crawford 1970) and since there are also marked differences in the development of the central and peripheral nervous system in mammalian species, our interest has centred on the fatty acids; we shall describe some of our findings here.

Dobbing has reviewed the timing of brain development in the rat (pp. 9-20). From some of the earlier studies on brain chemistry and development it was known that the maximum rate of brain growth was largely associated with myelination. As the myelin acids are mainly saturated and mono-unsaturated it might be thought that brain development would be independent of exogenous lipid factors. It is now well-established that the brain is also rich in long-chain polyunsaturated acids, and Svennerholm has suggested in this symposium (pp. 142-152) that diets low in polyunsaturated fat affect the development of saturated and mono-unsaturated (myelin-type) lipids. We have analysed the rat brain during the period before myelination and shown that 15 days after birth, when myelination has just begun, about 50% of the adult amounts of 20:4 (*n*–6) and 22:6 (*n*–3) have already accumulated (Sinclair and Crawford 1972).

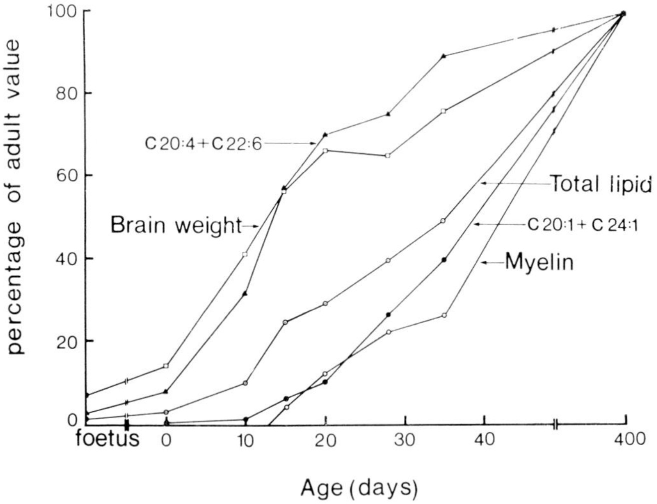


FIG. 4. Some parameters in developing rat brains expressed as a percentage of the adult values. The units are as follows: brain wet weight, mg; brain total lipid, mg; 20:4(*n*–6) + 22:6(*n*–3), mg/brain; 20:1 + 24:1, mg/brain; myelin, mg dry weight/brain. The figures for myelin were extrapolated from data given by Davison (1969).

The acids typical of myelin, such as nervonic acid (24:1) and eicosamonoenoic acid (20:1), are present in barely significant amounts at this time (Fig. 4).

These findings mean that the active period of brain cell development in the rat is associated with the accumulation of polyunsaturated fatty acids derived from linoleic and linolenic acids.

The milk lipids of the rat contain the parent and long-chain polyunsaturated fatty acids, a total of 26.3% of *n*–6 acids and 8.7% of *n*–3 acids being present. The $C_{20}$ and $C_{22}$ polyunsaturated fatty acids of rat milk may provide a source for the developing rat brain (Sinclair and Crawford 1972).

We also wanted to ascertain whether polyunsaturated fatty acids pass the placenta and reach the developing brain. To investigate foetal development we have used the guinea-pig, which has a long gestation period. In agreement with Professor Mead's findings we established that oral and subcutaneous administration of isotopically labelled linoleate or linolenate gave similar results. Table 1 illustrates that if the isotope was administered as the 18-carbon polyunsaturated acid, 18:3 (*n*–3), it was found in the maternal liver triglycerides and phospholipids as both the parent polyunsaturate and the long-chain derivative. The ratio of activity in the long-chain fraction to that in the parent $C_{18}$ fraction was higher in the foetal liver than in the maternal liver and the foetal brain contained significant amounts of activity only in the long-chain

TABLE 1

Incorporation of [$^{14}$C]linolenate in the guinea-pig foetus 18 hours after administration (c.p.m. per mg lipid)

| | | *Thin-layer fraction* | | |
|---|---|---|---|---|
| | | *Triglyceride* | *Phospholipid* | *Ratio of Δ3 to Δ5,6 in phospholipids* |
| Maternal | liver | 3400 | 532 | 1:7 |
| | plasma | 4661 | 393 | 1:6 |
| Foetal | liver | 2403 | 704 | 1:16 |
| | brain | 46 | 117 | 1:22 |

50 μCi of 1-$^{14}$C-labelled linolenate was administered orally to a 45-day pregnant guinea-pig.

fraction of the phospholipid. In other words, there appeared to be a progression of the fatty acid from a $C_{18}$ polyunsaturate to a $C_{20}$ or $C_{22}$ polyunsaturate as the acid is processed in the maternal liver, the placenta, the foetal liver and finally the foetal brain.

We would agree with Professor Mead that the existence of a brain barrier to lipids is doubtful and would extend this lack of barrier to the placenta and developing brain. We do not know why it is only the long-chain acids that are incorporated into the brain phospholipids. We could speculate that there is specific selection by the brain, or alternatively a particularly active chain-elongation system (Yatsu and Moss 1971).

## EXPERIMENTAL PRODUCTION OF LIPID DEFICIENCY

The rat is an especially convenient animal for the experimental production of lipid deficiency because of the ease with which it can be fed purified diets of different composition. Professor Paoletti has reported (pp. 121-132) the results of feeding pregnant rats with a fat-free diet for 5 days before delivery, and Dr Svennerholm has maintained rats on a low-fat diet (linoleic acid at 0.75% of the calories) from weaning before breeding them (pp. 141-152). There was some suggestion in the discussion that the results of the two experiments were not consistent (p. 156), but in fact these are two entirely different experimental designs. Because polyunsaturated fatty acids are tenaciously held by rat tissues, it is difficult to make rats completely deficient of these acids (Holman 1968). The effects of the deficiency on the pups will almost certainly be buffered to some extent by the presence of polyunsaturated acids in the rat milk. Although the deficient dams in Paoletti's experiments had less linoleic and arachidonic acids in their milk, the longer chain *n*–3 polyunsaturated acids are also present and long-chain $C_{20}$ and $C_{22}$ acids have been reported to be more effectively incorporated into phospholipids than the parent polyunsaturated $C_{18}$ acids (Mohrhauer and Holman 1963; Brenner and José 1965).

As we have shown that 50% of the brain polyunsaturated acids have accumulated by day 15 in the rat pup, it is likely that the deficiency induced in Paoletti's experiments may not exert its maximum effect until later. Svennerholm, on the other hand, exposed his rats to a long-term low-fat diet; this provides enough polyunsaturated fat to support breeding but a sufficiently low amount to induce an observable reduction in cerebrosides in the brain and an increase in 22:5(*n*–6) in the pups (see pp. 141-152).

We have gone to the other extreme, and have fed rats from weaning on a diet containing less fat than Svennerholm's diet (linoleic and linolenic acids at 0.33% of the calories). We then mate the rats, and would agree with Svennerholm that at this small intake of lipids we can expect a high mortality in the pups (only about 10% survive longer than two weeks). These are therefore different experiments from those of either Paoletti or Svennerholm. Whereas Svennerholm is examining the modifications which may occur, given sufficient lipid for survival and growth, we are examining the response to insufficient lipid for optimum reproduction.

We have found that the newborn pups of deficient dams have smaller brains than the oil-fed controls, but the same proportion of lipid in their brains. They have smaller livers and less lipid in the liver than the controls and there are significant changes in the pattern of fatty acids in the liver and brain lipids (Tables 2 and 3).

TABLE 2

Body, brain and liver weights and brain and liver lipids in newborn rats ($n = 11$)

| | *Control diet* | *Low-fat diet* | *P* |
|---|---|---|---|
| Birth weight (g) | 5.9 ± 0.1 | 4.5 ± 0.1 | < 0.001 |
| Liver weight (g) | 0.29 ± 0.01 | 0.24 ± 0.01 | < 0.025 |
| Liver lipid (mg/g fresh liver) | 45.6 ± 4.7 | 24.3 ± 2.3 | < 0.001 |
| Brain weight (g) | 0.29 ± 0.01 | 0.22 ± 0.01 | < 0.001 |
| Brain lipid (mg/g fresh brain) | 27.5 ± 0.8 | 27.9 ± 0.5 | > 0.05 |

The diets were fed to the dams from weaning to maturity. The control diet contained 6% of its calories as linoleic and linolenic acids and the low-fat diet, 0.33% as these acids; the ratio of linoleic to linolenic acid in each diet was 5:1.

TABLE 3

Liver and brain fatty acids in newborn rats (g/100 g of total tissue fatty acids)

| *Fatty acid* | *Liver (n = 5)* | | *Brain (n = 5)* | |
|---|---|---|---|---|
| | *Control diet* | *Low-fat diet* | *Control diet* | *Low-fat diet* |
| 18:2(*n*–6) | 12.3 ± 0.5 | 4.3 ± 0.7 | 2.2 ± 0.7 | 0.6 ± 0.1 |
| 18:3(*n*–3) + 20:1(*n*–9) | 1.3 ± 0.2 | 0.5 ± 0.09 | 0.2 ± 0.7 | 0.4 ± 0.06 |
| 20:3(*n*–9) | 0.3 ± 0.04 | 4.6 ± 1.1 | 0.3 ± 0.04 | 0.4 ± 0.07 |
| 20:4(*n*–6) | 16.2 ± 0.6 | 9.7 ± 0.8 | 11.9 ± 0.3 | 9.0 ± 0.6 |
| 22:4(*n*–6) | 1.3 ± 0.06 | 0.8 ± 0.1 | 2.7 ± 0.09 | 1.8 ± 0.08 |
| 22:5(*n*–6) | 0.4 ± 0.09 | 1.5 ± 0.1 | 1.7 ± 0.05 | 2.8 ± 0.3 |
| 20:5(*n*–3) | 3.0 ± 0.3 | 1.4 ± 0.07 | 0.4 ± 0.07 | 1.0 ± 0.2 |
| 22:5(*n*–3) | 3.5 ± 0.2 | 0.4 ± 0.1 | 0.4 ± 0.07 | 0.1 ± 0.02 |
| 22:6(*n*–3) | 14.5 ± 0.7 | 8.4 ± 0.8 | 12.2 ± 0.6 | 9.8 ± 0.3 |

We have also given the same low-fat diets to guinea-pigs and have found an interesting difference from the rat. Eicosatrienoic acid, 20:3 (*n*–9), is typical of fat deficiency in the rat, but the guinea-pig did not respond to the low-fat

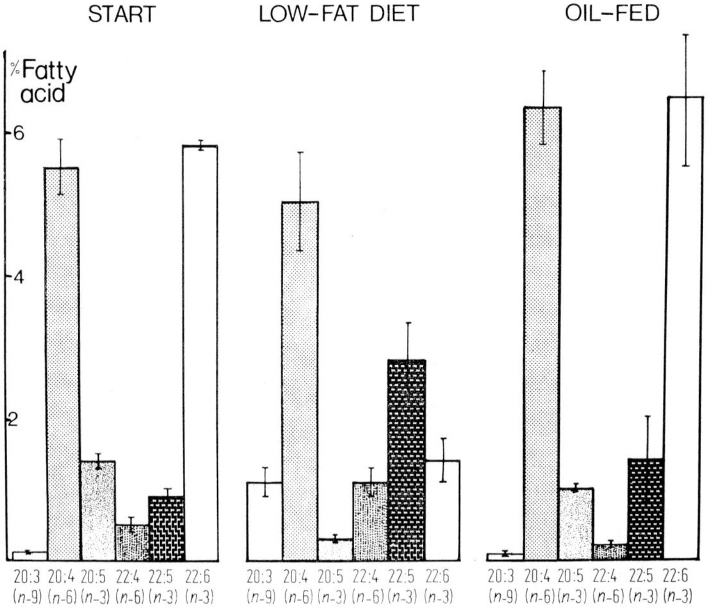


FIG. 5. Liver fatty acids in guinea-pigs fed a low-fat diet for 5 months. The animals were started on the diet at one month of age. The analyses represent means ± S.E.M. for six animals and the results are shown as the percentage of total liver fatty acids. Note the inversion in the ratio of 22:5 to 22:6 in the animals on the low-fat diet.

diet in the same manner (Fig. 5). After 5 months on the low-fat diet there was only a small rise in 20:3 (*n*–9), to about 1.3% of the fatty acids in the total liver lipids. Of particular interest was a fall in the long-chain *n*–3 acids. Normally the *n*–3, $C_{22}$ acids are dominated by docosahexaenoate, 22:6(*n*–3), but this acid fell markedly and the docosapentaenoate, mainly 22:5 (*n*–3), rose, reversing the relative significance of these two acids. Initially whole liver lipids were analysed (Crawford 1970) but we have recently repeated the experiment and found that the same principle applies to the ethanolamine and choline phosphoglycerides of the deficient guinea-pig liver.

These results suggest that different species may respond differently to lipid malnutrition and indicate the importance of examining the long-chain *n*–3 acids.

Our results on the progression of the parent polyunsaturated acids towards the long-chain fully desaturated constituents in the maternal and foetal liver in guinea-pigs, together with the marked changes in liver lipids of newborn rats from deficient dams, indicate the importance of the liver in the metabolic chain of events leading to the brain structural lipids.

## COMPARATIVE STUDIES OF FATTY ACIDS IN PHOSPHOLIPIDS

Clearly there are limitations to the use of laboratory animals if one wants to obtain information relevant to the human being. We have therefore made a comparative study to complement the information obtained from these experiments. In tissue phospholipids of small mammals the principal long-chain derivatives of the parent polyunsaturated acids are arachidonic, 20:4 (*n*–6), and docosahexaenoic acids, 22:6 (*n*–3). The same pattern occurs in the structural lipids from human tissues, as can be seen from published data on red cell lipids (Dodge and Phillips 1967).

The major *n*–3 derivative in the liver lipids of large herbivorous mammals was not docosahexaenoic acid but docosapentaenoic acid, 22:5 (*n*-3) (Crawford *et al.* 1970; Crawford 1970) (Table 4). The initial survey of large herbivorous mammals included ruminant species. As we had found that the proportion of 22:5 (*n*–3) was greater than that of 22:6 (*n*–3) in fat-deficient guinea-pigs, it might be thought that these large ruminants had become adapted to a marginally lipid-deficient diet; this would be consistent with the fact that much of the dietary polyunsaturated fatty acid is hydrogenated in the rumen. We therefore examined a non-ruminant species from the suids, the wart hog, *Phacochoerus aethiopicus*, and also found that the amount of 22:5 (*n*–3) exceeded that of 22:6 (*n*–3) (Crawford, Gale and Woodford 1970). Indeed, the lipids of the wart hog

TABLE 4

Polyunsaturated fatty acid content of ethanolamine phosphoglycerides from livers of some large herbivores (% of the total fatty acid)

| | *Ox calf* | *Eland* | *Buffalo* | *Wart hog* | *Horse* |
|---|---|---|---|---|---|
| 18:2(*n*–6) | 4.0 | 8.5 | 6.3 | 22.0 | 17.0 |
| 18:3(*n*–3) | 1.0 | 2.8 | 3.0 | 3.5 | 0.9 |
| 20:2(*n*–6) | 0.9 | 0.2 | 0.2 | 0.1 | 0.2 |
| 20:3(*n*–6) | 1.2 | 0.3 | 0.3 | 0.6 | 0.5 |
| 20:4(*n*–6) | 16.0 | 14.0 | 12.0 | 12.0 | 6.2 |
| 20:5(*n*–3) | 3.1 | 1.7 | 2.0 | 3.1 | 1.0 |
| 22:5(*n*–3) | 11.0 | 7.8 | 9.6 | 5.0 | 2.8 |
| 22:6(*n*–3) | 2.3 | 6.4 | 2.8 | 1.6 | 3.6 |

were little different from those of the ruminants in their long-chain polyunsaturated acids, but they had considerably more of the parent vegetable acids in their tissues and fewer saturated and mono-unsaturated acids. For example, linoleic acid accounted for 32% and linolenic acid for 5-6% of the fatty acids in muscle tissue from *Phacochoerus aethiopicus*, whereas figures of 15% and 4% respectively are typical of a large bovid ruminant such as *Syncerus caffer* (buffalo).

We have also analysed the liver lipids of a large carnivore, the hyaena. In contrast to the liver lipids of the Uganda kob, a herbivore from the same ecosystem, the hyaena had less of the parent vegetable fatty acids and more arachidonic acid, and docosahexaenoic acid was present in greater amounts than the *n*–3 docosapentaenoic acid (Fig. 6).

We have found the same dominance of docosahexaenoic acid in the liver ethanolamine phosphoglycerides from a leopard: docosahexaenoic acid constituted 18% of the fatty acids and docosapentaenoic acid only 2%. In other words, there appeared to be a progression in the proportion of long-chain acids and in the degree of unsaturation from the herbivore to the carnivore.

It is perhaps not generally appreciated that when one animal eats another, it is eating not only protein but also the phospholipids and their long-chain fatty acids. The lipids account for a major difference in the food structures of the herbivore and the carnivore. The herbivore eats only the parent $C_{18}$ polyunsaturated fatty acids, whereas the carnivore also eats the long-chain acids found in the phospholipids of the herbivore; there is effectively a progression of the acids through the food chain. This progression is represented diagrammatically in Fig. 7.

The large herbivore eats linoleic and linolenic acids and the combination of direct incorporation, chain-elongation and desaturation results in a profile of

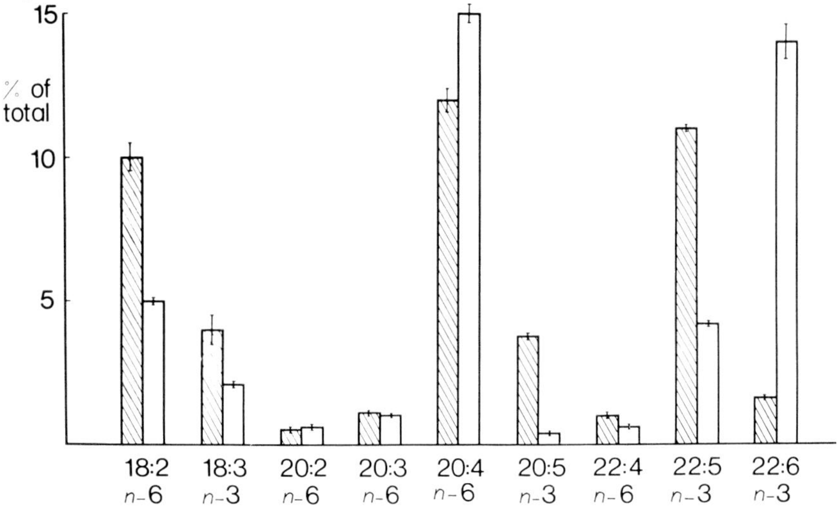


FIG. 6. Ethanolamine phosphoglycerides from livers of Uganda kob (hatched columns) and hyaena. Mean values ± S.E.M. for six adult male animals. Note the different amounts of 22:5(*n*-3) and 22:6(*n*-3).

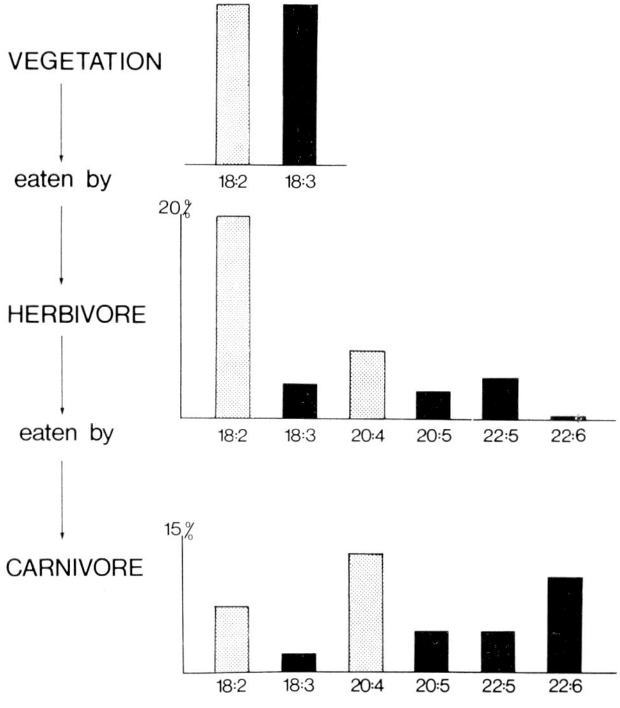


FIG. 7. Fatty acids in the food chain, to illustrate the progression of fatty acids from the vegetation through the herbivore to the carnivore. The height of the bars represents relative amounts of the different fatty acids at each point in the chain.

acids in the liver phosphoglycerides which includes both parent (vegetable) and long-chain derivatives but is weighted towards the parent acids. When the carnivore eats the herbivore it starts from a pattern that already includes the long-chain acids and the profile moves in favour of long-chain polyunsaturated acids with a simultaneous reduction in the parent acids. This change in the profile from herbivore to carnivore is of particular interest, because if we were to continue the progression, to reduce the parent acids to below 1 % and increase the long-chain acids correspondingly, we would have what is in effect the profile of the brain fatty acids. These are dominated by the long-chain acids and the parent acids are present in relatively insignificant amounts.

## THE QUALITATIVE CONTRAST BETWEEN HERBIVORE AND CARNIVORE

The large mammalian carnivores and herbivores (the 'Secundates' of Linnaeus) present a clear-cut biological contrast in the development of the central and peripheral nervous system. The ratio of brain to body weight is of the order of 0.05 % in the large herbivores whereas that of the carnivores is about 0.5 %. The visual system in the carnivore reaches a high degree of development, with night vision and remarkable control of the iris diaphragm; the response of the iris to bright light in the bovids is almost negligible. There are further contrasts in the development of the peripheral nervous system and vascular system in the carnivore, with the articulated claw as opposed to the hoof of herbivores. In general we see evidence of the development of attributes associated with the brain and its peripheral extensions in the carnivores, and the contraction of the same attributes in the herbivores.

Herbivores possess large amounts of muscle tissue, which could indicate an adequate supply of protein nutrients. On the other hand, the evidence of biohydrogenation, the presence of significant quantities of 20:3 (*n*–9) in liver lipids of newborn lambs (Noble, Steele and Moore 1970), and the difference in the ratio of 22:5 to 22:6 suggest a relative deficiency of polyunsaturated acids.

By contrast the carnivores have less bulk muscle but greater control of their limbs; they illustrate a greater degree of development of the lipid-rich tissues of the brain and peripheral nervous and vascular systems. (This same contrast between herbivores and carnivores is also seen in birds, where the flight of the buzzard, hawk or eagle, the vision of the vulture and the owl can be contrasted with the relatively simple activities of the pheasant.)

COMPARATIVE STUDIES OF BRAIN LIPIDS

Because we had found such clear-cut differences in the fatty acids in the liver of different mammalian species we felt it was important to establish whether these differences were reflected in the brain lipids. In general, we have consistently found the ethanolamine phosphoglycerides (PE) to be the fraction which contains the greatest amount of the long-chain polyunsaturated fatty acids, and have confined our analysis to this fraction. Although there were marked differences in the liver PE of the kob and hyaena, there was no difference in the PE of brain grey matter taken from the motor cortex (Fig. 8).

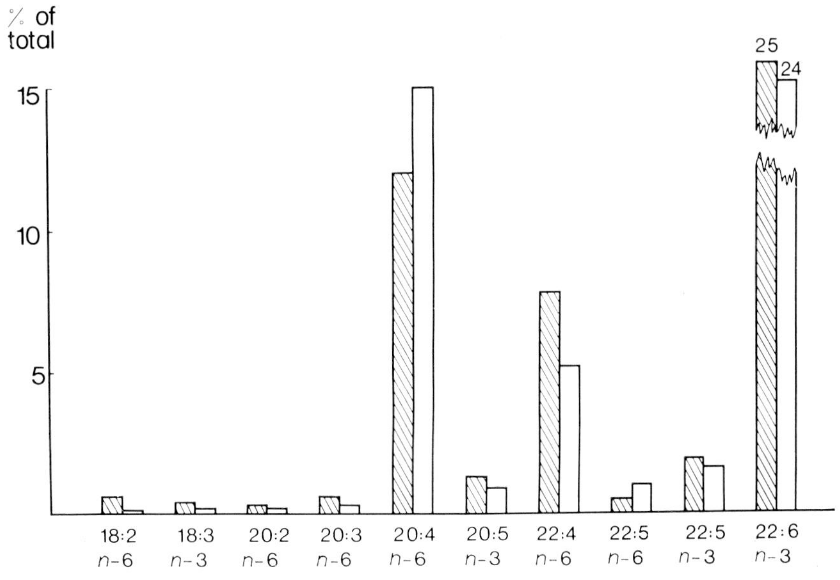


FIG. 8. Ethanolamine phosphoglycerides from brain grey matter of the kob (hatched columns) and hyaena. Note the similarity of these analyses despite the difference in the ratio of 22:5 to 22:6 in the liver (Fig. 6).

The brain PE from human grey matter (Fig. 9), taken from adults aged between 20 and 45 years, showed no substantial difference between European and African samples and no differences from the carnivores and herbivores.

We have now analysed the ethanolamine phosphoglycerides from liver in 23 different species of mammals and from brain grey matter in 15 of these. Although there were obvious species differences in the liver, summarized in

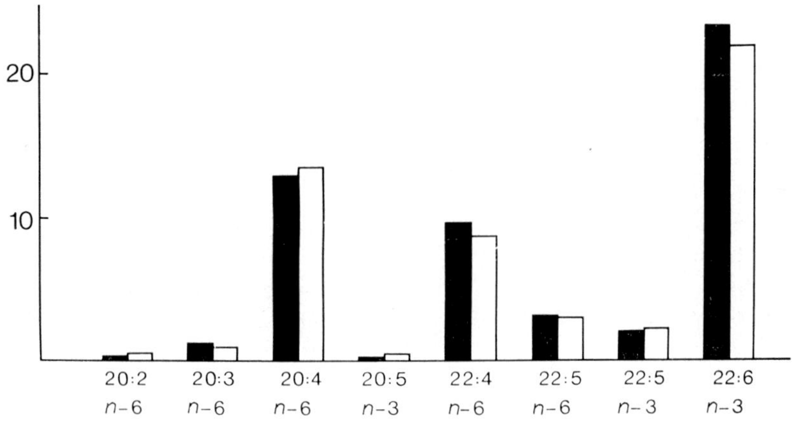


FIG. 9. Ethanolamine phosphoglycerides from grey matter of adult human brain. ■, European subjects; □, African subjects. The results are expressed as the percentage of total fatty acids.

Table 5, the brain PE fractions were essentially similar: linoleic and linolenic acids were less than 1% of the total fatty acids, 20:4 (*n*–6) was between 10 and 14%, 22:4 (*n*–6) between 6 and 9%, 22:5 (*n*–6) between 2 and 6%, 22:5 (*n*–3) between 0.5 and 2%, and 22:6 (*n*–3) between 18 and 29% and usually in the order of 24%.

We would not claim absolute identity of the brain PE fractions of different species but there is a remarkable similarity of the basic profile, despite wide deviations in the liver lipids. The inverted ratio of 22:5/22:6 in the liver lipids of the large herbivores was not reflected by any shift in the ratio of 22:5/22:6 in the brain; this always favoured the fully desaturated $C_{22}$ derivative of linolenic acid.

We must admit that in studying grey matter we are dealing with a mixture of cell types, but we consider this approach justified for an initial analysis because the high degree of instability of the long-chain polyunsaturated acids produces difficulties in complex isolation procedures.

In summary, it seems that there are wide variations in liver lipids of different mammals but that the ethanolamine phosphoglycerides of brain are similar. The brain fatty acids do not differ between species, but the size of the brain does. There is no reason to suggest any basic difference in the potential for lipid metabolism, because synthesis and oxidation of lipids occur in all species.

From these results one might be tempted to suggest that the closer the food structure enables the lipids to approach those of the brain, the greater the possibility of the development of the attributes of the lipid-rich nervous system.

TABLE 5

Examples of species variation in the polyunsaturated fatty acids of liver ethanolamine phosphoglycerides

| *Species* | *18:2(n–6)* | *18:3(n–3)* | *20:3(n–6)* | *20:4(n–6)* | *20:5(n–3)* | *22:4(n–6)* | *22:5(n–3)* | *22:6(n–3)* |
|---|---|---|---|---|---|---|---|---|
| Rat | | | | ++ | | | | ++ |
| Guinea-pig | | | | ++ | | | | ++ |
| Man | | | | ++ | | + | | ++ |
| Hyaena | ± | ± | | ++ | | | ± | ++ |
| Leopard | | | | ++ | | | | ++ |
| Lion | | | | ++ | | | + | + |
| Patas monkey | | | + | ++ | | | | ++ |
| Fruit-eating bat | | | | ++ | | | + | + |
| Wart hog | ++ | + | | ++ | + | | + | ± |
| Horse | ++ | + | | ++ | ± | | ± | ± |
| Elephant | | | + | + | | + | ++ | |
| Woodland buffalo | + | + | | ++ | + | | ++ | |
| Deer | | | | ++ | + | | ++ | |
| Eland | + | + | | ++ | + | | ++ | ± |
| Giraffe | + | + | | ++ | + | | ++ | |
| Kob | + | + | | ++ | + | | ++ | |

Some of the main characteristics of the polyunsaturated fatty acid profile of different mammalian species are summarized here. Despite species differences in the ethanolamine phosphoglycerides of liver, the profiles from brain grey matter were similar.

However, the species differences in structural lipids and differences within the food chains are likely to be only a part of a broader difference in food structure, about which we know very little. For example, the combination of growth rate and type of food lipids could be an important determinant of the ability of lipid synthesis to keep pace with protein synthesis; in large mammals such as the carnivores and man, the presence of long-chain polyunsaturated acids within the food could have made an important contribution to development. In other words, we are concerned with qualitative factors: the dog and the sheep both survive, but the quality of their lives is different. In broader evolutionary terms we could suggest the thesis that there was an interaction between genetics and food structure in the evolution of different species characteristics. This implies, as Dr Herschkowitz and Professor Bovet suggested earlier, that the response of the biological system to the exogenous environment could be development or degeneration. It also implies that genetics operate within certain limits imposed by the food structure.

Since there is evidence that malnutrition can affect human performance, it is likely that qualitative considerations similar to those we have discussed on a broad mammalian scale could also operate in man. This question is particularly important because it is the development of the brain which distinguishes man from other animals. This discussion could be briefly summarized by an analogy: the best blueprint of an architect is valueless without the building materials; given the materials and the tools, the quality of the building will be closely dependent on the quality of the materials used in its construction.

## SUMMARY

Wide variations have been found in the polyunsaturated fatty acids of liver lipids in 23 different mammalian species. Despite these variations, the fatty acids from the ethanolamine phosphoglycerides of brain grey matter are remarkably constant in the 15 mammalian species so far studied. In the brains of these species it was not the fatty acids which varied but the relative brain size.

Experiments on lipid deficiency are reported and the results are consistent with a role for polyunsaturated fatty acids in brain development.

The thesis is presented that the food structure was an important determinant in evolution.

## ACKNOWLEDGEMENTS

We wish to thank Unilever, Vlaardingen, for generous financial and technical assistance during the development of this work. We also thank the Uganda Game Department for cooperation in the collection of material. We are indebted to the late Mr N. M. Casperd of Makerere University of Uganda and to Mrs C. Lloyd, Mrs L. Springett, Miss J. Crocker and Mr G. Williams for their skilled technical assistance.

## References

BRENNER, R. R. and JOSÉ, P. (1965) *J. Nutr.* **85**, 196

COLLINS, F. D., SINCLAIR, A. J., ROYLE, A. J., COATS, J. P., MAYNARD, D. A. and LEONARD, R. F. (1970) In *Atherosclerosis* (Proc. 2nd Int. Symposium), p. 455, ed. R. J. Jones. Springer-Verlag, New York; see also (1971) *Nutr. Metab.* **13**, 150

COPPOCK, J. B. M. and DANIELS, N. W. A. R. (1962) *J. Sci. Food Agric.* **13**, 459

CRAVIOTO, J., PIÑERO, C., ARROYO, M. and ALCALDE, E. (1969) In *Nutrition in Preschool and School Age* (Swedish Nutr. Found. Symp. 7), pp. 85-98, ed. G. Blix. Almqvist & Wiksell, Uppsala

CRAWFORD, M. A. (1970) *FEBS Lett.* **11**, 117

CRAWFORD, M. A., GALE, M. M., SOMERS, K. and HANSEN, I. L. (1970) *Br. J. Nutr.* **24**, 393

CRAWFORD, M. A., GALE, M. M. and WOODFORD, M. H. (1970) *Int. J. Biochem.* **1**, 654

CRAWFORD, M. A., GALE, M. M., WOODFORD, M. H. and CASPERD, N. M. (1970) *Int. J. Biochem.* **1**, 295

DANIELLI, J. F. and DAVSON, H. (1935) *J. Cell Comp. Physiol.* **5**, 495-508

DAVISON, A. N. (1969) *Ann. Rev. Sci. Basis Med.* p. 220.

DODGE, J. T. and PHILLIPS, G. B. (1967) *J. Lipid Res.* **8**, 667

HITCHCOCK, C. and NICHOLS, B. W. (1971) In *Experimental Botany*, vol. 4, *Plant Lipid Biochemistry*. Academic Press, London and New York

HOLMAN, R. T. (1968) *Prog. Chem. Fats Other Lipids* **9**, 275

MOHRHAUER, H. and HOLMAN, R. T. (1963) *J. Lipid Res.* **4**, 151

NOBLE, R. C., STEELE, W. and MOORE, J. H. (1970) *Biochim. Biophys. Acta* **218**, 359

ROUSER, G., SIMON, G. and KRITCHEVSKY, G. (1969) *Lipids* **4**, 599

SCHENDEL, H. E. and HANSEN, J. D. L. (1959) *S. Afr. Med. J.* **33**, 1005

SIMON, G. and ROUSER, G. (1969) *Lipids* **4**, 607

SINCLAIR, A. J. and CRAWFORD, M. A. (1972) *J. Neurochem.* in press

YATSU, F. and MOSS, S. (1971) *J. Neurochem.* **18**, 1895

## Discussion

*Mead:* Your paper is extremely thought-provoking. A possible pitfall arises, however, from the tendency, noticeable throughout the symposium, for people to refer to phosphatidylethanolamine as a single compound when actually they are analysing the group of ethanolamine phosphoglycerides. When you compare 'phosphatidylethanolamine' from liver and brain, you are comparing two different compounds, because the ethanolamine phosphoglyceride of brain is largely phosphatid*al* ethanolamine. Considering this, it is not surprising to find mostly polyunsaturates in the ethanolamine phosphoglycerides of brain, because there are practically no saturated acids. The $\alpha$ position is occupied by an aldehydogenic group (the alkenyl ether) and is largely saturated. The fatty acid comes mainly from the $\beta$ position and is largely unsaturated. This is not true of the liver and no inferences can be made by comparing the two organs.

*Crawford:* We have examined both the phospholipid fractions and the saturated fatty acids and aldehydes in greater detail than we presented in the paper. I would agree that the brain is particularly rich in aldehydes by comparison with the liver, and the aldehydes themselves may be important, although it is generally thought that they can be made *de novo* by animal systems. Our paper was concerned with the polyunsaturated acids, where we are comparing the liver of one species with the liver of another and finding marked differences in the profile of the polyunsaturated acids; whereas when we compare the brain of one species with the brain of another we find a remarkable similarity. So the point is not that there is a difference between liver and brain (although a marked difference does exist) but that the liver profile varies and that of brain does not. For example, in the liver, the content of 22:5 can be greater than that of 22:6 or less, there can be a large proportion of $C_{18}$ polyunsaturated acids in the liver or relatively small proportions, but in large mammalian species we did not find these variations occurring in the brain grey matter. In other words it is not simply a question of 'polyunsaturates', but of the profile of the individual polyunsaturated acids. We may not be surprised that the brain is rich in polyunsaturated acids but it is interesting that it is the brain size which varies and not the polyunsaturates.

This fact raises the question of the relevance of the food chain. We have shown a progression from plants to liver and foetus and a similar progression from plants to herbivore to carnivore. Both progressions lead to an accumulation of the long-chain polyunsaturates which are found in brain cell structures. So we can compare the liver and brain in this sense of a progression of the profile of polyunsaturates. Interestingly, you obtain the same kind of answer if you simply analyse total fatty acids from liver and brain in large mammals within the context of their normal food chain, providing the animal is in health!

*Winick:* Dr Crawford pointed out the conceptual similarities between protein deficiency and deficiency of essential fatty acids. There is a basic difference, however. When an essential amino acid is deficient a reduced quantity of protein is made, because of a reduced rate of protein synthesis, but as far as we know that protein is of normal quality. We don't find a protein made that lacks that amino acid or contains a different amino acid. In fatty acid deficiency the reverse appears to be true: the synthesis of lipid doesn't change, but an abnormal lipid is made. So we may be dealing with two different types of mechanism, and we should focus on this change in the quality of lipids and 'turning-off' of synthesis in proteins, in order to elucidate the mechanisms.

*Crawford:* I would agree; the real interest in the lipids lies in the fact that unlike the proteins (Nolan and Margoliash 1968; Crawford *et al.* 1970), qualitative changes can occur, and we are beginning to see how subtle qualitative changes at a cell structural level can lead to gross morphological changes in the whole tissue and even the whole animal and possibly in evolution.

Dr Houtsmuller tells me that in polyunsaturated fatty acid deficiency he has observed changes in mitochondria, which is precisely what you would expect—subcellular qualitative changes which ultimately may be reflected macroscopically. This ability to change structure raises the most interesting questions. If you have protein deficiency or if you remove a limiting amino acid from the *in vitro* system, then it's 'no go', but in a lipid deficiency it may still be 'go' but the availability of lipids may define the direction in which to go. This is the difference between the dog and the sheep. They both survive but they have two different qualities of existence.

*Winick:* I look at this slightly differently, but I think we are saying the same thing. In an amino acid deficiency one is affecting the synthesis of the basic protein molecule; in essential fatty acid deficiency one is affecting something further along the pathway, perhaps. To say 'go' or 'no go' may not help me to design experiments in which I can look at the mechanism. But one might be able to ask questions about mechanisms if one asks how changes occur at the level of fitting fatty acids into the molecule. We might then proceed a step further and ask how altering the fatty acid composition of the diet changes the molecular configuration of certain brain lipids.

*Crawford:* Marshall and McLean (1971) have shown that certain polyunsaturated fats will induce cytochrome P-450. Mitochondrial enzymes in yeast are also induced by lipid (Wallace, Huang and Linnane 1968). Protein synthesis has been studied for many years; we are only just beginning to ask questions about the effects of lipid deficiencies on cellular structure and the enzyme systems. Daniels and Coppock (1962) found that if you reconstitute flour protein with lipid it is highly specific for the type of lipid which it accepts. So there is this possibility of interaction between protein and lipid, which up to now has not really been considered.

*Bernsohn:* Doesn't this reflect the fact that we know how protein molecules are assembled and we don't know how lipid membrane molecules are assembled?

*Crawford:* Yes. Protein systems have been studied for a much longer time.

*Chapman:* I consider the spectrum of fatty acids that are associated with membranes to have structural importance, for example in determining permeability processes, and in some cases for specific interactions with protein. I thought, however, that the so-called essential fatty acids as well as subserving some of these structural functions were also the precursors of prostaglandins and that the prostaglandins were then important for other biological interactions?

*Crawford:* Yes. Phospholipids with their component fatty acids are intimately involved in certain enzyme systems and may be part of the active centre (Attwood, Graham and Wood 1971). During metabolism they are converted into prostaglandins. Just as in proteins there are pharmacologically active metabolic offshoots of amino acids such as noradrenaline and 5-hydroxytryptamine, the prostaglandins are an offshoot of the structural components in the lipid.

*Mead:* The reversal of the ratio of 22:5 and 22:6 fatty acids that you find between the liver of a herbivore and a carnivore is very intriguing. If you wanted to study this phenomenon in a cellular or subcellular system, you could add a great excess of a polyunsaturated precursor to the system, and it would inhibit its own conversion. If, on the other hand, you simply added saturated fatty acids to the system, you would not inhibit to nearly the same extent. In the one case you might go to perhaps 22:5 and in the other case to 22:6.

I think that the carnivore, at least if you take him out on the African veldt, is getting mostly saturated fatty acids from his prey, whereas the herbivore, always excluding the ruminant, is consuming largely plant (or polyunsaturated) fatty acids. Perhaps this could explain the results.

*Crawford:* This is a common misconception. If you take meat from the free-living species which the carnivores, and for that matter the Africans, eat (when they get the chance) and stain it for triglyceride with Sudan Red, you will see small patches of lipid store. If you do this with English market beef you see a massive staining (Crawford 1969). This is basically an infiltration of saturated and mono-unsaturated fat as triglyceride. If you analyse the total fat from the beef you will in consequence find a predominantly saturated pattern, but if you analyse the meat from free-living species you obtain a polyunsaturated pattern because you are analysing structural lipid, including the phospholipids. If you isolate muscle cells from beef you find that they, like any other muscle cells, contain phospholipids and polyunsaturated fatty acids; but these are swamped by the massive amounts of saturated triglycerides which are the product of 'intensification' and 'high energy feeds' and are in the biological sense artificial (Crawford *et al.* 1970).

*Mead:* Would you say then that the carnivore is getting as highly unsaturated fat in its diet as the herbivore?

*Crawford:* The herbivore and carnivore eat different lipids. The herbivore eats the two parent plant acids, whereas the carnivore also eats the long-chain polyunsaturated fatty acids derived from the parent polyunsaturates and found in the phospholipids of the herbivore's tissues. Furthermore, the carnivore not only eats 'meat' but also eats kidneys, intestines, lungs and other membrane-rich organs, together with the liver which is particularly rich in structural lipid and contains a store of lipid-soluble and other nutrients. In other words, these are quite different food structures: the presence of the long-chain polyunsaturated fatty acids in the food structure of the carnivore provides a food pattern which is identifiably much closer to that found in the brain.

I am quite certain that the issue has been clouded by the idea that the fats of animal meat are saturated. When we published our findings that the fatty acid profile of meat of the buffalo was rich in polyunsaturated acids (Crawford 1968; Crawford, Gale and Woodford 1969) some people would not believe the results, and people are still confused about the issue (e.g. Yudkin 1971), and refer to the meat that African hunters or nomads eat as being 'fatty' and rich in saturated fat. The matter becomes simple if you analyse what the animals are eating and analyse the animals themselves. In our view the ruminant is a classical essential fatty acid-deficient animal (see, for example, its tough epidermis) that has adapted to a food structure which is relatively deficient in polyunsaturates, because the microorganisms in the ruminant's stomach act anaerobically to hydrogenate a significant proportion of the polyunsaturated fats that the animal eats. So it seems to us that ruminants have solved the problem of a protein supply but have sacrificed their lipids. They lay down about two or three times as much protein in 9 months as we do in 20 years. What they do not do is to lay down the lipid-rich tissues of the brain and nervous system. Protein synthesis may be accelerated in fast-growing mammals but lipid synthesis may be left behind, so that there is an incomplete pattern of incorporation into the phospholipids at the time that cell structures are put together.

The carnivore is at the opposite extreme from the herbivore. It eats much the same protein constituents as the herbivore but the lipids are from animal cells.

*Mead:* The ruminant is not a ruminant in early life of course; when does the change take place?

*Crawford:* That's true: during foetal development all mammals are effectively carnivorous. This is when brain development takes place, and both the carnivorous food structure and brain development may be extended during lactation.

## References

ATTWOOD, D., GRAHAM, A. B. and WOOD, G. C. (1971) *Biochem. J.* **123**, 875
CRAWFORD, M. A. (1968) *Lancet* **1**, 1329
CRAWFORD, M. A. (1969) *Lancet* **2**, 1419
CRAWFORD, M. A., GALE, M. M., SOMERS, M. and HANSEN, I. L. (1970) *Br. J. Nutr.* **24**, 393
CRAWFORD, M. A., GALE, M. M. and WOODFORD, M. H. (1969) *Biochem. J.* **115**, 25
CRAWFORD, M. A., GALE, M. M., WOODFORD, M. H. and CASPERD, N. (1970) *Int. J. Biochem.* **1**, 295
DANIELS, N. W. A. R. and COPPOCK, J. B. M. (1962) *J. Sci. Food Agric.* **13**, 459
MARSHALL, W. J. and MCLEAN, A. E. M. (1971) *Biochem. J.* **122**, 569
NOLAN, C. and MARGOLIASH, E. (1968) *Ann. Rev. Biochem.* **37**, 727-790
WALLACE, P. G., HUANG, M. and LINNANE, A. D. (1968) *J. Cell Biol.* **37**, 207
YUDKIN, J. (1971) *Br. J. Hosp. Med.* **5**, 666

# Looking back

ALEXANDER VON MURALT

*Nestlé Foundation, Lausanne*

There we were—all of us together for three days in a conference room—a congenial and stimulating group of scientists, bound by the spell of the world-wide problems of malnutrition, hunger and poor socio-economic conditions, discussing one of the issues: the developing brain. We felt that more should be known about the devastating effects of malnutrition and of inadequate parental care on the mental development of children. We tried to evaluate the knowledge and to find answers to urgent problems. And now, as I write this two months later, it all seems to be so distant and one wonders whether there will be a response to our aim to stimulate further research, to improve the teaching in this field and to change the sometimes passive attitude of governments in developing countries towards the problems of malnutrition; very often they are not aware of the extent to which the mental retardation produced by malnutrition and lack of parental care can affect the future of their countries, whose development depends in the last issue not on foreign aid, but on the initiative and intelligence of their own people!

On the last afternoon of the symposium, all the participants made concise statements about the results of our gathering, as seen by them. The transcripts of these opinions, the discussions and the papers are in front of me and it is now my task to bring together some of the highlights of this meeting as loyally as possible—and yet it is unavoidable that my personal touch will show through.

## 'GROWTH SPURT' OF THE DEVELOPING BRAIN

See pages 2, 9-19

The development of the central nervous system occurs in phases, which follow a precise sequence, different in the various brain regions, different in timing and different from one animal species to another. The morphological events in the developing brain coupled with the biochemical events, which occur in phase or out of phase, can be followed step by step in animal experiments. The complex sequences of brain development have different time scales in every brain area and are complicated by the migration of cells from one area to the other. In each species of laboratory animal, at a special period, the development of the brain enters a dramatic phase where the increase in brain weight and the speeding up of other important developmental processes rises to a peak or an elevated plateau (in the graphical representation of velocity against time) and then falls off to the previous growth rate. This is called the 'growth spurt'. The unsatisfactory aspect of such studies resides in the uncertainty of the extrapolation from experimental evidence found in laboratory animals to the development of the human brain, which has a very much higher organizational pattern. As far as we know today, the 'growth spurt' in humans starts at the end of the second foetal trimester, reaches a maximum before birth and falls off at a slower rate, tapering to the normal growth rate in the course of the first 18 months after birth.

In all species, the 'growth spurt' begins at the time when the development of neurons has reached the adult number, and gives rise to a very considerable multiplication of glial cells, which in term of numbers is much greater than the 'pre-growth spurt' multiplication of neurons. Then follows the formation of myelin, incorporated in the glial cells, known as the period of myelination. If the right conditions for the formation of this essential electrical insulating material, inserted between the excitable neuronal structures, are not fulfilled, a once-and-for-all opportunity for a normal development and function of the brain is missed.

## THE CONCEPT OF 'VULNERABILITY'

See pages 1-2, 9-29, 199-212

During organogenesis, there are very precise moments of an increased 'vulnerability' of the developing body towards harmful agents. This concept originated mainly from the sad experiences in the field of teratology, where the damage occurring at a specific 'vulnerable' period during gestation leads to irreversible disturbances of shape and form of the newborn. From these and other observations, it was concluded that the developing brain also has a 'vulnerable' period for which the term 'sensitive' proposed by Dobbing seems more appropriate. Evidence that the 'sensitivity' of the brain is closely related to the 'growth spurt' is accumulating. Any external measures which restrict the normal growth of the animal during the period of 'growth spurt' produce permanent, irrecoverable deficits and distortions in the developing brain. Malnutrition in every form, by restricting growth, has such an effect, especially protein-calorie malnutrition. Before we can understand the mechanism of this growth-restricting insult on the developing brain, we must have a deeper insight into the mechanisms controlling *normal* brain growth—an insight that is lacking today. Feeding a diet deficient in one or several critical components to laboratory animals is always a rewarding experimental design for the scientist; but in order to understand its effects on the developing brain, we must know more about the genetic control, the biosynthetic enzymes concerned in the production of proteins and lipids in the brain and the distribution of their incorporation into the various functional structures.

The specific high 'sensitivity' of the brain during the 'growth spurt' is a well-established fact, but it should not overshadow the possible discovery of other phases of minor, but eventually equally important 'sensitivities' of the developing brain. So far, we have only measured the things which have been easy to isolate out of an interwoven sequence of developmental processes. At the present state of our knowledge, it is safer to promote the notion that the brain may be more or less 'sensitive' or 'vulnerable' to external nutritional deficits at various periods or even during the whole time of brain development. It is specifically 'vulnerable' during the 'growth spurt'.

## MYELIN

See pages 31-37, 57 composition; 73-90 biosynthesis; 5, 37-57, 270-273 membrane structure

In the adult human brain, one half of the lipids are built into myelin, with a preponderance of cerebrosides and cholesterol. Gangliosides occur mainly in the neuronal and synaptic structures. Several methods for isolating myelin by differential centrifugation and gradient density centrifugation are available for the preparation of myelin in relatively pure form. The most characteristic lipid component is cerebroside and its 3-sulphate ester, sulphatide. Phosphatidal-ethanolamine is the most abundant among the phospholipids, and of special interest is polyphosphoinositide. About 70% of the dry weight of the separated myelin is lipid; 30% is protein. There is a proteolipid protein (chloroform-methanol soluble) which is important for the structural incorporation of the lipids and a basic protein of the membrane of the oligodendroglial cells. A third minor protein which appears in isolated myelin (Wolfgram) might be a contaminant from other sources. The enzyme activity of myelin is comparatively small. An aminopeptidase and cathepsins are present and supposedly have a physiological function. The enzyme 2′:3′-cyclic nucleotide 3′-phosphatase is a useful 'enzyme marker' present in myelin.

Myelin prepared from white matter of the brain contains more saturated and longer-chain fatty acids than grey matter, in which the proportion of myelin is small. Myelin is compact and has good electrical insulating properties (high resistance), together with a limited permeability for water, ions and organic molecules. The cholesterol content of myelin seems to be the main factor controlling its physical-chemical properties. The inhibition of chain motion in phospho- and sphingolipids in liquid crystalline condition depends on the degree of unsaturation of the lipid. It is greatest at the end of the chain, nearest to the polar group. Absence or reduction of the cholesterol will increase the fluidity within the myelin structure. There is evidence that the maintenance of special physical-chemical properties of myelin, in particular a certain degree of fluidity, is important for its function in the brain and in myelinated peripheral nerves. This is achieved, even if the availability and incorporation of certain fatty acids vary. Compensatory effects, keeping the overall fluidity of the membrane the same, maintain the physical-chemical properties of myelin. We assume that this is of functional significance.

The stability of myelin increases with age, presumably by a successive replacement of the shorter-chain fatty acids, which are present during brain development, by longer-chain fatty acids. We have to revise our notions about the so-called metabolic stability of myelin and that the incorporation of labelled fatty acids into myelin is less important than into all other subcellular fractions. There is good evidence available that between sterols recycling occurs and that two metabolic pools exist in myelin: a rapidly exchanging pool and a more persistent pool, with a slow turnover rate. Despite the rapid exchange of cholesterol and lecithin, the degradation of most lipids is slow, because the brain is able to re-utilize them.

Myelin is formed as an extrusion of the membrane of the oligodendroglial cell in the central nervous system and of the Schwann cell in the peripheral nervous system. At the start of this biosynthesis, there is a premyelinating phase where an 'early myelin' is deposited, containing cholesterol esters, which are not present in the adult myelin. It was suggested that these cholesterol esters might serve as an intermediary in the intracellular transport of fatty acids when lipogenesis becomes maximal. This 'early myelin' has relatively little cerebroside, a higher phospholipid concentration and shorter chains of fatty acids, which are more saturated than those of mature myelin.

In the developing human peripheral nervous system, myelination is seen in the sciatic nerve at about 18 weeks of menstrual age, and traces of cerebroside appear at about 20 weeks. The adult concentration of cerebroside is already reached by 32 weeks, so the biosynthesis of myelin is rapid, once it has started.

The high diversity of unsaturation, length and physical-chemical properties in the lipids and their organized incorporation into the myelin sheaths of axons and the myelin-containing membranes of white and grey matter, forces us also to revise the static concept of the Davson-Danielli-Robertson model of membrane structure. In this model, the lipids are supposed to be arranged in a bilayer as two radially oriented rows of rods of identical length between two axial protein sheaths. The polar ends of these rods are fixed in the protein layers on the outside and inside of the membrane and the non-polar tails face each other in the middle of the bilayer. From the fluidity of myelin, and the great variety of chain lengths of the fatty acids and of their degrees of unsaturation, it is apparent that the membrane structure must be much more dynamic than the model. The mutual strong lipid–lipid interactions and the bonds between lipids and the protein backbone of the membrane, the presence of hydrophobic bonds and the variations in fluidity are only compatible with a revised membrane model.

It is always helpful to devise new models for the membrane structure, but they must be based on solid data. Modern X-ray analysis is so advanced that it would be highly desirable to repeat with modern techniques the work of Schmitt and his collaborators on the structure of the myelin sheath of peripheral nerves, done more than 35 years ago. This would give a reliable basis for the design of dynamic models of the membrane.

## MYELIN-DEFICIENT MUTANTS

See pages 91-105 mainly Quaking; 111, 116-117 mainly Jimpy

Two myelin-deficient mutant mice, Quaking and Jimpy, show severe neuropathological symptoms, such as abnormal gait, tremor and seizures, which start at the time of myelination in mice, around the 10th or 12th day after birth. The Quaking mutation is an autosomal recessive and the Jimpy an X-linked recessive mutation. Genes involved in the formation of myelin must therefore be located on at least two different chromosomes. Quaking mice, unlike Jimpy mutants, have a normal lifespan and therefore comparisons can be made with normal mice as a control. What happens to the process of myelination in these mice? Before the onset of myelination, their glial cells multiply more than normally; the oligodendroglial cells lie in rows among myelinating fibres, but they are qualitatively abnormal, so the number of myelin lamellae is reduced and their compaction does not occur. In Jimpy mice, there is a lack of myelinating glia, indicating a block at an earlier step in the sequential events leading up to myelination.

Jimpy mice show a normal development up to about 11 days but die before the age of 30 days. The percentage of cerebroside and sulphatide in the brain of Jimpy mice is negligible, correlating with a very early impairment of myelin formation.

Quaking mice, which live longer, have a considerable lack of myelin lipids, including plasmalogens, cholesterol, cerebrosides and proteolipids in the brain. The cerebrosides, sulphatides and sphingomyelin, which they can synthesize, are deficient in long-chain fatty acids with 24 carbon atoms. In normal animals, these long-chain fatty acids have a key role in the formation and stability of myelin and its normal function. The loss of metabolic differentiation in the oligodendroglial cells seems to be responsible for the neuropathological symptoms of Quaking mice and several enzymes of cerebroside and sulphatide metabolism are affected. Membrane proteolipids of myelin are also diminished in Quaking mice, so there is a considerable biochemical distortion at the base of the neurological disturbance. Interestingly, myelination of the peripheral nervous system is not affected in mutant mice. This has to be interpreted as a different location of the gene involved in the formation and deposition of myelin by Schwann cells. This may also be the reason why a marked difference in the development of the central and peripheral nervous system is observed in many mammalian species.

It seems that there are three systems in the brain responsible for the elongation of fatty acids: the soluble system, providing palmitic and some stearic acid; the mitochondrial system, which elongates saturated and unsaturated fatty acids; and the microsomal system, which at the time of myelination in the developing brain has a marked predilection for the elongation of saturated fatty acids. It seems likely that in Quaking mice, the impairment occurs mainly in the microsomal system.

One has to be cautious about connecting the neuropathological symptoms only with the deficiency of myelination, which is easy to observe in these mutant mice. The excitable membranes of neurons appear to contain the same cerebrosides and sulphatides as those of the oligodendroglial cells, so if the synthesis of the normal membrane components is impaired, it could affect both the neuronal and the glial development and produce neurological disturbances in this way, especially since the neuronal fraction of the brain has a more active metabolism during the phase of brain development.

INCORPORATION OF FATTY ACIDS AND LIPIDS IN THE BRAIN

See pages 59-72, 159-178, 179-197, 199-212, 267-292

The incorporation of lipid fatty acids in the brain originates from three sources: synthesis within the brain; synthesis in other organs of the body and transport through the blood to the brain; and passage from the gut, with or without modifications, through the blood to the brain.

Radioactive labelling permits a great variety of transport and incorporation studies which have shown that the so-called 'blood–brain barrier' is practically passed without any resistance, not only by fatty acids but even by lipids. It was unanimously felt at this symposium that the notion of a blood–brain barrier is obsolete. It is probable that a large portion, if not the whole frontier between the brain structures and the capillaries of the vascular distribution system in the brain, is lined by astrocytes. Since these glial cells have an active metabolism, the possibility of a triple transport and storage mechanism from the blood to the astrocytes must be taken into account: passive transport along a concentration gradient, active transport against the gradient, and synthetic activity within the astrocytes.

In the premyelination phase of brain development, the synthesis of lipids in the brain is very active. As the lipid content of the developing brain rises, the synthesis of lipids falls inversely to this rise to a level of steady-state synthesis. In the rat brain, this happens between birth and the first 30 days.

Fatty acids incorporated into the brain undergo many changes: chain elongation, desaturation, hydroxylation, chain degradation and resynthesis. The essential fatty acids (EFA), linoleic (18:2(*n*–6)) and linolenic (18:3(*n*–3)), pass from the blood to the brain with a high incorporation rate, measured at 24 hours after administration either by injection into the carotid artery or by feeding. This explains their dominance as precursors of the fatty acids in the brain in comparison to all other tissues. Linoleic acid is elongated into longer chains and is thus the only dietary precursor for polyunsaturated fatty acids of the *n*-6 series, and linolenic acid is elongated into the polyunsaturated acids of the *n*-3 series. In the absence of these essential precursors, the corresponding polyunsaturated acids in the brain cannot be synthesized to any extent. It seems to be safe to state that a deficiency of essential fatty acids leads to profound functional disturbances. The analysis of brain lipids has shown that the ethanolamine phosphoglycerides are the fraction which contains the greatest amount of the long-chain polyunsaturated fatty acids. The grey matter of brain from 15 mammalian species showed a remarkable similarity of the profile of polyunsaturated fatty acids, which gave the following figures:

| *Polyunsaturated fatty acid* | *Name* | *% of total fatty acids of ethanolamine phosphoglyceride fraction* |
|---|---|---|
| 18:2(*n*–6) | linoleic | < 1 |
| 18:3(*n*–3) | linolenic | < 1 |
| 20:4(*n*–6) | eicosatetraenoic | 10-14 |
| 22:4(*n*–6) | docosatetraenoic | 6- 9 |
| 22:5(*n*–6) | docosapentaenoic | 2- 6 |
| 22:5(*n*–3) | docosapentaenoic | 0.5- 2 |
| 22:6(*n*–3) | docosahexaenoic | 18-29 |

Data from text of Crawford and Sinclair, p. 284

The remarkable similarity of this profile among species is not reflected when polyunsaturated fatty acids in the liver are analysed, so the brain as such has a well-defined incorporation and synthesis pattern.

Labelled acetate injected into the carotid artery is incorporated into a great number of brain lipids within 15 seconds. Even in adult brain, the synthesis of fatty acids from acetate and their incorporation into lipids is very rapid. The controlling factor governing the rate of incorporation and of fatty acid discrimination seems to be at the transacylase level. One cannot help feeling that we know very little about how the multiplicity of molecular species within the structural lipids, among which there are about 70 different phospholipids, is controlled in such a way that the mutual relations within a given brain sample are found to be fairly constant.

The mitochondrial pathway, responsible for elongation, using acetyl-CoA, converts palmitic acid as the most active fatty acid entering this pathway, and mono-unsaturated acids into the long-chain fatty acids of the sphingolipids. The microsomal elongation and desaturation system uses malonyl-CoA for elongation and its products are incorporated by ester-linkage in more metabolically active phospholipids.

A relatively new and useful technique for studying the incorporation of fatty acids is the cultivation of brain tissue *in vitro*. Brain explants remain metabolically active for several days in a serum-free medium and synthesize lipids from precursors added to the medium, but the total fatty acid uptake varies considerably between experiments. The relative amount of label incorporated, however, is nearly constant. Palmitic acid was found to be incorporated to the greatest extent into the phospholipid fraction and a chain elongation of palmitic to stearic acid occurred in the explants. In the neutral lipid fraction, triglycerides took up most of the label and, among the phospholipids, choline and ethanolamine phosphoglycerides accounted for about 60% of the total phospholipid radioactivity.

Experiments *in vitro* and *in vivo* show that embryonic chick brain can synthesize polyunsaturated fatty acids before the period of active myelination. In the developing brain (10 days postnatally in the rat), labelled acetate is incorporated into phosphoglyceride fatty acids of glial cells much more rapidly than into neurons. At 21 days, however, when myelination has come to an end, the ratio of incorporation into glial cells and neurons is reversed, but at a much lower level of activity. The biosynthesis of polyunsaturated fatty acids in developing brain is therefore connected with myelination in various temporal phases.

Another aspect is provided by the study of demyelinating diseases. It was postulated that a suboptimal availability of *n*–3 fatty acids during the period of rapid deposition of myelin or a defect in the metabolic pathway leading to the biosynthesis of docosahexaenoic acid (22:6(*n*–3)) and the lipids derived from it, during the active myelination period, might lead to the formation of a myelin unable to maintain its structural stability which would ultimately break down. The very long time interval between the period of myelination and the manifestations of a demyelinating disease could be attributed to the slow turnover rate of myelin. The hypothesis is attractive, but the long delay between the hypothetical cause and the onset of the disease means that extremely well-controlled vertical studies are needed in order to substantiate it.

## MALNUTRITION AND THE DEVELOPING BRAIN

See pages 107-119, 121-140, 141-157, 273-279

In recent years it has become apparent that malnutrition not only delays the maturation of the brain, but that reversible and irreversible damage of the brain structure may be the consequence. The word 'malnutrition' defines all forms of *insufficient* nutrition*. The ambiguity that overfeeding is also bad (Latin, *male*) for the organism is excluded by the definition given above. The deficiency in nutrition can be a general reduction of calories, of proteins, of lipids, of vitamins, or of trace nutrients. Generally, it is a combination of several deficiencies and this is a drawback, because the term 'malnutrition' is very often used without any indication of the deficiencies in nutrients which have produced malnutrition.

There are various techniques available for producing malnutrition in laboratory animals. The most widely used experimental procedure is the increase of the size of the suckling litter so that the pups are weaned at about half

* See *The Concise Oxford Dictionary of Current English.*

their normal weight for age. A second procedure starts by underfeeding the mother animal during pregnancy, which results in stunted offspring. These stunted pups, as well as a normal control group of newborns, are cross-fostered at birth to well-fed and undernourished lactating females, the litter size being standardized.

A third procedure starts even earlier by feeding the experimental diet to rats from weaning up to mating (90 days), through gestation and lactation. At the day of birth of the second generation, all litters are reduced to six and are then used as the dietary groups.

Complete deficiency in essential fatty acids (EFA) in the diet affects the fertility of the dam and the survival of the offspring. A complete lack of dietary fat or only a difference in the ratio of linoleic acid to linolenic acid between the control and the experimental diets introduce a number of factors which render the interpretation of the results uncertain. It is obvious that the study of the nutritional effects of a diet deficient in essential fatty acids is much more difficult than studies in protein, amino acid or vitamin deficiencies.

The best experimental design seems to be not an exclusion but a reduction of the concentration of linoleic + linolenic acids in the diet and the maintenance of a fixed ratio between these two acids, in both the experimental and control diets; this is important, because the relative percentage of 22:5(*n*–6) and 22:6(*n*–3) fatty acids in brain lipids is strongly influenced by a change in the dietary linoleate/linolenate ratio, but independent within a wide range of the amounts of EFA in the food.

In protein-calorie malnutrition, which is always the consequence of a food composition low in protein and in lipids, a deficiency of myelin lipids and a delay in their formation is the most characteristic nutritional effect on brain development. When low and high levels of protein were combined with low and high levels of essential fatty acids in the diet, the following results were obtained: body weight developed normally in the high-protein groups and was stunted in the low-protein groups. High protein and low EFA gave a slightly smaller body weight than high protein and high EFA, but in the low-protein group growing at a much lower rate, there was no difference between high or low nutritional EFA.

With regard to brain weight, the observations depend on the experimental design. If the pregnant animals are fed beginning one week before delivery with a fat-free diet, the brain weight of the EFA-deficient offspring is reduced. After nutritional rehabilitation, brain and body weight catch up with the controls. If the animals are fed a high-protein, low-EFA diet, there is no change in brain weight. It appears, therefore, that as long as the protein matrix of the brain develops normally and as long as there is a certain supply of EFA, the brain weight is not affected. If the EFA supply is cut off temporarily, the brain weight is reduced, but returns to normal values under rehabilitation.

Protein, phospholipids, cholesterol and total fatty acids of brain were found to be the same in high and low EFA groups. Only the cerebrosides were significantly lower, whereas the gangliosides, measured as *N*-acetylneuraminic acid, showed no differences between the two groups. In the more radical experiments with a fat-free diet of the dam, the fatty acid composition of brain phospholipids is affected. The three major lipid fatty acid families derived from the precursors oleate (*n*–9), linoleate (*n*–6) and linolenate (*n*–3) change as follows: 20:3(*n*–9) and 22:3(*n*–9) increase, (*n*–6) decrease after 10 days and (*n*–3) are affected only after 6 months, which shows again how difficult it is to produce a deficiency in linolenate.

In an acute deficiency of polyunsaturated fatty acids, the rats desaturate and elongate oleic acid to 20:3(*n*–9) and 22:3(*n*–9), but the enzyme systems are unable to introduce double bonds between the 9 position and the methyl end. This explains the increase in trienes of the (*n*–9) type. Supposedly, these trienes functionally replace the (*n*–6) and (*n*–3) families in the long run. The accumulation of 20:3(*n*–9) fatty acids is always a sign of a deficiency in the supply of linoleic and arachidonic acids in experimental nutritional designs in the rat. In the guinea-pig, low-fat diets produce only a very small rise of 20:3(*n*–9), but there is a fall in the long-chain (*n*–3) acids. This shows that various species of laboratory animals respond differently to EFA malnutrition.

What do we know about humans, especially children living and growing under poor socio-economic conditions? Severe malnutrition leads to a diminished brain weight and in the brain a diminished content of DNA and reduced concentrations of cholesterol and cerebrosides. One is entitled to ascribe these changes primarily to protein-calorie malnutrition, but also to a deficiency in fat supply.

A very alarming new aspect came up in the symposium. Protein-calorie malnutrition in children is usually treated by feeding high-protein diets, which may contain insufficient amounts of fatty acids, especially of the polyunsaturated type. The rehabilitation of the brain structures, damaged by malnutrition, is coupled with a higher requirement for polyunsaturated fatty acids, so the treatment can induce an EFA deficiency. It is vital that fundamental work be done on the relationship of protein synthesis to the enhanced need for polyunsaturated fatty acids, leading ultimately to membrane formation in the brain. It is interesting that the 20:3(*n*–9) fatty acid, derived by elongation from oleic acid, is not found in children suffering from kwashiorkor (protein-calorie malnutrition), but this fatty acid appears during the curative feeding of a high-protein diet! The supply of protein in these cases apparently stimulates protein synthesis to such an extent that it outruns the lipid synthesis.

Normal brain development depends on the exact sequence of the developmental phases, and the metabolic reactions regulate the cellular events. They are primarily determined by the genome, so the genetic regulation of brain development must also be considered under the influence of malnutrition. Genes code for the formation of enzyme proteins and determine their catalytic functions; they control the intracellular sites and the timing of activation and de-activation during development. Exogenous factors, such as malnutrition, can alter the activity of enzymes and can interfere with protein synthesis and protein structure, and thus also interfere with the incorporation of the right lipids in the various brain structures. It is possible that already in the very early phases of foetal life the brain is 'sensitive' to adverse nutritional influences on the genetic regulation of development.

On the whole, it can be said that malnutrition provokes disturbances in the protein and lipid structure of the developing brain. Nutritional rehabilitation of the lipid structure seems easier than rehabilitation of the protein structure, which suffers permanent damage mainly if the insult occurred during the 'growth spurt'.

## NUTRITIONAL ASPECTS

See pages 213-225, 282-292

From the practical point of view, it is desirable to appraise the minimal requirements in the lipid fraction of the maternal and infant diet needed for a normal development of the human brain.

Among the fatty acids, linoleic acid is of chief importance for optimal brain development, since it is the unreplaceable precursor for the (*n*–6) fatty acids in lipids. In the prenatal period, very little lipid passes through the placenta and therefore the difference in fatty acid composition of maternal and foetal blood is considerable, which makes an appraisal of the optimal amount of linoleic acid in the diet of the pregnant mother difficult. To be on the safe side, a level of 2% of calories is recommended. After birth, the supply depends either on breast milk or on a formula. Breast milk normally contains enough linoleic acid and in the milk of Japanese mothers, the concentration rises to as much as 5% of calories, due to soya which is a major part of the Japanese diet. In Sweden, the general consumption of fat is 42% of calories and the content of linoleic acid in pooled breast milk is 3% of calories.

In human nutrition, the role and importance of linolenic acid as an essential fatty acid is often questioned. From the physiologists' point of view, the presence of this fatty acid in maternal milk at a percentage of 1.2% is more convincing evidence for its importance than any number of animal experiments which attempt to show that it is not 'essential'.

So, linoleic acid and linolenic acid together provide approximately 5% of calories, which may also be considered as a guideline for baby food. But there is another point which has to be considered. If the diet contains linoleic acid, its auto-oxidation must be prevented. Vitamin E is able to protect the unsaturated fatty acids in the body from oxidation by maintaining an adequate anti-oxidation potential. Its function is the protection of the fatty acids of the *n*–6 family, and also the pentaenes and hexaenes of the linolenic type. Interestingly, the brain has the lowest vitamin E level of all organs (0.25 mg tocopherol/100 g tissue).

The lipid fraction of a formula diet may also contain adverse factors for the growth of the child. The dietary level of cholesterol should be low in baby food, although neither adverse nor favourable effects of cholesterol on brain maturation have been observed. Saturated fatty acids (mainly in animal fats) increase the cholesterol level in blood and both factors together may accelerate the development of an initial deficiency in essential fatty acids.

Very interesting are the studies reported on herbivores and carnivores in Africa (pp. 282-286). The brain to body weight ratio of the large herbivores is ten times lower than in carnivores. The herbivore covers its requirement of linoleic acid by eating seeds, bark and leaves, and its requirements of linolenic acid mainly from leaves. The profile of polyunsaturated fatty acids in the lipids of the liver shows a dominance of the 18:2 family, falling off over 18:3, 20:4, 20:5, 22:5 to 22:6.

The carnivore feeding on a herbivore eats among other nutrients all the phospholipids with their long-chain fatty acids, which results in a profile in favour of the long-chain polyunsaturated acids and a reduction of the precursor fatty acids in its liver. Are these differences reflected in the brain? Between the kob and the hyaena there was no difference in the ethanolamine phosphoglyceride (EPG) in the grey matter of their brains. This shows that the selection and incorporation of fatty acids in the brain is independent of the concentrations of fatty acids in the pool. This is also the reason for the similarity of the EPG fractions in the grey matter of 15 mammals examined (see p. 284).

## MALNUTRITION AND MENTAL RETARDATION

See pages 3-4, 130-131, 227-248, 249-265

We heard that in Colombia two-thirds of the children under 5 years of age, altogether 2 million children, are malnourished, and the same is probably true for a great number of countries in the third world. This brought the full weight of our responsibility towards many millions of undernourished children, with all its drastic and tragic reality, into the symposium.

From all that has been said so far about the influence of malnutrition on the developing brain, it is obvious that one should start to examine the nutrition of a child at the prenatal period; in other words one has to start with the examination of the pregnant mother with regard to her nutritional status and her placental metabolism, which is now possible by measuring the placental lactogenic hormone in the blood of the mother. Previously this was not possible and it must be said that in the observations of mental retardation of malnourished children, very elaborate psychological methods have been used, but the causal connection between mental retardation and malnutrition remains uncertain. The opposite must be said about the animal experiments, where the effects of malnutrition on the brain biochemistry have been studied with elaborate modern methods, but where the testing of the effects of these changes on behaviour is not equivalent to the high precision of the biochemical work. I am fully aware of the great difficulties of such work and this remark is not meant to be a criticism, but rather a stimulus for future experimental designs.

Groups of rats, kept on a diet deficient in EFA for 90 days, were submitted to a behavioural test together with control animals (see p. 130). The test was a conditioned-avoidance response and the performance of the EFA-deficient rats was significantly lower after the third, fourth and fifth session. The most striking symptom was the inability to retain the learned information, a symptom also described by Caldwell and Churchill (1966; see p. 140 for reference).

After protein-calorie malnutrition, the impairment of behaviour in laboratory animals is known to be permanent and remains so after nutritional rehabilitation. The problem of whether an EFA deficiency alone during the 'vulnerable' period of the brain has such a permanent effect, even after nutritional rehabilitation, remains open. It must be said that in animal experiments, the environment, the handling of the test animals and even the humidity in the rooms has an influence on their performance. In order to arrive at a solid basis in this field, coordination of the experimental design of behavioural experiments on laboratory animals with studies of the damaging effects of malnutrition on the brain is highly desirable.

The evidence in humans that early malnutrition causes mental retardation is complicated by the influence of the poor socio-economic environment, which is always coupled with malnutrition. It is further complicated by the problems of a cross-cultural evaluation of human intelligence and, worst of all, if we assume that the developing brain is most 'vulnerable' to malnutrition, the time which elapses between the insult and the psychological evaluation of its effect on brain function is at least several years. This introduces a number of almost uncontrollable new environmental factors, both restrictive and compensatory, which in conjunction lead ultimately to mental retardation. All these entities have an effect on the brain and its function, and since they usually occur together they are the cause. The practical problem of fighting mental retardation produced by these external influences is whether the improvement of nutrition is more important than the improvement of the socio-economic environment. Experience in Africa has shown that an improvement of the earning power had no effect on the poor nutrition—on the contrary, the surplus was invested in alcoholic beverages!

A valuable experimental design is based on the experience that siblings have a high correlation of psychological scores. They have the same genetic background, they live under the same socio-economic conditions and by and large they are exposed to the same epidemiological risks. In areas where malnutrition prevails one can find families where one child is malnourished and a sibling is well-nourished. This paired-sibling model of the Harvard-I.C.B.F.-Cornell Project has already given promising preliminary results (pp. 237-243).

The study on the cross-cultural evaluation of human intelligence (pp. 254-260), comparing malnourished with well-nourished children, showed that one of the immediate effects of early severe malnutrition was the inability to habituate to a novel stimulus and to recognize a transformation of that stimulus. Here again the socio-economic environment and its influence on emotional behaviour complicates the relationships and it is apparent that the study of the influence of malnutrition on mental development is complex. It is, however, so worthwhile that an increased research effort in diverse cultural regions can warmly be recommended. For the future, it is important to define the nutritional insult in such studies as clearly as possible: age of onset, duration of the insult, severity and type of insult (calorie-malnutrition, protein-calorie malnutrition, deficiency in essential fatty acids, imbalance in the diet, vitamin deficiency, deficiency in trace nutrients). It is also important to characterize the defects in behaviour more broadly.

The somewhat critical attitude towards the problem of whether malnutrition *per se* causes mental retardation in humans or not should not block, but rather stimulate further research, in view of the tremendous importance of the fact that millions of children are malnourished and suffer from mental retardation. Whether it is the cause *per se* or whether it is a summation with other aggravating factors is of secondary importance in view of the huge problems of developing countries and the population explosion.

## IN CONCLUSION

I would like to make it very clear that this summary could only be written because of the generosity of the participants at the symposium in allowing me to use their discussion remarks and statements freely, and sometimes literally, in order to round off the picture they have drawn. The authors of important statements can be found from the page references given in this summary, a procedure by which I have tried to make the text easily readable. I hope that I have rendered the opinions of the contributors to the symposium with a fair amount of accuracy without quoting their names. On behalf of the organizers of this symposium, may I extend our gratitude to all those who have carried the burden of preparing their remarkable papers, of contributing at the meeting, and of reviewing their discussion remarks, thus building the backbone of this book.

# Index of contributors

*Entries in* **bold** *type indicate papers; other entries are contributions to discussions*



Indexes prepared by William Hill.

# Subject index